T0227359

Cutaneous Melanoma

Guest Editor

WILLIAM W. DZWIERZYNSKI, MD, FACS

CLINICS IN PLASTIC SURGERY

www.plasticsurgery.theclinics.com

January 2010 • Volume 37 • Number 1

SAUNDERS an imprint of ELSEVIER, Inc.

W.B. SAUNDERS COMPANY
A Division of Elsevier Inc.

1600 John F. Kennedy Boulevard • Suite 1800 • Philadelphia, Pennsylvania 19103-2899

http://www.theclinics.com

CLINICS IN PLASTIC SURGERY Volume 37, Number 1
January 2010 ISSN 0094-1298, ISBN-13: 978-1-4377-1861-4

Editor: Barbara Cohen-Kligerman
Developmental Editor: Theresa Collier

Clinics in Plastic Surgery (ISSN 0094-1298) is published quarterly by Elsevier Inc., 360 Park Avenue South, New York, NY 10010-1710. Months of issue are January, April, July, and October. Periodicals postage paid at New York, NY and additional mailing offices. Subscription prices are $384.00 per year for US individuals, $551.00 per year for US institutions, $193.00 per year for US students and residents, $436.00 per year for Canadian individuals, $644.00 per year for Canadian institutions, $495.00 per year for international individuals, $644.00 per year for international institutions, and $244.00 per year for Canadian and foreign students/residents. To receive student/resident rate, orders must be accompanied by name of affiliated institution, date of term, and the *signature* of program/residency coordinator on institution letterhead. Orders will be billed at individual rate until proof of status is received. Foreign air speed delivery is included in all *Clinics* subscription prices. All prices are subject to change without notice. **POSTMASTER:** Send address changes to *Clinics in Plastic Surgery*, Elsevier Health Sciences Division, Subscription Customer Service, 3251 Riverport Lane, Maryland Heights, MO 63043. **Customer Service: 1-800-654-2452 (US and Canada). From outside of the United States and Canada, call 314-447-8871. Fax: 314-447-8029. E-mail: JournalsCustomerService-usa@elsevier.com (for print support); JournalsOnlineSupport-usa@elsevier.com (for online support).**

Reprints. For copies of 100 or more of articles in this publication, please contact the Commercial Reprints Department, Elsevier Inc., 360 Park Avenue South, New York, New York 10010-1710. Tel.: (+1) 212-633-3812; Fax: (+1) 212-462-1935; E-mail: reprints@elsevier.com.

Clinics in Plastic Surgery is covered in *Current Contents, EMBASE/Excerpta Medica, Science Citation Index, MEDLINE/ PubMed (Index Medicus), ASCA, and ISI/BIOMED.*

Printed and bound in the United Kingdom
Transferred to Digital Print 2011

Contributors

GUEST EDITOR

WILLIAM W. DZWIERZYNSKI, MD, FACS
Professor of Plastic Surgery, and Program
Director of Plastic and Reconstructive Surgery
Residency Program, Department of Plastic
Surgery, Medical College of Wisconsin,
Milwaukee, Wisconsin

AUTHORS

MARK W. BOSBOUS, MD
Resident, Department of Plastic Surgery,
Medical College of Wisconsin, Milwaukee,
Wisconsin

MELISSA P. CHIANG, MD, JD
Assistant Clinical Professor, Department of
Dermatology, Medical College of Wisconsin,
Milwaukee, Wisconsin

YOUNGHOON R. CHO, MD, PhD
Department of Plastic Surgery, Medical
College of Wisconsin, Milwaukee, Wisconsin

MACKENZIE D. DALY, MD
Resident, Department of Radiation Oncology,
Medical College of Wisconsin, Milwaukee,
Wisconsin

WILLIAM W. DZWIERZYNSKI, MD, FACS
Professor of Plastic Surgery, and Program
Director of Plastic and Reconstructive Surgery
Residency Program, Department of Plastic
Surgery, Medical College of Wisconsin,
Milwaukee, Wisconsin

MATTHEW G. FLEMING, MD
Associate Professor of Dermatology and
Pathology, Department of Dermatology,
Medical College of Wisconsin, Milwaukee,
Wisconsin

NINA GARLIE, PhD
Research Scientist and Cell Lab Director,
Immunotherapy Program, Aurora St Luke's
Medical Center, Milwaukee, Wisconsin

THOMAS J. HORNYAK, MD, PhD
Investigator, Dermatology Branch, Center for
Cancer Research, National Cancer Institute,
National Institutes of Health, Bethesda,
Maryland

CHRISTOPHER J. HUSSUSSIAN, MD
Clinical Assistant Professor, Department
of Plastic and Reconstructive Surgery,
Medical College of Wisconsin, Milwaukee,
Wisconsin

J. ALEX KELAMIS, MD
Resident, Johns Hopkins University, and
University of Maryland Plastic Surgery
Residency Program, Baltimore, Maryland

JEFFREY H. KOZLOW, MD
Section of Plastic and Reconstructive Surgery,
University of Michigan, Ann Arbor, Michigan

DAVID L. LARSON, MD
Chairman and George J. Korkos Professor of
Plastic Surgery, Department of Plastic Surgery,
Medical College of Wisconsin, Milwaukee,
Wisconsin

JEFFREY D. LARSON, MD
Resident, Department of Surgery, Section
of Plastic Surgery, University of Wisconsin,
Madison, Wisconsin

SCOTT D. LIFCHEZ, MD
Chief, Section of Plastic Surgery,
Johns Hopkins Bayview Medical Center;
Assistant Professor, Department of Surgery,
Johns Hopkins University School of Medicine,
Baltimore, Maryland

VALERIE B. LYON, MD
Assistant Professor, Department of
Dermatology; Assistant Professor, Department
of Pediatrics, Medical College of Wisconsin,
Children's Hospital of Wisconsin, Milwaukee,
Wisconsin

MARCELLE NEUBURG, MD
Professor of Dermatology, Department of
Dermatology, Medical College of Wisconsin,
Milwaukee, Wisconsin

RILEY S. REES, MD
Section of Plastic and Reconstructive
Surgery, University of Michigan, Ann Arbor,
Michigan

CHRISTOPHER J. SCHULTZ, MD
Professor, Department of Radiation Oncology,
Medical College of Wisconsin, Milwaukee,
Wisconsin

VINOD B. SHIDHAM, MD, FIAC, FRCPath
Professor, Department of Pathology, Medical
College of Wisconsin, Milwaukee, Wisconsin;
Executive Editor and Editor-in-Chief,
CytoJournal

JAIME H. SHUFF, MD
Resident, Department of Radiation Oncology,
Medical College of Wisconsin, Milwaukee,
Wisconsin

MALIKA L. SIKER, MD
Resident, Department of Radiation Oncology,
Medical College of Wisconsin, Milwaukee,
Wisconsin

WAYNE K. STADELMANN, MD, FACS
Private Practice, Stadelmann Center for Plastic
Surgery, Concord, New Hampshire

JONATHAN TREISMAN, MD
Section Chief, Medical Oncology,
Immunotherapy Program; Medical Consultants,
Inc, Aurora St Luke's Medical Center,
Milwaukee, Wisconsin

Contents

The first part of this review examines the reliability of histologic diagnosis in pigmented lesions, as measured by concordance studies and medicolegal analysis. It emphasizes the role of clinicians in maximizing that reliability, by providing adequate clinical descriptions, using appropriate biopsy technique, and critically interpreting pathology reports. It identifies those entities that are especially problematic, either because they cannot be reliably recognized by the histopathologist or because their histology is a poor guide to their biologic behavior. The second part of the review is a guide to some of the more difficult and controversial pigmented lesions, including dysplastic nevus, spitzoid nevi and melanomas, cellular blue nevus, animal-type melanoma, and deep penetrating nevus.

The Spitz nevus is a relatively common skin lesion in children and is less commonly seen in adults. The lesion is defined by the presence of distinctive-appearing spindle or epithelioid cells on light microscopy in a recognizable nevus-like pattern. Spitz lesions share features with melanoma on light microscopic examination. When Spitz features are atypical or typical features are absent, distinction from melanoma can be difficult. A spectrum of pathology of Spitz lesions can be found from lesions that are benign and typical to lesions that are atypical with melanoma-like features and frank melanoma. There is significant interobserver variation in interpretation of Spitz lesions. The lack of uniformly applied criteria for distinction of light microscopic grades and the confusion in diagnostic terminology demonstrate the difficulty in the pathologic interpretation of these lesions. Exciting progress has been made recently in ancillary testing that will likely be helpful in determining in more detail the biologic nature of these lesions, in better differentiating the benign Spitz lesions from malignant lesions, and in eventually improving treatment recommendations.

Lentigo maligna is an overgrowth of atypical melanocytes at the dermal–epidermal junction also known as melanoma in situ. Left untreated, these lesions can continue to grow, resulting in dermal invasion and progression to lentigo maligna melanoma. Many operative and nonoperative treatments have been developed with the goals of preserving function and cosmesis while at the same time addressing the diffuse nature of these lesions. Previous recommendations have led plastic surgeons to commonly perform wide local excision with 5 mm margins. More recent literature has suggested that in many cases this treatment can result in high recurrence rates.

This has led to margin control procedures becoming the treatment of choice for these lesions.

of diagnosing nodal metastatic disease, with the ability to detect smaller and smaller volumes of tumor in the sentinel lymph nodes (SLNs) biopsied using immunohisto-chemical staining, has impacted the accurate staging and stratification of melanoma patients. The role that elective lymph node dissection now plays in staging the melanoma patient and determining subsequent treatment has been greatly diminished in favor of less morbid and less invasive techniques that have a higher degree of accuracy in detecting occult nodal disease. This article explores what has driven the advent of selective or SLN biopsy, the rationale behind obtaining a preoperative lymphoscintigram, the technical details of the SLN biopsy procedure, and the refinement in the pathologic detection of ever smaller volumes of tumor in nymph node tissue removed. The role that these new modalities have played in changing the dynamic field of melanoma care is emphasized.

The pathologic evaluation of sentinel lymph nodes for melanoma metastases is not without significant challenges. It is affected by significant variation in approaches, which may compromise the final interpretation, leading to nonrepresentative spurious results. This article discusses various approaches along with recommended dos and don'ts for optimum evaluation of sentinel lymph nodes for melanoma metastases.

The primary management of lymph nodes involved with metastatic melanoma is regional lymphadenectomy. Axillary or inguinal node complete lymph node dissection (CLND) is performed after an occult metastasis is found by sentinel lymph node biopsy, or after a clinically apparent regional lymph node metastasis. CLND completely removes all lymph-node-bearing tissue in a nodal basin. This procedure continues to be controversial. No randomized prospective studies have yet determined the survival advantage of CLND. The National Comprehensive Cancer Network recommends that all patients with stage III melanoma have a CLND.

This article provides a review of the current medical management of patients with high-risk and metastatic cutaneous melanoma, including a review of the use of adjuvant interferon therapy and a discussion of adjuvant treatments under evaluation. The use of standard chemotherapeutic agents for metastatic disease is discussed, with an emphasis on developmental therapeutics using targeted agents. This discussion includes a review of the immune therapy for metastatic melanoma, including newer immunomodulatory agents and cellular therapeutics that are expected to significantly impact the care of these patients.

Cutaneous melanoma is a disease that often has an aggressive and unpredictable course. It was historically thought to be a radioresistant neoplasm; however, substantial radiobiologic and clinical evidence has emerged to refute this notion. Improved local control has been demonstrated with the use of adjuvant radiation therapy delivered to the primary site or regional lymphatics in patients with high-risk clinical or pathologic features. Despite improved local control, high-risk cutaneous melanoma often spreads systemically, leading to poor survival. In the setting of systemic progression, radiation therapy can frequently palliate symptomatic sites of metastatic disease.

Primary surgical treatment should be considered for patients with metastatic melanoma. Because of the poor response of melanoma to chemotherapy or radiation therapy, surgery can be the best approach to quickly eliminate detectable disease and return the patient to normal activities. In properly selected patients, surgery can lead to significant palliation and prolongation of survival. This article reviews the principles of patient selection and the potential benefits of surgical management of melanoma metastatic to various sites. Novel adjuvant therapies are being developed to augment the benefits of surgical treatment of advanced melanoma in the future.

The future of melanoma research is promising. Specific mechanisms leading to oncogenic transformation in melanoma development have been identified, and are likely to produce new targets for melanoma therapy. Also, advances in melanoma research will result from melanoma investigators co-opting approaches used to study other malignancies in which progress has been made more rapidly. Systematic roadblocks limiting advances in melanoma research relative to other malignancies are being addressed in a formal manner. The public and public officials are increasingly becoming aware of the need for more dedicated efforts to address the challenges of research on this malignancy.

Clinics in Plastic Surgery

THE CLINICS ARE NOW AVAILABLE ONLINE!

Access your subscription at:
www.theclinics.com

Preface

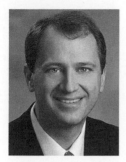

William W. Dzwierzynski, MD, FACS
Guest Editor

It has been almost 10 years since an issue of *Clinics in Plastic Surgery* was dedicated to the diagnosis and treatment of malignant melanoma. Since that time, significant changes in the diagnosis and treatment of melanoma have occurred. In 2000, at the time of the last issue, elective lymph node dissection was still being performed and sentinel lymph node biopsy was in its infancy. Sentinel lymph node biopsy has now become the standard of care in melanoma. The staging system was totally revamped in 2002, taking into account the significance of ulceration and the information gained during sentinel node biopsy. Although the treatment of melanoma still remains surgical, new research into immunotherapy gives hope for further medical therapies.

With more than 60,000 patients being diagnosed each year with malignant melanoma, plastic surgeons will continue to see patients with this disease. Treatment of this disease involves a coordinated effort of many specialists. These include plastic surgeons, dermatologists, dermatopathologists, nuclear medicine physicians, radiation oncologists, medical oncologists, surgical oncologists,

and primary care specialists. Plastic surgeons have a long history of involvement in the care of patients with melanoma. The plastic surgeon must continue to be pivotal in the care of patients with melanoma, coordinating care among the specialists and being integral in all aspects of surgery and follow-up.

I hope this issue of *Clinics in Plastic Surgery* serves both as a compendium of information for the surgical management of patients with melanoma and also as a reference source for physicians and patients researching treatment options, current therapies, and further innovations.

William W. Dzwierzynski, MD, FACS
Professor of Plastic Surgery
Medical College of Wisconsin
8700 Watertown Plank Road
Milwaukee, WI 53226, USA

E-mail address:
billd@mcw.edu

Clin Plastic Surg 37 (2010) xi
doi:10.1016/j.cps.2009.08.007
0094-1298/09/$ – see front matter © 2010 Elsevier Inc. All rights reserved.

Pigmented Lesion Pathology: What You Should Expect from Your Pathologist, and What Your Pathologist Should Expect from You

Matthew G. Fleming, MD

KEYWORDS

- Melanoma • Nevus • Pathology
- Dysplastic nevus syndrome
- Nevus, epithelioid and spindle cell

The diagnosis and treatment of melanoma and related neoplasms is difficult and dangerous for all concerned. In the typical scenario, a lesion is identified by a dermatologist or other clinician as sufficiently atypical to warrant biopsy; a dermatopathologist or general pathologist renders the "gold standard" (ie, histologic) diagnosis, and stages the lesion and the patient is referred to a surgeon (and oncologist if necessary) for treatment appropriate to the stage of his disease.

In this sequence, several things can go wrong. The patient may not seek care while the lesion is curable; the practitioner to whom he initially presents may fail to recognize it; the pathologist may misdiagnose it; and the surgeon may misinterpret and therefore fail to act appropriately on the pathologist's report. These errors would usually lead to undertreatment, but overtreatment of, for example, a mildly atypical dysplastic or spitzoid lesion, can also lead to unnecessary morbidity and cost.

That these problems are real, and bear especially on pathology, is attested by the experience of a large pathology insurer, that melanoma is responsible for more malpractice claims than any other diagnostic entity,[1] a frequency disproportionate to the prevalence of this disease (13% of claims[1] but only 4%–5% of cancers[2]). Errors can and should be minimized at each stage of the pipeline. Patients can benefit from public education programs that emphasize melanoma prevention and detection, while the accuracy of screening personnel can be improved by novel diagnostic modalities such as dermoscopy. Pathologists can benefit from technical controls and consultation, within their own laboratories.[3,4] However, these measures do not address the problems that may arise at the interface between clinical and pathologic practice. What clinicians do—how they obtain and submit specimens—influences the accuracy of the pathology report they will in turn receive. The quality of that report (the accuracy and completeness of staging information, for example) then feeds back to the treating clinician. Some reports may contain terms, such as dysplastic nevus, nevus with architectural disorder and cytologic atypia, atypical Spitz tumor, atypical blue nevus, and melanocytoma, that are frankly mystifying to the clinician, who may not even understand whether they refer to a benign or malignant diagnosis.

In this review, we will tread the interface between clinical and pathologic practice, which holds the promise of the most fruitful diagnostic

Department of Dermatology, Medical College of Wisconsin, 8701 Watertown Plank Road, Milwaukee, WI 53226, USA
E-mail address: mfleming@mcw.edu

Clin Plastic Surg 37 (2010) 1–20
doi:10.1016/j.cps.2009.07.003

and therapeutic collaborations, but also carries the risk of serious error. We will review data on the reliability of pathologic diagnosis in melanoma and other pigmented lesions; discuss measures that may be taken by the clinician to help maximize that reliability; and review some of the more confusing diagnoses in pigmented lesion pathology, such as those mentioned above.

RELIABILITY OF HISTOLOGIC DIAGNOSIS OF MELANOCYTIC NEOPLASMS
Interobserver Concordance

There are several studies of interobserver concordance in the histologic diagnosis of melanocytic neoplasms. For the most part they are not encouraging. One of the first and most cited was part of the Consensus Development Conference on the Diagnosis and Treatment of Early Melanoma, convened by the National Institutes of Health (NIH).[5] Thirty-seven cases, submitted as "classic" examples of melanoma and nevi, were reviewed by 7 panelists selected for their publications and recognized expertise in pigmented lesion pathology. There was complete concordance in only 13 of the cases, with almost complete concordance (none or 1 dissenter) in 23 (64%). When the diagnoses were grouped into benign, intermediate, and malignant categories, the k value was 0.50, indicating only moderate agreement.[5] (One of the panelists subsequently commented that the cases were in fact not "classic".[6])

A somewhat similar experiment was performed in 2000 at the 21st Symposium of the International Society of Dermatopathology.[7] Seventy-one "difficult" melanocytic neoplasms were reviewed by a panel of 6 experts. Complete agreement was achieved in 49% of cases, with almost complete agreement (only 1 dissenter) in another 31%.[7] Although 1 of the participants described the experience as producing "the impression of watching a slow-motion multivehicle accident,"[8] these results are probably not that bad, considering the "difficult" nature of the cases. Further, there was excellent concordance in several areas traditionally regarded as problematic, including desmoplastic melanomas and nevi, recurrent melanomas and nevi, and nevoid melanoma.[7] Spitz nevi and other childhood lesions were responsible for much of the discordance.[7]

These studies are somewhat difficult to interpret because of questions involving case selection (just how "classic" were the cases in the first study[5] and how "difficult" were they in the second?).[7] Two studies from Italy are of interest because they employed unselected, sequential accessions.[9,10] In the first study, 100 melanomas and 20 nevi were evaluated by 4 dermatopathologists.[9] There was complete agreement in 76% of cases, with a k value for the diagnosis of melanoma of 0.61. k values for melanoma features were fairly low; for example, 0.76 for Breslow depth. The second Italian study measured concordance for 13 histologic features in 64 melanomas evaluated by 9 dermatopathologists.[10] k values were quite high, greater than 0.75 for 10 out of the 13.

Concordance has been assessed for specific subsets of melanocytic neoplasms. As already mentioned, childhood lesions are especially problematic. Eighty-five childhood melanomas were examined by a panel of 8 expert dermatopathologists, divided into 4 pairs.[11] There was complete agreement within each pair for only 39% of cases. When, as a control, 20 adult melanomas and 15 nevi were evaluated by the same mechanism, there was complete agreement for all cases.

Thirty spitzoid lesions were collected by a panel of 10 dermatopathologists, and then categorized by the members of the panel as Spitz nevus, atypical Spitz nevus, melanoma, or indeterminate.[12] Seventeen of the 30 lesions were regarded by at least some members of the panel as displaying features of Spitz nevus, but in only 1 case was there agreement by a majority of panelists on that diagnosis. That case eventuated in metastasis and death.

Atypical cellular blue nevus (CBN) is another problematic entity. A collection of these lesions was examined in a set that included typical CBN, common blue nevi, and melanomas, by a panel of 10 experienced dermatopathologists.[13] A majority selected the correct diagnosis in only 38% of cases; average sensitivity for the diagnosis of atypical CBN was 35%; and overall k value was 0.25.[13]

One hundred and forty-nine nevi were classified as dysplastic, banal, or intermediate by a panel of 6 dermatopathologists, divided into pairs.[14] There was 56% concordance, with a k value of 0.34. When intermediate and dysplastic categories were pooled, the k value rose to 0.49. Intraobserver concordance was also measured. Interestingly, it was 85% for the same slide and 78% for recuts.[14]

Concordance is only moderate for margin assessment in lentigo maligna and lentigo maligna melanoma. These tumors occur on sun-exposed skin, which may have a baseline of increased melanocyte density and atypia. When 5 pathologists evaluated excision margins from these lesions, there was only 72% agreement with the original pathologic diagnosis (as involved or not), and the k value was 0.4 to 0.5 for agreement within the panel.[15]

All of these studies investigated concordance among experienced dermatopathologists, generally academic dermatopathologists with a record of publication in the area. Concordance among general pathologists in melanoma diagnosis is much worse.[16]

Be Kind to Your Pathologist

Faced with these dismal statistics, what should be done? First, cheer up: they probably overstate the problem. In reviewing some of this work, Glusac expressed his opinion "that experts would disagree significantly (benign vs malignant) on less than 1% of randomly selected melanocytic neoplasms." Although concrete evidence for this view is lacking, it probably is substantively correct.

Second, recognize that the clinician is not a passive bystander in the process of histologic diagnosis, but rather an active participant with a great deal of influence over its outcome. The clinician can contribute through expert clinical assessment, clear communication of clinical observations to the laboratory, optimal biopsy technique, and judicious interpretation of the final pathology report.

A case from my practice briefly illustrates these principles. A tiny (1 mm) specimen was submitted by a generalist without any clinical information. It was entirely ulcerated, so that the epidermal component of the lesion, if any, could not be evaluated. At the base of the ulcer a small number of melanocytes were observed. They were somewhat atypical, but this could be explained by proximity to the ulcer, and the findings were regarded as most consistent with traumatized nevus. A second experienced dermatopathologist concurred with this interpretation. Two weeks after the case was completed, a call was received from ancillary staff at the referring practice. The staff member said that the referring physician was entirely satisfied with my diagnosis, but would I be interested to learn that the specimen had been obtained from a 2-cm black plaque?

With respect to clinical assessment, it is obvious that lesions susceptible to unequivocal clinical diagnosis will not be biopsied at all. Nevertheless, skilled clinical evaluation, even when it is not conclusive, reduces the opportunity for histologic error. There are differences in the ability of clinicians to evaluate pigmented lesions,[17–19] and most of us have room for improvement. (Dermatologists, for example, do as well or better than other practitioners,[18,19] but are only about 64% to 80% accurate in the clinical diagnosis of melanoma.[20,21]) For most practitioners the introduction of dermoscopy would be the quickest route to improved screening accuracy. This technique employs a simple hand-held instrument (the dermatoscope) that provides a low (approximately 10×) magnification view of the skin, with crosspolarization or immersion oil to eliminate specular reflectances from the skin surface. Structures from the epidermis to the deep papillary dermis can be visualized. The dermoscopy literature is immense and encompasses several different approaches to the interpretation of dermoscopic imagery. Nevertheless, practitioners can realize substantial improvements in clinical screening accuracy after a day or less of dermoscopic training.[22–24] In expert hands, dermoscopy improves the mean log odds ratio for the diagnosis of melanoma from 2.7 to 4.0, in effect increasing screening accuracy by 49%, according to a meta-analysis of 27 studies.[25]

To be most useful, clinical information must be generously shared with the pathologist. The pathology submission slip has been called "one of the most underutilized documents in medicine."[3,26] As a minimum, age, sex, site, and relevant clinical history should be included. Site is important because nevi from the "special sites" frequently display architectural irregularities that may create some resemblance to melanoma. These sites include acral locations, genitals, breast, scalp, ear, flexural regions, and the conjunctiva.[27] History should include recent change, trauma, sun exposure, phototherapy, and personal or family history of melanoma and dysplastic nevus syndrome. Trauma[28] and ultraviolet (UV) light exposure[29,30] (either natural or from phototherapy) can produce pagetoid spread and other changes that can be misinterpreted as evidence of melanoma. (For this reason it has been suggested that biopsy of traumatized or UV-irradiated lesions be deferred for 4 weeks, unless there is strong clinical evidence for melanoma.[31]) If a biopsy of the lesion was taken previously this should also be recorded, because surgery and subsequent reparative change can also distort nevus architecture,[32] and sampling errors can occur in a lesion that was removed in stages. For example, a previous specimen might contain melanoma, whereas the current specimen reveals only precursor nevus. For previously biopsied lesions, the pathologist will in many instances want to review the original specimen, and the clinician should facilitate this by providing the necessary information.

A description of the lesion's clinical appearance should also accompany the specimen. The "ABCDE" screening criteria[33] might provide a framework for this description, as they are easily learned and applied. If the lesion is clinically heterogeneous (eg, if it contains a "black dot"),[34] this should be communicated, as it would stimulate the pathologist to section through the block if initial sections are negative for melanoma. Results of dermoscopic examination, if performed, should be recorded. If the pathologist, but not the clinician, has dermoscopic expertise (entirely possible if the former is a dermatologist/dermatopathologist), dermoscopic photographs might be transmitted to the laboratory. They would be especially valuable for heterogeneous lesions (eg, melanoma originating in nevus). Dermoscopy and histopathology are complementary in such cases, because the former visualizes the entire lesion in the horizontal plane (parallel to the skin surface), whereas the latter visualizes only a limited number of vertical planes through it. Dermoscopy can guide sectioning toward the most suspicious area, or at least ensure that multiple sections are obtained. Four cases of melanoma originating in nevus, which would have been misdiagnosed without dermoscopy, have been reported.[35,36] More generally, in a series of 301 nevi and melanomas, the submission of dermoscopic images caused the pathologic diagnosis to be revised in 11 equivocal cases, 8 from melanoma to nevus and 3 from nevus to melanoma.[37] When this series was evaluated by pathologists at 2 centers, the addition of dermoscopic images improved concordance between the centers from a k value of 0.81 to 0.88.[37] Lesions that are histologically equivocal also tend to be dermoscopically equivocal,[38] so correlation between the 2 modalities is important.[39]

Biopsy technique is critical for accurate histologic evaluation. The guidelines of the American Academy of Dermatology (AAD)[40] and the National Comprehensive Cancer Center (NCCN)[41] call for removal of the entire lesion with narrow (1–3 mm) margins, at the initial encounter. The AAD guidelines specify that "an incisional biopsy technique is appropriate when the suspicion for melanoma is low, when the lesion is large, or when it is impractical to perform an excision,"[40] whereas the NCCN states that "full thickness incisional or punch biopsy of the clinically thickest portion of the lesion is acceptable, in certain anatomic areas (eg, palm/sole, digit, face, ear) or for very large lesions."[41] Partial biopsy should be avoided, when at all possible, because it can lead to errors in diagnosis and staging, and possibly a worse clinical outcome.

One study evaluated the accuracy of partial biopsy by comparing the initial and final histologic diagnoses in a series of 63 lesions obtained from patients with dysplastic nevus syndrome.[42] Punch biopsies were obtained from 41 of these lesions, and shave biopsies from the remainder; all were then re-excised, and the excision and biopsy specimens compared. In 12 of the lesions obtained by punch biopsy, but only 1 of the shaved lesions, there was diagnostic discordance between the biopsy and excision specimens. In 2 cases the punch biopsy specimen was interpreted as nevus but excision revealed melanoma; in 1 case a melanoma interpreted as in situ in the punch biopsy specimen was found to be invasive in the excision specimen; and in 1 case shave biopsy revealed in situ melanoma but invasive disease (Breslow depth 2.85 mm) was found in the excision specimen.[42]

In a series of 1784 histologically diagnosed melanomas, melanoma had not been clinically suspected in 503. Of these, diagnosis was compromised in 31 and histologic staging was impossible in 62 because of inadequate biopsy technique.[43] For 10 specimens (5 punch biopsy specimens, 5 shaves) the diagnosis of melanoma was completely missed, and established only at a later date by rebiopsy.[43]

Diagnostic certainty was evaluated subjectively in a retrospective study of 525 specimens with a pathologic diagnosis of certain or probable melanoma.[44] Of these specimens, 37% had been obtained by excision, 36% by punch biopsy, 9% by shave biopsy, 4% by deep shave biopsy, and 14% by unknown technique. The pathologic diagnosis was regarded as certain in 65% of cases, and at least somewhat doubtful in the remainder (35%). In 25%, uncertainty was the unavoidable result of equivocal pathologic findings, but in 9% inadequate specimen width was partially or entirely responsible for the uncertainty. In no case was uncertainty caused by inadequate depth. Comparing specimen types, 23% of punches, 21% of shaves, 11% of deep shaves, and 9% of excisions were assigned the lowest category of diagnostic certainty.[44]

The investigators in this study suggested that subtotal biopsy can contribute to diagnostic uncertainty in many ways. Some pathologic features–such as size, symmetry, and margination (abrupt vs indistinct lateral boundaries)–cannot be evaluated unless the full breadth of the lesion is visible.[44] Some features are assessed at a smaller scale but may vary within the tumor, so that an accurate summary judgment requires the entire lesion. These features include spacing between epidermal melanocytes, size and shape of nests, pagetoid spread, and cytology.[44] Maturation (diminishing melanocyte size with depth) and deep mitotic activity, which are especially important for spitzoid and other nodular tumors, cannot be evaluated in superficial specimens. Heterogeneous lesions, consisting of both melanoma and precursor nevus, are of course especially problematic in partial specimens. The investigators illustrate 1 such case, in which punch biopsy through the thickest part of the lesion would have sampled only nevus and missed the surrounding melanoma.[44] Sampling only the regressed area in a partially regressed melanoma can create similar difficulties.[4]

Several studies have compared Breslow depth in initial partial biopsy and subsequent re-excision specimens of invasive melanoma. Ng and colleagues[45] found concordance in 88% of 145 such cases. For 28 of 30 superficial shave biopsy specimens, 34 of 37 deep shave biopsy specimens, and 33 of 41 punch biopsy specimens, Breslow depth in the biopsy specimen was equal to or greater than the depth in the re-excision specimen.[45] Concordance was thus lower (80%) for punch biopsy than for shave, and was only 53% for the subset of punch biopsy specimens with involved margins. However, punch biopsied tumors were thicker than shaved lesions.[45] In similar work, Stell and colleagues[46] compared 224 melanomas, evaluated initially by excisional, shave, or punch biopsy. Shave biopsy specimens had a significantly higher proportion of involved deep margins than punch or excision specimens (22%, 7%, and 2%, respectively). However, re-excision increased the Breslow depth in a much higher proportion of punch biopsied than shaved cases (26% vs 4%), and this resulted in significant upstaging (higher T score) in many more punched than shaved cases (12% vs 2%).[46]

These studies suggest that shave biopsy might be preferable to punch biopsy if partial biopsy cannot be avoided, although differences between the tumors sampled by the 2 procedures (punched lesions were generally deeper than those shaved) casts some doubt on this conclusion. They also support the recommendations of the NCCN and AAD for complete initial excision. In addition to the diagnostic and staging errors found in these studies to result from partial biopsy, a further concern has been that cutting through the tumor might facilitate metastasis by providing vascular access or displacing tumor into deeper tissue layers. Some studies have shown initial partial biopsy to adversely affect survival,[47] but many have not.[48] In any case, it is likely to be unhealthy for the practitioner, if not the patient. Of all medical malpractice claims involving melanoma submitted between 1995 and 2001, the tumor had been biopsied by shave, punch, or incisional technique in 83% of cases,[49] whereas complete excisional biopsy was performed in only 17%.[49]

Despite their ample justification, the guidelines are not being followed—at least not in England, where compliance was recently investigated.[50] Of 100 melanoma patients referred to a plastic surgery practice, 50 were referred without biopsy and of the rest there were 17 excisional, 20 punch, 3 shave, and 1 incisional biopsies and 1 curettage. Punch biopsies were more common than excisions for patients referred by both dermatologists and generalists. Almost all of the punch biopsied lesions were small and/or from sites (trunk and extremities) where excision with primary closure would have been feasible, and in almost all these cases melanoma had been suspected clinically. Breslow depth could be determined in only 45% of the punch biopsy specimens. The investigators speculate that the punch biopsies were performed because they were "more accessible to the outpatient setting."[50]

Shave biopsy remains a reasonable approach for pigmented lesions with a convincingly benign clinical appearance, because it has been demonstrated in several studies to produce the best cosmetic outcome.[48] NCCN guidelines regard it as "acceptable when the index of suspicion is low."[41]

The clinician's responsibility does not, of course, end with the submission of the specimen. Discordance between clinical and pathologic diagnoses should always be pursued.[4] Although pathologic examination is traditionally regarded as the diagnostic gold standard for pigmented lesions, it is subject to error for all the reasons described earlier, and its conclusions cannot be accepted uncritically. Even if an optimal (complete excisional) specimen was submitted, the initial sections may not be representative of the entire lesion, revealing, for example, only nevus in a specimen that also contains melanoma.[4,35,36,44] Most pathologists will step-section specimens clinically suspected of melanoma, when the initial sections do not show it; but in some cases this may be done only at the clinician's request.[4,49] When the initial specimen was suboptimal (partial), the appropriate response to clinicopathologic discordance is to remove the remainder of the lesion.

The clinician should note elements in the pathology report that express diagnostic uncertainty, such as "consistent with," "suggestive of," "atypical melanocytic neoplasm," and so forth. According to Crowson, "the more frequent scenario in litigation … is that a lesion with a metastatic potential has been considered … benign *without any equivocation or caveats applied in the pathology report*" [italics mine].[4] In some cases, even if the specimen was optimal and sectioned exhaustively, the pathologic condition itself will be equivocal. Treatment of such cases must be individualized and may test the experience and judgment of the pathologist and clinician.

Finally, diagnostic terminology varies among pathologists and the clinician should become familiar with that used by his or her pathologist(s).

PROBLEM DIAGNOSES
Dysplastic Nevus

Some of the more confusing and controversial diagnostic terms and entities are addressed in the following sections.

The dysplastic nevus is perhaps *primum inter pares* among controversial entities in pigmented lesion pathology. Disputed issues include the diagnostic terminology that should be applied to this entity, the reproducibility and significance of histologic grading, and the biologic status of the lesion as fully benign or in some way intermediate between benign and malignant. Related questions address the primacy of clinical or histologic features for diagnosis, prevalence, and clinical management (should a dysplastic nevus diagnosed in a partial biopsy be re-excised, and if so, does this apply to all such nevi or only to particular histologic grades?).

The dysplastic nevus was described in 1978 by Clark, as the "B-K mole," a nevus with distinctive clinical and histologic features occurring at high density in individuals with the "B-K mole syndrome." These were members of 6 families afflicted by multiple melanomas.[51] Subsequently Clark's group proposed the term "dysplastic nevus," because they regarded the entity as a stage in the evolution of melanoma, analogous to lesions recognized as carcinoma precursors.[52] In the next decade, it became apparent that nevi with similar clinical and histologic characteristics occur sporadically, as single lesions or in small numbers, in patients with no relevant family history. It also became apparent that these lesions are common,[53,54] with about 20% of nevi meeting histologic criteria for dysplasia.[53,55] Clearly, most of these will not evolve to melanoma. Writing in the late 1980s, the influential dermatopathologist A.B. Ackerman asserted that the dysplastic nevus is in fact "the most common nevus," and, when sporadic, poses no risk of progression ("wholly benign").[56] He further complained that the clinical and histologic criteria proposed for the recognition of dysplastic nevus and dysplastic nevus syndrome could not be reproducibly applied.[56] He proposed renaming the entity "Clark nevus," to avoid the unjustifiably negative implications of its original designation.[57]

An NIH Consensus Conference held in 1992 had a slightly more muted response.[58] It recognized a "10-fold difference in estimates of ... frequency," but attributed this to variation in the application of histologic criteria for diagnosis. These criteria had included certain architectural features and mild ("random"[51]) cytologic atypia.

The 1992 Consensus Conference uncoupled architecture and cytology, regarding architecture as constant but cytologic atypia as variable and in some cases absent.[58] In their view, the histologic architecture of a lesion places it within the spectrum of dysplastic nevus, whereas its cytology defines the position it occupies within that spectrum. Consistent with this understanding, and to avoid the controversy that then attended the term "dysplastic nevus," the NIH recommended that the lesion be renamed "nevus with architectural disorder." This (subsequently amended to "nevus with architectural disorder and cytologic atypia") should be the preferred histologic diagnosis, and accompanied by a comment specifying the degree of cytologic atypia.[58]

This history has left a legacy of confusion. In a 2004 survey of the membership of the American Society of Dermatopathology and the AAD, Shapiro and colleagues[59] found that no single diagnostic term was preferred by a majority of dermatopathologists. "Dysplastic nevus" was the most common term, used by 39% of dermatopathologists, whereas some variant of "nevus with architectural disorder" was used by 28%, and "Clark's nevus" by 10%. These terms are essentially synonymous, but 4% of dermatopathologists use the term "atypical nevus," 2.7% "compound nevus," 1.5% "compound nevus with extension of the junctional component," and 1% "atypical melanocytic hyperplasia."[59] For these dermatopathologists, presumably, the dysplastic nevus is not a histopathologic entity. Thirty-three percent of the 39% of dermatopathologists calling these lesions "dysplastic nevus" scored them for the degree of dysplasia (as mild, moderate, or severe). Of those preferring "nevus with architectural disorganization" what proportion rated them for cytologic atypia (in accordance with NIH recommendations) was apparently not investigated.[59] The dermatologists were slightly more consistent: 62% used "dysplastic nevus."

Shapiro and colleagues[59] questioned whether those using older language were unaware of the NIH terminology or actively opposed to it. The language can be criticized for lack of specificity; that is, dysplastic nevi are not just disorganized and cytologically atypical but have specific architectural and cytologic features; alternatively, some nevi with "architectural disorganization and cytologic atypia" are not dysplastic (eg, traumatized, sun-exposed, and halo nevi). In addition, it seems that all dysplastic nevi are cytologically atypical,[54] and that cytologic atypia should not be the sole basis for grading dysplasia.[60] There is evidence that the severity of architectural abnormality and the degree of cytologic atypia are highly correlated.[60–63]

Nevertheless, recent work suggests that the Consensus Conference was justified in trying to define a spectrum of histologic dysplasia. DNA content[64] and microsatellite instability[65] were found to increase with the degree of dysplasia. Dysplasia also correlates with melanoma risk. Arum-Uria and colleagues[60] examined all of the dysplastic nevi accessioned to a single laboratory between 1989 and 1996. There were 6275 nevi belonging to 4481 patients. For each nevus the degree of dysplasia was rated as mild, moderate, or severe according to combined architectural and cytologic criteria. Patients were classified according to their most dysplastic nevus. Of the 4481 patients, the worst nevus was mildly dysplastic in 2504, moderately dysplastic in 1657, and severely dysplastic in 320 patients. Pathology submission slips were examined to determine whether the specimen had been obtained from a patient with a history of melanoma. Such a history was reported for 5.7%, 8.1%, and 19.7% of patients with mildly, moderately, and severely dysplastic nevi, respectively.[60]

Approaching this question from the opposite direction, Shors and colleagues[66] examined the most clinically atypical nevus in 80 melanoma patients and 80 spousal controls. The nevi were graded as mildly, moderately, or severely dysplastic by a panel of 13 dermatopathologists, who had not previously met to agree on rating criteria. Most (82%) of the nevi were rated mildly dysplastic. The presence of a severely dysplastic nevus was significantly associated with melanoma, with an odds ratio of 2.6. This correlation remained significant after adjustment for the number of nevi and many other known melanoma risk factors.[66]

These studies point to differences within the group of histologically recognizable dysplastic nevi, a concept that may help to reconcile the conflict, noted earlier, between the clear epidemiologic association of dysplastic nevus and melanoma, in some settings, and the frequency of the diagnosis.

One difficulty with Shors' study[66] was that, whereas the consensus dysplasia score predicted the presence or absence of melanoma, the scores of individual pathologists generally did not. Of the 13 dermatopathologists, only 1 pathologist's scores correlated significantly with melanoma risk.[66] There was no statistical analysis or other evaluation to determine whether this was a chance association, or reflected greater experience or the application of unique diagnostic criteria by this dermatopathologist. If the latter, then accurate grading of histologic dysplasia might be a teachable skill.

In Shors' study, the k value for agreement among the 13 pathologists was only 0.28.[66] Other work showed somewhat better concordance in rating dysplasia. In 1 study, 30 dysplastic nevi were graded as mild, moderate, or severe by 3 experienced dermatopathologists and 2 dermatopathology fellows, divided into pairs.[62] Concordance among the pairs of experienced dermatopathologists was 35% to 58%, for k values of 0.38 to 0.47. Concordance among the trainees was lower (16%–65%). Twenty common nevi and 10 melanomas were also included in the study, and concordance for the diagnosis of dysplastic nevus was 69% to 80% ($k = 0.53$–0.71) for the experienced dermatopathologists and 61% to 88% ($k = 0.55$–0.84) for the trainees. Apparently, less experience is required to recognize dysplastic nevi than to grade them. Concordance was 90% for the distinction between dysplastic nevus and melanoma and was better for the distinction between severely dysplastic nevus and melanoma than among the lesser grades of dysplasia.[62]

The frequency of various diagnoses rendered by 2 dermatopathologists in evaluating 2631 melanocytic neoplasms was compared.[67] Although concordance between the 2 was not investigated, they assigned a remarkably similar proportion of cases to mildly, moderately, and severely dysplastic categories. One regarded 8.8%, 7.0%, and 2.7% of melanocytic lesions as mildly dysplastic, moderately dysplastic, and severely dysplastic nevi, respectively, and the comparable percentages for the other dermatopathologist were 12.0%, 6.8%, and 1.6%. Interestingly, the 2 dermatopathologists articulated different formal criteria for the diagnosis of dysplastic nevus, with only 1 requiring cytologic atypia. Note that in this study, as in those of Arum-Uria and colleagues[60] and Shors and colleagues,[66] only a small minority of nevi were judged to be severely dysplastic.

There are other studies of concordance in the histologic diagnosis of dysplastic nevus. Clemente reported 92% concordance among a panel of 6 dermatopathologists, in distinguishing among 114 examples of banal nevus, dysplastic nevus, and melanoma.[68] Most discordance involved the distinction between severely dysplastic nevus and melanoma. The panel had agreed in advance on diagnostic criteria for dysplastic nevus. In a similar but smaller study, there was 87% agreement among 10 dermatopathologists in distinguishing dysplastic nevus from banal nevus and melanoma.[69]

Other recent research confirms that Clark was correct in placing dysplastic nevus on the spectrum from banal nevus to melanoma. Unlike ordinary nevi, dysplastic nevi share genetic lesions (such as loss of heterozygosity at 1p36,[70,71] 9p22-21,[70–72] and 17p13[72]) with melanoma. They are intermediate between banal nevus and melanoma in DNA content,[64,73–75] immunohistochemical labeling fraction for proliferation markers,[76–78] and telomerase activity.[78] Microsatellite instability is present in dysplastic nevi, at a frequency only slightly lower than in melanoma, but absent in other nevi.[65,79] Severely dysplastic nevi show more microsatellite instability than lower grades.[65] Mismatch repair proteins are reduced in dysplastic nevi, to a level intermediate between that in banal nevus and melanoma.[80] These findings suggest that dysplastic nevi manifest the same kind of genetic instability as has been observed in premalignant and early malignant lesions in other cell lineages.[65] Dysplastic nevi serve as an epidemiologic marker of melanoma risk in familial melanoma kindreds[81] and in patients without a family history but large numbers of nevi.[82] Dysplastic nevus remnants have been found in 7% to 60% of unselected melanomas[83,84] and up to 80% of familial melanomas,[81] suggesting that Clark was also correct that the lesion itself constitutes part of at least 1 important pathway to melanoma formation.

In conclusion, the dysplastic nevus remains a problem, but it can and must be recognized. It is simply unacceptable for pathologists to apply nonspecific diagnostic terms such as "compound nevus" (as did almost 10% of dermatopathologists in Shapiro's survey). The lesions should be graded (basically as mild, moderate, or severe). The reliability of this grading will not be perfect, but it should be attempted, as histologic grade correlates with melanoma risk and biologic markers of malignancy. Although dysplastic nevi are moderately common, only a small proportion will be rated as severely dysplastic.[60,66,67]

Should the diagnosis of dysplastic nevus lead to re-excision for a partially biopsied nevus? Although some authorities have recommended re-excision in all such cases,[4] in my opinion it is a question that each practitioner must answer for himself, because it involves trade-offs between risk, inconvenience, and cost in which the risk cannot be precisely quantified and the risk tolerance of the practitioner and the patient must be accommodated. For the reasons described earlier, in my practice dysplastic nevi are graded, and an explicit recommendation to re-excise accompanies reports of incompletely removed, severely dysplastic examples. Margin information

is provided for mildly dysplastic nevi, but it seems reasonable not to re-excise such lesions, and few experienced clinicians do so.

It may be that in the future there will be markers to help establish the significance of an individual lesion, in the same way that immunohistochemical staining for mismatch repair proteins can be performed to determine whether an individual sebaceous adenoma is a manifestation of Muir-Torre syndrome or is sporadic.[85,86] Meanwhile, the clinician must, of course, consider clinical and histologic findings in his assessment of the patient and in therapeutic planning for individual lesions.[53,54,87,88]

Spitzoid Lesions

Like dysplastic nevi, spitzoid neoplasms can be arranged along a spectrum, extending in this case from a fully benign lesion (Spitz nevus) to a fully malignant lesion (spitzoid melanoma). Intermediate positions within the specimen are occupied by the "atypical Spitz nevus" and "atypical Spitz tumor" (or "spitzoid tumor of uncertain malignant potential" [STUMP]).[89] These intermediate entities are regarded as posing some risk of malignant behavior, but less than that of histologically unequivocal melanomas. The term "atypical Spitz nevus" has been applied to lesions regarded as probably, but not certainly, benign, whereas "atypical Spitz tumor" or STUMP reflects greater diagnostic uncertainty.[89] Many investigators have not distinguished between atypical Spitz nevus and tumor, but recognize only a single intermediate category.[90–92]

But what explains the unpredictable behavior of the intermediate lesions? Are they discrete biologic entities, whose behavior is indeterminate because they have traversed only the initial stages of progression toward full-fledged malignancy, and may or may not complete the remainder? Or do the intermediate terms describe not discrete entities, but a heterogeneous mixture of completely benign and completely malignant tumors, which are confounded because they cannot be distinguished histologically? In the first interpretation, the "atypical Spitz nevus" would be a less advanced entity than the "atypical Spitz tumor"; in the second interpretation, a sample of "atypical Spitz nevi" simply contains a higher proportion of benign tumors than a sample of "atypical Spitz tumors."

As Lee has written, "What is not clear in all of these [equivocal] designations is whether the issue is the inability of the histopathologist to discriminate between benign and malignant, in which case they represent euphemisms for 'I don't know', or whether the issue is that these difficult lesions actually lie somewhere between the spectrum of benign and malignant in accordance with the multistep theory of carcinogenesis."[93] If the latter is correct, and true biologic intermediates exist, how many are there? Two ("atypical Spitz nevus" and "atypical Spitz tumor"), more than 2, or only 1? How can the intermediates be recognized? And there are more questions. Do we even really know what to expect from the polar entities (typical Spitz nevus and spitzoid melanoma), based on analogies to common nevi and melanomas? There is some molecular evidence that the spitzoid lesions constitute a distinct lineage separate from that of ordinary nevi and melanomas.[90] H-ras activation occurs in about a quarter of Spitz nevi,[89,94–97] but they infrequently reveal B-raf or N-ras mutations.[89] The opposite profile is observed in other melanocytic neoplasms. In most common nevi, dysplastic nevi, and melanomas, B-raf and N-ras mutations are common, whereas H-ras abnormalities are rare.[89] H-ras mutations have been identified in atypical Spitz nevi and in a single spitzoid lesion suspicious for melanoma.[98] The presence of B-raf or N-ras mutations in a minority of Spitz nevi, atypical Spitz tumors, spitzoid melanoma,[89] and in a majority of spitzoid melanomas in 1 study,[98] does cast some doubt on a separate progression pathway for spitzoid lesions, however.

There are case reports of histologically typical Spitz nevi that metastasized.[12] It may be that the pathologic diagnosis was simply wrong, but maybe it was correct; maybe even typical Spitz nevi are not always (only almost always) as harmless as, for example, intradermal nevi. At the other end of the spectrum, it seems increasingly clear that there is a group of spitzoid neoplasms that would classically be regarded as malignant but do not behave as typical melanomas, because they are capable of nodal but not distant metastases (see later discussion). Can these be distinguished from the smaller group of spitzoid malignancies that do metastasize widely?

As the plethora of questions suggests, histopathologists have not been successful in predicting the behavior of spitzoid lesions. Cerroni speaks of the "frustration of a seemingly never-ending search for ... morphologic criteria that would allow dermatopathologists to reliably and repeatably differentiate spitzoid tumors that behave in a benign fashion from those that will eventually metastasize ... these criteria simply do not exist."[99] As mentioned earlier, melanoma is the single largest cause of malpractice claims against pathologists,[1] and 29% of such claims involve melanoma misdiagnosed as Spitz nevus.[1] In a concordance study mentioned earlier, 31 spitzoid lesions were diagnosed by a panel of 10 dermatopathologists as Spitz nevus, atypical Spitz nevus, melanoma, or uncertain.[12] Seventeen of the 31 were diagnosed as melanoma by 6 or more of the 10 panelists, and of these, 13 eventuated in local recurrence, metastasis, or death. The remaining 14 cases received other diagnoses from most of the panelists, but 10 of these cases also resulted in local recurrence, metastasis, or death.[12] The 1 case that received a majority diagnosis of typical Spitz nevus was fatal.[12]

As mentioned, there is molecular evidence for a lineage of spitzoid tumors. In practical terms, a tumor, whether nevus or melanoma, is regarded as spitzoid because of its cytologic characteristics. All spitzoid tumors are composed of large epithelioid and/or spindle-shaped melanocytes with large, open, variable nuclei and abundant, lightly pigmented cytoplasms.[100] There are, of course, architectural and cytologic differences within the spectrum of spitzoid tumors that provide the criteria for histologic diagnosis. These differences have been reviewed in detail elsewhere.[91,92,100,101] As discussed, their reliability is far from perfect, especially for the intermediate lesions. It is generally accepted that the polar entities (Spitz nevus and melanoma) can be recognized with good if not perfect reliability,[102] whereas intermediate lesions have been more problematic.

Several modalities have been explored as a diagnostic adjunct in the histologic diagnosis of spitzoid neoplasms. One of these is immunohistochemistry. Proliferative activity can be assessed by immunohistochemical staining with antibodies such as MIB-1 that stain cells in or past the late G1 phase of the cell cycle. The proliferation fraction is the proportion of cells staining with such antibodies, and it is greater for melanoma than Spitz nevus.[89] Unfortunately, all studies have shown some degree of overlap (at a proliferation fraction of approximately 2%–6%).[103] Worse, it is the histologically equivocal lesions that tend to have an intermediate proliferation fraction,[104] so the technique is least useful where it is most needed.

Spitz nevi resemble common nevi in displaying a zonal pattern of reaction with HMB-45 antibody, staining in the epidermis and upper dermis, but not the deep dermis. Melanomas stain throughout.[105,106] Similar differences in zonal staining are observed with bcl-2[106] and cyclin D1 antibodies.[107] Unfortunately there is some overlap, and atypical spitzoid lesions have not been studied.

An antibody to p53 (which probably labels only the mutant form of this suppressor gene product) stains a higher proportion of melanomas than Spitz nevi.[105,108] There are differences in staining for fatty acid synthase among Spitz nevus, atypical Spitz nevus, and melanoma, with little overlap among the 3 groups.[104] Differences in staining for a number of cell cycle regulators, including p-16, p-27, Rb, cyclin A, and cyclin B1, have been reported.[108–111]

As mentioned, about a quarter of Spitz nevi reveal characteristic abnormalities in H-ras, consisting of gene duplication and, in some cases, mutation.[94–97] Duplication of H-ras can be detected by a variety of molecular techniques, including comparative genomic hybridization (CGH),[94–96] array-based comparative genomic hybridization,[97] fluorescence in situ hybridization (FISH),[94,95] and multiplex ligation-dependent probe amplification (MLPA).[112,113] These techniques fail to demonstrate any cytogenetic abnormalities in the three-quarters of Spitz nevi with normal H-ras copy number. By contrast, they show multiple chromosomal abnormalities in the vast majority of melanomas.[96,97,112,114] In 1 series of 132 melanomas, for example, 96% displayed chromosomal gain or loss by CGH.[96]

There is preliminary evidence that these molecular techniques may be of practical value as a diagnostic adjunct for histologically indeterminate spitzoid tumors. Bauer and Bastian described 2 such equivocal lesions evaluated by CGH.[115] One revealed no cytogenetic abnormalities, and was judged benign, whereas the other displayed the multiple chromosomal gains and losses typical of melanoma. Harvell and colleagues[116] examined 16 recurrent Spitz nevi by CGH and/or FISH. Twelve were normal, in 2 there was 11p (H-ras) amplification, in 1 multiple chromosomal gains and losses, and in 1 gain of 1q and loss of 9p.[116] After an average 4.8 years of follow-up, there was no further evidence of disease in all but the last case, which eventuated in nodal metastasis.[116] Takata and colleagues[113] applied MLPA to 16 atypical spitzoid lesions. Of these, 13 revealed no abnormalities, but in 3 there was a reduced copy number of the cyclin-dependent kinase inhibitor 2A gene (CDKN2A). This was detected in 0 of typical Spitz nevi but 12 of 22 melanomas.[113]

These modalities are new and have not yet been thoroughly evaluated. They must be applied to many more lesions, and their results correlated to both histopathology and clinical outcome. Nevertheless, preliminary results are encouraging.

In 2000, Kelley and Cockerell[117] advised sentinel node biopsy for histologically equivocal melanocytic neoplasms, including equivocal spitzoid tumors, more than 1 mm in thickness. Thinner tumors could be treated by simple excision.[117] They argued that because the tumors were equivocal, their treatment should accommodate the worst possibility (melanoma), and this meant sentinel lymphadenectomy followed by completion lymphadenectomy if the sentinel node was positive. They argued further that the procedure could play a diagnostic, as well as therapeutic role because sentinel node involvement would push the diagnostic compass toward melanoma, whereas its absence would favor benignity.[117]

There have subsequently been a number of case reports and small series describing atypical spitzoid lesions managed in exactly this manner.[118–124] Recently, however, several of the world's most prominent dermatopathologists, including Philip LeBoit,[125] Mark Wick,[126] and Klaus Busam,[127] have strongly criticized the approach. They question the fundamental assumption that nodal involvement by an equivocal melanocytic neoplasm implies melanoma: "So what do the melanocytes in the lymph node … prove? To some, everything—a sure diagnosis of melanoma. To me, nothing." (LeBoit[125]). Normal tissue elements, including breast epithelium and mesothelium, can sometimes be found in nodes, apparently as a result of passive lymphatic transport.[127] The same mechanism apparently also explains nodal nevi,[128] which are common. Nodal nevi have been observed, for example, in 3% to 22% of melanoma patients and 0.33% of patients with breast cancer undergoing sentinel lymphadenectomy.[128] The critical issue is their frequency in association with benign Spitz nevi, and this is unknown. As LeBoit suggested, only a series of sentinel lymphadenectomies in patients with unequivocally benign Spitz nevi would establish the necessary baseline frequency, and this experiment will never be performed.[125]

There are, of course, histologic differences between nodal nevi and nodal deposits of melanoma. The former tend to involve the nodal capsule and trabeculea, the latter the parenchyma. However, melanoma can involve the capsule[127] and nevi can involve the parenchyma.[127,129] Nodal nevi are smaller and less cytologically atypical than metastases. However, the cytology of nodal deposits tends to resemble that of the primary, and the latter is at least somewhat atypical in the case of an atypical spitzoid neoplasm. Conversely, bland cytologic features do not entirely exclude melanoma.[127] Diagnosis might be facilitated by various immunohistochemical markers, including Melan-A to label melanocytes, HMB-45 to identify malignant melanocytes, and MIB-1 to assess proliferation rate, which is higher in melanoma than nevus. All of these procedures have limitations that can lead to both over- and underdiagnosis of melanoma.[127]

Busam and Pulitzer[127] have emphasized the remarkable fact that no patient with an atypical spitzoid neoplasm and positive sentinel node has subsequently developed distant metastasis,[118–124] even when completion lymphadenectomy revealed additional nodal involvement. The significance of this observation is limited by short follow-up times,[127] and it might even be marshalled as support for the procedure. More fundamentally, it invites comparison with conventional melanoma, in which half of patients with positive sentinel nodes would experience distant metastasis. It suggests that these atypical spitzoid lesions are either benign or malignant but incapable of distant metastasis. The latter possibility was suggested by Smith and colleagues[130] who reported as "malignant Spitz nevus" a series of 32 tumors with distinctive (atypical) histologic characteristics and an apparent capacity for nodal, but not distant, metastasis. Six of their cases had nodal involvement (manifest not just histologically but as clinical adenopathy), but no further extension occurred after an average of 6 years of follow-up.[130] A meta-analysis demonstrating 88% 5-year survival for spitzoid melanoma diagnosed in the first 10 years of life, despite a mean thickness of 4.67 mm, is consistent with the concept of limited malignancy.[131] Other organ systems provide examples of similarly limited malignancies, such as papillary carcinoma of the thyroid, and an explanation for this behavior has been proposed.[101]

In summary, histopathologists can recognize typical Spitz nevi with good reliability, although lesions regarded as such by competent dermatopathologists have occasionally metastasized. For this reason, it is reasonable to completely excise every Spitz nevus, even histologically typical examples.[127] At the other extreme, an unequivocal histologic diagnosis of spitzoid melanoma can also be accepted. Such a lesion should be treated like any other melanoma, although there is evidence suggesting much more favorable outcomes.

For lesions that fall into the intermediate categories of atypical Spitz nevus, atypical spitzoid tumor, STUMP, and so forth, the limitations of histologic analysis must be kept in mind. Immunohistochemical labeling for proliferation markers, HMB-45, bcl-2, and other moieties have revealed differences between Spitz nevus and melanoma, but overlaps and lack of experience with intermediate spitzoid lesions limit their usefulness.

Molecular techniques such as CGH may, in some cases, be highly informative: H-ras (11p) duplication without other chromosomal abnormalities strongly implies benignity; no chromosomal abnormality also implies nevus but can occur in melanoma; and multiple chromosomal gains and losses constitute strong evidence for melanoma. In uncertain cases a sentinel node biopsy can be performed, but a number of authorities have argued against it and the approach is unsupported by outcomes research. If a nodal deposit is observed it should be assessed for size, location, cytology, and perhaps staining for HMB-45 and other markers. The mere fact of nodal involvement should not be accepted as conclusive evidence for malignancy and complete justification for therapeutic interventions such as completion adenectomy and adjuvant chemotherapy.

Cellular Blue Nevi

As with Spitz nevi, there is a spectrum of CBN, extending from a fully benign nevus, to an intermediate category ("atypical cellular blue nevus," ACBN), to the fully malignant pole ("malignant cellular blue nevus," MCBN). All of these are uncommon; the great majority of blue nevi encountered in ordinary clinical practice are common blue nevi, which are relatively small (<1 cm diameter); distributed on the dorsal hands and feet, buttocks, scalp, and face; and histologically straightforward.[132] CBN are somewhat larger and often located on the sacrococcygeal area, buttocks, or distal extremities.[133] They are more complex histologically, manifesting 3 distinct histologic patterns.[133]

The term "malignant cellular blue nevus" is generally applied to melanoma originating within a CBN, that is, a melanoma with a histologically identifiable blue nevus remnant.[134,135] However, it has also been used for melanomas originating within common blue nevi (thought to be very rare)[135]; for melanomas originating within other dermal melanocytoses, such as nevus of Ota[134]; and for melanomas resembling CBN but not associated with a nevus remnant.[135] In older work, it was suggested that MCBN is a discrete entity, separate from melanoma.[135,136] This concept was supported by molecular analysis of a single case, which failed to reveal loss of heterozygosity at any of 8 genes frequently abnormal in melanoma, such as 9p21, whereas all of 28 melanomas evaluated by the same procedure were genetically abnormal.[137] Subsequently, however, all of 7 MCBN evaluated by CGH revealed cytogenetic abnormalities typical of melanoma, especially losses of chromosome 9 and gains of chromosome 20.[138] An additional case revealed mutation at 3p26, which is fairly common in conventional melanoma.[139] Clinically, MCBN is large (>2 cm) and almost always located on the scalp.

Compared with other melanomas, MCBN exhibits unusually aggressive clinical behavior. In the largest series, 10 of 12 cases metastasized and 8 were fatal.[140] In a series of 10 cases, of the 7 for which follow-up information was available there was distant metastasis in 4 and local recurrence in the rest.[135] Of 6 cases, 2 were fatal and 2 spread regionally and to nodes.[141] Other small series and case reports describe a metastatic rate of approximately 80%.[142]

The atypical CBN is an entity with clinical features of ordinary CBN (size <2 cm, location on the extremities, trunk, buttocks, and scalp),[143] but histologic features overlapping with malignant CBN.[13,133,143–145] These features may include larger size, asymmetry, infiltrative architecture, hypercellularity, mitotic activity, and cytologic atypia.[13,133,143–145] Most investigators have indicated that the severity of these features is what distinguishes ACBN from MCBN, but some have suggested that atypical mitotic figures are unique to MCBN,[143] or that cytologic atypia is focal in ACBN but diffuse in MCBN.[134,146]

Early work showed that ACBN could be recognized despite its histologic overlap with MCBN. Tran and colleagues[143] reviewed 16 cases that had been diagnosed by a single expert as atypical CBN. On review, 7 of these were reclassified as deep penetrating nevus (DPN) (see later discussion). The other 9 displayed fairly uniform histologic characteristics and, most importantly, had not recurred after an average 42 months of follow-up.[143]

A recent study was far less encouraging. Twenty-six lesions in the spectrum of CBN, including 8 CBN, 11 ACBN, 6 MCBN, and 1 ordinary blue nevus, were evaluated by a panel of 14 expert pathologists.[13] At least 4 years of follow-up was available for all cases, and for each outcome was consistent with pathologic diagnosis (no progression for the CBN and ACBN, metastasis or death for half of the MCBN). The correct diagnosis was rendered by a majority of panelists in only 38% of cases. A majority recognized only 2 (18%) of ACBN, 3 (37%) of CBN, and 4 (67%) of MCBN.[13] k values were extremely low: 0.02, 0.20, and 0.52 for ACBN, CBN, and MCBN, respectively.[13] In a much earlier study of CBN, 16% had been originally misdiagnosed as melanoma.[147]

The role of genomic analysis in diagnosing equivocal blue nevi remains to be determined. As mentioned, chromosomal abnormalities resembling those of ordinary melanoma were identified by CGH in 7 of 7 MCBN.[138] The same study found chromosomal abnormalities in 3 of 11 ACBN, and in 2 of these the abnormality (loss of 3q) was not typical of melanoma.[138]

Sentinel lymphadenectomy would be a particularly unrewarding diagnostic adjunct for this group of lesions. Nodal extension occurs in about 5% of ordinary CBN,[147,148] and frequently involves the subcapsular sinuses and parenchyma, rather than the capsule.[133,136,148] Nodal disease may be even more common in ACBN. Of 11 cases, 3 involved sentinel or regional nodes but did not recur after a mean 4.4 years of follow-up.[13] Interestingly, blue nevi can occur primarily in nodes,[148,149] and have been found in various other tissues, including mouth, lung, prostate, cervix, and muscle.[136]

In summary, the CBN define a problematic histologic spectrum analogous to the spitzoid tumors. As with the spitzoid tumors, polar diagnoses (ordinary CBN and MCBN) are probably reliable, but intermediate examples should be treated with respect. Tran and colleagues[143] advised that all ACBN be excised with 1-cm margins, followed by careful clinical surveillance, and it is difficult to argue with this recommendation.

Animal-type Melanoma

Animal- or equine-type melanoma is a rare and equivocal entity that overlaps histologically with several types of blue nevi. It was named for its clinical and histologic resemblance to a dermal malignancy that affects elderly, darkly colored (especially gray) horses, called equine melanotic disease. These are dark nodules whose appearance is accompanied by spontaneous depigmentation of the horse, from gray to white. They are often indolent, and even after widespread metastasis are rarely fatal.[150]

The putative human analog presents as a heavily pigmented nodule or, less commonly, plaque, about 1 cm in diameter. It occurs much earlier than other melanomas, at a median age of 28 years,[151] 39 years,[150] and 24 years,[152] in the 3 reported series. It seems to be much less aggressive than other melanomas. Of the 84 cases reported by 2007, sentinel lymphadenectomy was performed in 63%, and 41% of the sentinel nodes were positive.[153] Nevertheless, only 2% of patients died of their disease, after 0.5 to 17 years of follow-up.[153] Because of the low frequency of distant metastasis and death, several investigators have suggested that this is a uniquely low-grade or indolent form of melanoma,[134,150,151] and have compared it to the spitzoid neoplasms (described earlier) that are apparently capable of lymphatic but not distant metastasis.[135,151,154]

Histologically, the entity is characterized by very heavy pigmentation and a distinctive architecture. These are large and deep tumors, with dense, sheetlike dermal deposits toward the center, and infiltration of the dermis, subcutis, and sometimes adnexae at the periphery. Many display little or no necrosis, mitotic activity, or cytologic atypia,[134,150–152] and thus may lack conventional criteria for malignancy.[152] The degree of mitotic activity and cytologic atypia appears not to correlate with the likelihood of lymphatic metastasis.[151]

Because of the deceptively bland cytology and low mitotic rate, this lesion can be confused with several types of nevi, including CBN, other blue nevi, darkly pigmented Spitz nevus, pigmented spindle cell nevus, and DPN.[134,146,152] It can also be confused with several other forms of melanoma, including malignant blue nevus, melanoma regressing with melanophage deposition,[134,152] and perhaps primary dermal melanoma. Zembowicz and colleagues[151] who reported the largest series of 41 cases, found it to be indistinguishable from epithelioid blue nevus, an unusual type of nevus that is associated with Carney syndrome but can also occur spontaneously. They proposed a new term, pigmented epithelioid melanocytoma, as a "provisional histologic entity encompassing ... both animal-type melanoma and epithelioid blue nevus."[151] Cases have subsequently been reported as pigment epithelioid melanocytoma,[153–155] but not all have welcomed this nomenclature,[146,156] and some continue to insist that animal-type melanoma and epithelioid blue nevus can and must be distinguished.[146] Other terminology has been proposed, including pigmented synthesizing melanoma,[150,157] and, in older literature, pilar neurocristic hamartoma (because of the tumor's tendency to infiltrate around follicles and other adnexae).[152,158,159]

It has been uniformly recommended that animal-type melanoma be managed like other melanomas, with wide local excision and sentinel lymphadenectomy.[134,151,152,154,155,157] The depth of these tumors and their uncertain biologic potential probably underlies the recommendation for sentinel lymphadenectomy, which was in fact performed in most reported cases. However, given the high frequency of sentinel node involvement (41%[153]), but rarity of distant metastasis and death, a positive sentinel node clearly does not have the same prognostic implications for animal-type as for other forms of melanoma, and the value of sentinel lymphadenectomy in the management of this condition has recently been questioned.[153,156]

Deep Penetrating Nevus

DPN overlaps somewhat with animal-type melanoma, because it is deep, may be moderately pigmented, contains both epithelioid and spindle-shaped melanocytes, and characteristically infiltrates adnexae. Further, there is usually inflammation, a degree of cytologic atypia, and, in some cases, mitotic activity.[160–164] For these reasons, misdiagnosis as melanoma is not uncommon.[164] The lesion may also be confused with various benign entities, including blue nevus, CBN, pigmented Spitz nevus, and combined nevus.[160,161]

Fortunately, DPN (also known as plexiform spindle cell nevus [161]) has a characteristic clinical presentation, as a heavily pigmented, smooth-surfaced, dome-shaped nodule, <1 cm diameter, located on the upper body of an adolescent or young adult.[160–164] It also has a distinctive histologic architecture,[160–162] with a wedge-shaped, symmetric configuration, deeper than it is wide. Also, cytologic atypia and mitotic activity, although present in many cases, are much milder than in most melanomas.[160,162–164]

Mehregan and colleagues[165] reported a much lower proliferation fraction, measured by immunohistochemistry, in a small series of DPN, compared with melanoma. Roesch and colleagues[166] confirmed the difference in mean labeling fractions, but found it to be an unreliable basis for diagnosis because of overlap between the 2 groups. They also investigated Rb, metalloproteinases, and integrin β3 and demonstrated that immunohistochemical staining for dipeptidyl peptidase IV reliably distinguishes melanoma and DPN. This peptidase is a cell surface marker found in normal melanocytes and nevus cells, but not melanoma.[166] Subsequently they used a microarray containing 47,000 genes to screen transcripts from DPN and nodular melanoma.[167] A difference in ataxia-telangiectasia mutated gene transcripts motivated immunohistochemical staining for the product of this gene, which was found to reliably distinguish DPN and melanoma.[167] Commercially sourced antibodies were used in both studies, but unfortunately they are not available in routine clinical practice.

DPN exhibits reliably benign clinical behavior, as no recurrences were observed in several large series, which included atypical and incompletely excised examples.[160,164] (However, a single case of "malignant deep penetrating nevus," with axillary but not distant metastasis, has been briefly described.[168]) The main problem seems to be the possibility of histologic misdiagnosis. How frequently this occurs, and the direction of the error (DPN misdiagnosed as melanoma or melanoma misdiagnosed as DPN) is unknown, because diagnostic concordance and other reliability metrics have not been estimated for DPN and its simulants, as they have for spitzoid lesions and CBN (see earlier discussion). Because of the possibility of histologic underdiagnosis, most dermatopathologists recommend that an incompletely removed DPN be re-excised.

Atypical Melanocytic Hyperplasia

This is merely a descriptive term referring to epidermal features that might occur in early or nondiagnostic examples of melanoma, but could also be observed in lentigines, nevi, or even normal skin as a result of physical trauma or UV exposure. They include increased melanocyte density and architectural disorganization, with melanocytes arranged not in nests but as single cells within, or in some cases above, the epidermal basal layer. Melanocytic atypia is generally absent or slight, because severe cytologic atypia in combination with these architectural features would generally result in an unequivocal diagnosis of melanoma (except perhaps for a tiny specimen whose size alone might preclude diagnostic certainty).

SUMMARY

Nevi and melanomas continue to present formidable challenges to the histopathologist. In most practices, the great majority of such lesions will be unequivocal examples of common entities, and can be reliably diagnosed by an experienced dermatopathologist. Formal studies of diagnostic concordance have not, however, been entirely reassuring, especially with regard to some diagnostic categories, such as the spitzoid tumors. No doubt some of the variance simply results from the subjective nature of histopathologic analysis, but it is also clear that histology is not a perfect guide to clinical behavior. Better tools are needed, and they seem to be arriving, in the form of molecular diagnostics such as CGH. Meanwhile, the clinician can contribute by cultivating his own diagnostic skills (perhaps incorporating new modalities such as dermoscopy), submitting adequate specimens, communicating clearly with the laboratory, and intelligently interpreting pathology reports. In my opinion it is critical that practitioners avoid 2 oversimplifications: that all pigmented lesions may be divided into 2 homogeneous categories,

benign (nevus) and malignant (melanoma); and that a positive sentinel node justifies assignment to the latter group. Some of the problematic entities described earlier, such as spitzoid and animal-type melanomas, appear to be low-grade malignancies capable in most cases of lymphatic but not distant metastasis; whereas others, such as malignant CBN, seem to be more high-grade than other melanomas. Some benign lesions, in particular dysplastic nevi, also must be graded, as their clinical associations and appropriate management vary with the degree of dysplasia. The status of these complex entities will become more certain as clinical experience accumulates and their molecular mechanisms are worked out.

REFERENCES

1. Troxel DB. Medicolegal aspects of error in pathology. Arch Pathol Lab Med 2006;130: 617–9.
2. American Cancer Society. Surveillance research, leading sites of new cancer cases and deaths – 2008 estimates. Available at: http://www.cancer.org/downloads/stt/CFF2008M&F_Sites.pdf. Accessed October, 2008.
3. Glusac EJ. Under the microscope: doctors, lawyers, and melanocytic neoplasms. J Cutan Pathol 2003;30:287–93.
4. Crowson AN. Medicolegal aspects of neoplastic dermatology. Mod Pathol 2006;19:S148–54.
5. Farmer ER, Gonin R, Hanna MP. Discordance in the histopathologic diagnosis of melanoma and melanocytic nevi between expert pathologists. Hum Pathol 1996;27:528–31.
6. Ackerman AB. Serious limitations of a method. Am J Dermatopathol 2001;23:242–3.
7. Cerroni L, Kerl H. Tutorial on melanocytic lesions. Am J Dermatopathol 2001;23:237–41.
8. LeBoit PE. The 21st colloquium of the International Society of Dermatopathology. Symposium on melanocytic lesions. Am J Dermatopathol 2001;23: 244–5.
9. Corona R, Mele A, Amini M, et al. Interobserver variability on the histopathologic diagnosis of cutaneous melanoma and other pigmented skin lesions. J Clin Oncol 1996;14:1218–23.
10. Urso C, Rongioletti F, Innocenzi D, et al. Interobserver reproducibility of histological features in cutaneous malignant melanoma. J Clin Pathol 2005;58:1194–8.
11. Wechsler J, Bastuji-Garin S, Spatz A, et al. Reliability of the histopathological diagnosis of malignant melanoma in childhood. Arch Dermatol 2002;138:625–8.
12. Barnhill RL, Argenyi ZB, From L, et al. Atypical Spitz nevi/tumors: lack of consensus for diagnosis,

discrimination from melanoma, and prediction of outcome. Hum Pathol 1999;30:513–20.

13. Barnhill RL, Argenyi Z, Berwick M, et al. Atypical cellular blue nevi (cellular blue nevi with atypical features): lack of consensus for diagnosis and distinction from cellular blue nevi and malignant melanoma ("malignant blue nevus"). Am J Surg Pathol 2008;32:36–44.

14. Piepkorn MW, Barnhill RL, Cannon-Albright LA, et al. A multiobserver, population-based analysis of histologic dysplasia in melanocytic nevi. J Am Acad Dermatol 1994;30:707–14.

15. Florell SR, Boucher KM, Achman SA, et al. Histopathologic recognition of involved margins of lentigo maligna excised by staged excision. An interobserver comparison study. Arch Dermatol 2003;139:595–604.

16. Cook MG, Clarke TJ, Humphreys S, et al. A nationwide survey of observer variation in the diagnosis of thin cutaneous malignant melanoma including the MIN terminology. J Clin Pathol 1997;50:202–5.

17. Chen SC, Bravata DM, Weil E, et al. A comparison of dermatologists' and primary care physicians' accuracy in diagnosing melanoma: a systematic review. Arch Dermatol 2001;137:1627–34.

18. Chen SC, Pennie ML, Kolm P, et al. Diagnosing and managing cutaneous pigmented lesions: primary care physicians versus dermatologists. J Gen Intern Med 2006;21:678–82.

19. Osborne JE, Chave TA, Hutchinson PE. Comparison of diagnostic accuracy for cutaneous malignant melanoma between general dermatology, plastic surgery, and pigmented lesion clinics. Br J Dermatol 2003;148:252–8.

20. Grin CM, Kopf AW, Welkovich B, et al. Accuracy in the clinical diagnosis of malignant melanoma. Arch Dermatol 1990;126:763–6.

21. Morton CA, Mackie RM. Clinical accuracy of the diagnosis of cutaneous malignant melanoma. Br J Dermatol 1998;138:283–7.

22. Binder M, Puespoeck-Schwarz M, Steiner A, et al. Epiluminescence microscopy of small pigmented lesions: short-term formal training improves the diagnostic performance of dermatologists. J Am Acad Dermatol 1997;36:197–202.

23. Westerhoff K, McCarthy WH, Menzies SW. Increase in the sensitivity for melanoma diagnosis by primary care physicians using skin surface microscopy. Br J Dermatol 2000;143:1016–20.

24. Argenziano G, Puig S, Zalaudek I, et al. Dermoscopy improves accuracy of primary care physicians to triage lesions suggestive of skin cancer. J Clin Oncol 2006;24:1877–82.

25. Kittler H, Pehamberger H, Wolff K, et al. Diagnostic accuracy of dermoscopy. Lancet Oncol 2002;3: 159–65.

26. McCalmont TH. The clinical context: a tool for fine-tuning objective histologic diagnosis of cutaneous pigmented lesions. In: LeBoit PE, editor. Malignant melanoma and melanocytic neoplasms, Pathology: state of the art reviews, vol. 2–2. Philadelphia: Hanley and Belfus; 1994. p. 143–80.

27. Hosler GA, Moresi JM, Barrett TL. Nevi with site-related atypia: a review of melanocytic nevi with atypical histologic features based on anatomic site. J Cutan Pathol 2008;35:889–98.

28. Tronnier M, Hantschke M, Wolff HH. Presence of suprabasal melanocytes in melanocytic nevi after irritation of them by tape stripping. Dermatopathol Pract Concept 1997;3:6–8.

29. Tronnier M, Wolff HH. UV-irradiated melanocytic nevi simulating melanoma in situ. Am J Dermatopathol 1995;17:1–6.

30. Tronnier M, Wolff HH. Ultraviolet irradiation induces acute changes in melanocytic nevi. J Invest Dermatol 1995;104:475–8.

31. Pharis DB, Zitelli JA. Sunburn, trauma, and the timing of biopsies of melanocytic nevi. Dermatol Surg 2001;27:835–6.

32. Park HK, Leonard DD, Arlington JH, et al. Recurrent melanocytic nevi: clinical and histologic review of 175 cases. J Am Acad Dermatol 1987;17:285–92.

33. Rigel DS, Friedman RJ, Kopf AW, et al. ABCDE – an evolving concept in melanoma detection. Arch Dermatol 2005;141:1032–4.

34. Bologna JL, Lin A, Shapiro PE. The significance of eccentric foci of hyperpigmentation ("small dark dots") within melanocytic nevi. Analysis of 59 cases. Arch Dermatol 1994;130:1013–7.

35. Bauer J, Metzler G, Rassner G, et al. Dermatoscopy turns histopathologist's attention to the suspicious area in melanocytic lesions. Arch Dermatol 2001;137:1338–40.

36. Ferrara G, Argenziano G, Cerroni L, et al. A pilot study of a combined dermoscopic pathological approach to the telediagnosis of melanocytic skin lesions. J Telemed Telecare 2004;10:34–8.

37. Bauer J, Leinweber B, Metzler G, et al. Correlation with digital dermoscopic images can help dermatopathologists to diagnose equivocal skin tumors. Br J Dermatol 2006;155:546–51.

38. Ferrara G, Argenziano G, Soyer HP, et al. Dermatoscopic and histopathologic diagnosis of equivocal melanocytic skin lesions: an interdisciplinary study on 107 cases. Cancer 2002;95:1094–100.

39. Soyer HP, Massone C, Ferrare G, et al. Limitations of histopathologic analysis in the recognition of melanoma. A plea for a combined diagnostic approach of histopathologic and dermoscopic evaluation. Arch Dermatol 2005;141:209–11.

40. Sober AJ, Chuang TY, Duvic M, et al. Guidelines of care for primary care melanoma. J Am Acad Dermatol 2001;45:579–86.

41. National Comprehensive Cancer Network: clinical practice guidelines in oncology. Melanoma 2009; 1. Available at: http://www.nccn.org/professionals/physician_gls/PDF/melanoma.pdf. Accessed October, 2008.

42. Armour K, Mann S, Lee S. Dysplastic naevi: to shave or not to shave? A retrospective study of the use of the shave biopsy technique in the initial management of dysplastic nevi. Australas J Dermatol 2005;46:70–5.

43. Witheiler DD, Cockerell CJ. Sensitivity of diagnosis of malignant melanoma: a clinicopathologic study with a critical assessment of biopsy techniques. Exp Dermatol 1992;1:170–5.

44. Pariser RJ, Divers A, Nassar A. The relationship between biopsy technique and uncertainty in the histopathologic diagnosis of melanoma. Dermatol Online J 1999;5:4.

45. Ng PC, Barzilai DA, Ismail SA, et al. Evaluating invasive cutaneous melanoma: is the initial biopsy representative of the final depth? J Am Acad Dermatol 2003;48:420–4.

46. Stell VH, Norton HJ, Smith KS, et al. Method of biopsy and incidence of positive margins in primary melanoma. Ann Surg Oncol 2006;14:893–8.

47. Austin JR, Byers RM, Brown WD, et al. Influence of biopsy on the prognosis of cutaneous melanoma of the head and neck. Head Neck 1996;18:107–17.

48. Tran KT, Wright NA, Cockerell CJ. Biopsy of the pigmented lesion—when and how. J Am Acad Dermatol 2008;59:852–71.

49. Sullivan M. How to protect yourself from melanoma claims. Skin Allergy News 2005;24–5.

50. Tadiparthi S, Panchani S, Iqbal A. Biopsy for malignant melanoma – are we following the guidelines? Ann R Coll Surg Engl 2008;90:322–5.

51. Clark WH, Reimer RR, Green M, et al. Origin of familial malignant melanoma from heritable melanocytic lesions. 'The B-K mole syndrome'. Arch Dermatol 1978;114:732–8.

52. Green MH, Clark WH Jr, Tucker MA, et al. Precursor naevi in cutaneous malignant melanoma: a proposed nomenclature [letter]. Lancet 1980;2:1024.

53. Piepkorn M, Meyer LJ, Goldgar D, et al. The dysplastic melanocytic nevus: a prevalent lesion that correlates poorly with clinical presentation. J Am Acad Dermatol 1989;20:407–15.

54. Klein LJ, Barr RJ. Histologic atypia in clinically benign nevi: a prospective study. J Am Acad Dermatol 1990;22:275–82.

55. Meyer LJ, Goldgar DE, Cannon-Albright LA, et al. Number, size, and histopathology of nevi in Utah kindreds. Cytogenet Cell Genet 1992;59:167–9.

56. Ackerman AB. What naevus is dysplastic, a syndrome and the commonest precursor of malignant melanoma? A riddle and an answer. Histopathology 1988;13:241–56.

57. Ackerman AB, Milde P. Naming acquired melanocytic nevi. Common and dysplastic, normal and atypical, or Unna, Miescher, Spitz, and Clark. Am J Dermatopathol 1992;14:447–53.

58. Goldsmith LA, Askin FB, Chang AE, et al. Early Melanoma NIH Consensus Development Panel. NIH Consensus Conference. Diagnosis and treatment of early melanoma. JAMA 1992;9:1314–9.

59. Shapiro M, Chren MM, Levy RM, et al. Variability in nomenclature used for nevi with architectural disorder and cytologic atypia (microscopically dysplastic nevi) by dermatologists and dermatopathologists. J Cutan Pathol 2004;31:523–30.

60. Arumi-Uria M, McNutt SN, Finnerty B. Grading of atypia in nevi: correlation with melanoma risk. Mod Pathol 2003;16:764–71.

61. Barnhill RL, Roush GC, Duray PH. Correlation of histologic architectural and cytoplasmic features with nuclear atypia in atypical (dysplastic) nevomelanocytic nevi. Hum Pathol 1990;21:51–8.

62. Duncan LM, Berwick M, Bruijn JA, et al. Histopathologic recognition and grading of dysplastic melanocytic nevi: an interobserver agreement study. J Invest Dermatol 1993;100(3 Suppl):318–21.

63. Shea CR, Vollmer RT, Prieto VG. Correlating architectural disorder and cytologic atypia in Clark (dysplastic) melanocytic nevi. Hum Pathol 1999;39:500–5.

64. Schmidt B, Weinberg DS, Hollister K, et al. Analysis of melanocytic by DNA image cytometry. Cancer 1994;73:2971–7.

65. Hussein MR, Sun M, Tuthill RJ, et al. Comprehensive analysis of 112 melanocytic skin lesions demonstrates microsatellite instability in melanomas and dysplastic nevi, but not in benign nevi. J Cutan Pathol 2001;28:343–50.

66. Shors AR, Kim S, White E, et al. Dysplastic naevi with moderate to severe histological dysplasia: a risk factor for melanoma. Br J Dermatol 2006;155:988–93.

67. Smoller BR, Egbert BM. Dysplastic nevi can be diagnosed and graded reproducibly: a longitudinal study. J Am Acad Dermatol 1992;27:399–402.

68. Clemente C, Cochran AJ, Elder DE, et al. Histopathologic diagnosis of dysplastic nevi: concordance among pathologists convened by the world health organization melanoma programme. Hum Pathol 1991;22:313–9.

69. Wit PEJ, Hof-Grootenboer B, Ruiter DJ, et al. Validity of the histopathological criteria used for diagnosing dysplastic naevi. Eur J Cancer 1993;29:831–9.

70. Böni R, Zhuang Z, Albuquerque A, et al. Loss of heterozygosity detected on 1p and 9q in

microdissected atypical nevi. Arch Dermatol 1998; 134:882–3.

71. Hussein MR, Roggero E, Tuthill RJ, et al. Identification of novel deletion loci at 1p36 and 9p22-21 in melanocytic dysplastic nevi and cutaneous malignant melanoma. Arch Dermatol 2003;139:816–7.

72. Park WS, Vortmeyer AO, Pack S, et al. Allelic deletion at chromosome 9p21(p16) and 17p13(p53) in microdissected sporadic dysplastic nevus. Hum Pathol 1998;29:127–30.

73. Fleming MG, Wied GL, Dytch HE. Image analysis cytometry of dysplastic nevi. J Invest Dermatol 1990;95:287–91.

74. Newton JA, Camplejohn RS, McGibbon DH. The flow cytometry of melanocytic skin lesions. Br J Cancer 1988;58:606–8.

75. Berman DM, Wincovitch S, Garfield S, et al. Grading melanocytic dysplasia in paraffin wax embedded tissue by the nuclei acid index. J Clin Pathol 2005;58:1206–10.

76. Takahashi H, Strutton GM, Parsons PG. Determination of proliferating fractions in malignant melanomas by anti-PCNA/cyclin monoclonal antibody. Histopathology 1991;18:221–7.

77. Kanter L, Blegen H, Wejde J, et al. Utility of a proliferation marker in distinguishing between benign naevocellular naevi and naevocellular naevus-like lesions with malignant properties. Melanoma Res 1995;5:345–50.

78. Rudolph P, Schubert C, Tamm S, et al. Telomerase activity in melanocytic lesions: a potential marker of tumor biology. Am J Pathol 2000;156:1425–32.

79. Palmieri G, Ascierto PA, Cossu A, et al. Assessment of genetic instability in melanocytic skin lesions through microsatellite analysis of benign naevi, dysplastic naevi, and their metastases. Melanoma Res 2003;13:167–70.

80. Hussein MR, Roggero E, Sudilovsky EC, et al. Alterations of mismatch repair protein expression in benign melanocytic nevi, melanocytic dysplastic nevi, and cutaneous malignant melanomas. Am J Dermatopathol 2001;23:308–14.

81. Carey WP Jr, Thompson CJ, Synnestvedt M, et al. Dysplastic nevi as a melanoma risk factor in patients with familial melanoma. Cancer 1994;74:3118–25.

82. Naeyert JM, Brochez L. Dysplastic nevi. N Engl J Med 2003;349:2233–40.

83. Hastrup N, Osterlind A, Drzewiecki KT, et al. The presence of dysplastic nevus remnants in malignant melanomas: a population-based study of 551 malignant melanomas. Am J Dermatopathol 1991;13:378–85.

84. Rhodes AR, Harrist TJ, Day CL, et al. Dysplastic melanocytic nevi in histologic association with 234 primary cutaneous melanomas. J Am Acad Dermatol 1988;9:563–74.

85. Marazza G, Masouye I, Taylor S, et al. An illustrative case of Muir-Torre syndrome: contribution of immunohistochemical analysis in identifying indicator sebaceous lesions. Arch Dermatol 2006;142:1039–42.

86. Chhibber V, Dresser K, Malalingham M. MSH-6: extending the reliability of immunohistochemistry as a screening tool in Muir-Torre syndrome. Mod Pathol 2008;21:159–64.

87. Roush GC, Barnhill RL. Correlation of clinical pigmentary characteristics with histopathologically-confirmed dysplastic nevi in nonfamilial melanoma patients: studies of melanocytic nevi IX. Br J Cancer 1991;64:943–7.

88. Roesch A, Burgdorf W, Stolz W, et al. Dermatoscopy of "dysplastic nevi": a beacon in diagnostic darkness. Eur J Dermatol 2006;16:479–93.

89. Da Forno PD, Fletcher A, Pringle JH, et al. Understanding spitzoid tumors: new insights from molecular pathology. Br J Dermatol 2007;158:4–14.

90. Piepkorn M. The Spitz nevus is melanoma. Am J Dermatopathol 2005;27:367–9.

91. Barnhill RL. The spitzoid lesion: the importance of atypical variants and risk assessment. Am J Dermatopathol 2006;28:75–83.

92. Barnhill RL. The spitzoid lesion: rethinking spitz tumors, atypical variants, 'Spitzoid melanoma', and risk assessment. Mod Pathol 2006;19:S21–33.

93. Lee JB. Spitz nevus versus melanoma: limitation of the diagnostic methodology exposed. Eur J Dermatol 2006;16:223–4.

94. Bastian BC, Wesselmann U, Pinkel D, et al. Molecular cytogenetic analysis of Spitz nevi shows clear differences to melanoma. J Invest Dermatol 1999;113:1065–9.

95. Bastian BC, LeBoit PE, Pinkel D. Mutations and copy number increase of HRAS in spitz nevi with distinctive histopathologic features. Am J Pathol 2000;157:967–72.

96. Bastian BC, Olshen AB, LeBoit PE, et al. Classifying melanocytic tumors based on DNA copy number changes. Am J Pathol 2003;163:1765–9.

97. Harvell JD, Kohler S, Zhu S, et al. High-resolution array-based comparative genomic hybridization for distinguishing paraffin-embedded Spitz nevi and melanomas. Diagn Mol Pathol 2004;13:22–5.

98. Dijk MC, Bernsen MR, Ruiter DJ. Analysis of mutations in B-RAF, N-RAS, and HRAS genes in the differential diagnosis of Spitz nevus and spitzoid melanoma. Am J Surg Pathol 2005;29:1145–51.

99. Cerroni L. A new perspective for Spitz tumors? Am J Dermatopathol 2005;27:366–7.

100. Urso C. A new perspective for Spitz tumors? Am J Dermatopathol 2005;27:364–5.

101. Mooi WJ, Krausz T. Spitz nevus versus Spitzoid melanoma. Diagnostic difficulties, conceptual controversies. Adv Anat Pathol 2006;13:147–56.

102. Cerroni L. Spitzoid tumors. A matter of perspective? Am J Dermatopathol 2004;26:1–3.

103. Vollmer R. Use of Bayes rule and MIB-1 proliferation index to discriminate Spitz nevus from malignant melanoma. Am J Clin Pathol 2004;122: 499–505.

104. Kapur P, Selim MA, Roy LC, et al. Spitz nevi and atypical Spitz nevi/tumors: a histologic and immunohistochemical analysis. Mod Pathol 2005;18: 197–204.

105. Bergman R, Dromi R, Trua H, et al. The pattern of HMB-45 antibody staining in compound Spitz nevi. Am J Dermatopathol 1995;17:542–6.

106. Kanter-Lewensohn L, Hedblad MA, Wejde J, et al. Immunohistochemical markers for distinguishing Spitz nevi from malignant melanomas. Mod Pathol 1997;10:917–20.

107. Nagasaka T, Lai R, Medeiros LJ, et al. Cyclin D1 overexpression in Spitz nevi: an immunohistochemical study. Am J Dermatopathol 1999;21: 115–20.

108. Stefanaki C, Stefanaki K, Antoniou C, et al. Cell cycle and apoptosis regulators in Spitz nevi: comparison with melanomas and common nevi. J Am Acad Dermatol 2007;56:815–24.

109. Sparrow LE, Eldon MJ, English DR, et al. p-16 and p21WAF1 protein expression in melanocytic tumors by immunohistochemistry. Am J Dermatopathol 1998;20:255–61.

110. Maldonado JL, Timmerman L, Fridyand J, et al. Mechanisms of cell-cycle arrest in Spitz nevi with constitutive activation of the MAP-kinase pathway. Am J Pathol 2004;164:1783–7.

111. Wang YL, Uhara H, Yamazaki Y, et al. Immunohistochemical detection of CDK4 and p-16 proteins in cutaneous malignant melanoma. Br J Dermatol 1996;134:269–75.

112. Dijk MC, Rombout PD, Boots-Sprenger SH, et al. Multiplex ligation-dependent probe amplification for the detection of chromosomal gains and losses in formalin-fixed tissue. Diagn Mol Pathol 2005;14: 9–16.

113. Takata M, Lin J, Takayanagi S, et al. Genetic and epigenetic alterations in the differential diagnosis of malignant melanoma and spitzoid lesion. Br J Dermatol 2007;156:1287–94.

114. Bastian BC, LeBoit PE, Hamm H, et al. Chromosomal gains and losses in primary cutaneous melanoma detected by comparative genomic hybridization. Cancer Res 1998;58:2170–5.

115. Bauer J, Bastian BC. Distinguishing melanocytic nevi from melanoma by DNA copy number changes: comparative genomic hybridization as a research and diagnostic tool. Dermatol Ther 2006;19:40–9.

116. Harvell JD, Bastian BC, LeBoit PE. Persistent (recurrent) Spitz nevi. A histopathologic, immunohistochemical, and molecular pathologic study of 22 cases. Am J Surg Pathol 2002;26: 654–61.

117. Kelley SW, Cockerell CJ. Sentinel lymph node biopsy as an adjunct in the management of histologically difficult to diagnose melanocytic lesions: a proposal. J Am Acad Dermatol 2000; 42:527–30.

118. Lohmann CM, Coit DG, Brady MS, et al. Sentinel node biopsy in patients with diagnostically controversial Spitzoid melanocytic tumors. Am J Surg Pathol 2002;26:47–55.

119. Su LD, Fullen DR, Sondak VK, et al. Sentinel lymph node biopsy for patients with problematic Spitzoid melanocytic lesions: a report on 18 patients. Cancer 2003;97:499–507.

120. Roaten JB, Partrick DA, Pearlman N, et al. Sentinel lymph node biopsy for melanoma and other melanocytic tumors in adolescents. J Pediatr Surg 2005;40:232–5.

121. Gamblin TC, Edingtion H, Kirkwood JM, et al. Sentinel lymph node biopsy for atypical melanocytic lesions with Spitzoid features. Ann Surg Oncol 2006;37:1664–70.

122. Urso C, Borgognoni L, Saieva C, et al. Sentinel lymph node biopsy in patients with "atypical Spitz tumors". A report on 12 cases. Hum Pathol 2006; 37:816–23.

123. McArthur GJ, Banwell ME, Cook MG, et al. The role of sentinel node biopsy in the management of melanocytic lesions of uncertain malignant potential (MUMP). J Plast Reconstr Aesthet Surg 2007;60: 952–4.

124. Murali R, Sharma RN, Thompson JF, et al. Sentinel lymph node biopsy in histologically ambiguous melanocytic tumors with Spitzoid features (so-called atypical Spitzoid tumors). Ann Surg Oncol 2008;15:302–9.

125. LeBoit PE. What do these cells prove? Am J Dermatopathol 2003;25:355–6.

126. Wick MR. Melanocytic lesions with features of Spitz nevus. Hum Pathol 2006;37:779–80.

127. Busam KJ, Pulitzer M. Sentinel lymph node biopsy for patients with diagnostically controversial spitzoid melanocytic tumors. Adv Anat Pathol 2008; 15:253–62.

128. Patterson JW. Nevus cell aggregates in lymph nodes. Am J Clin Pathol 2004;121:13–5.

129. Biddle DA, Evans HL, Kemp BL, et al. Intraparenchymal nevus cell aggregates in lymph nodes: a possible diagnostic pitfall with malignant melanoma and carcinoma. Am J Surg Pathol 2003;27: 673–81.

130. Smith K, Skelton H, Lupton G, et al. Spindle cell and epithelioid cell nevi with atypia and metastasis (malignant Spitz nevus). Am J Surg Pathol 1989;13: 931–9.

131. Pol-Rodriquez M, Lee S, Silvers DN, et al. Influence of age on survival in childhood spitzoid melanomas. Cancer 2007;109:1579–83.

132. McKee PH, Calonje E, Granter SR. Pathology of the skin:1299–1300. 3rd edition. Elsevier Mosby; 2005.

133. Temple-Camp CRE, Saxe N, King H. Benign and malignant cellular blue nevus. A clinicopathologic study of 30 cases. Am J Dermatopathol 1988;10: 289–96.

134. Magro CM, Crowson AN, Mihm MC. Unusual variants of malignant melanoma. Mod Pathol 2006; 19:S41–70.

135. Granter SR, McKee PH, Calonje E, et al. Melanoma associated with blue nevus and melanoma mimicking cellular blue nevus. A clinicopathologic study of 10 cases on the spectrum of so-called 'malignant blue nevus'. Am J Surg Pathol 2001; 25:316–23.

136. Lambert WC, Brodkin RH. Nodal and subcutaneous cellular blue nevi: a pseudometastasising pseudomelanoma. Arch Dermatol 1984;120: 367–70.

137. Ariyanayagam-Baksh SM, Baksh FK, Finkelstein SD, et al. Malignant blue nevus. A case report and molecular analysis. Am J Dermatopathol 2003;25: 21–7.

138. Maize JC, McCalmont TH, Carlson JA, et al. Genomic analysis of blue nevi and related dermal melanocytic proliferations. Am J Surg Pathol 2005;29:1214–20.

139. Zyrek-Betts J, Micale M, Lineen A, et al. Malignant blue nevus with lymph node metastases. J Cutan Pathol 2008;35:651–7.

140. Connelly J, Smith JL. Malignant blue nevus. Cancer 1991;67:2653–7.

141. Aloi F, Pich A, Pippione M. Malignant cellular blue nevus. A clinicopathological study of 6 cases. Dermatology 1996;192:36–40.

142. Özgür F, Akyürek M, Kayikçioğlu A, et al. Metastatic malignant blue nevus: a case report. Ann Plast Surg 1997;39:411–5.

143. Tran TA, Carlson JA, Basaca PC, et al. Cellular blue nevus with atypia (atypical cellular blue nevus): a clinicopathologic study of nine cases. J Cutan Pathol 1998;25:252–8.

144. Avidor I, Kessler E. Atypical blue nevus – a benign variant of cellular blue nevus. Presentation of three cases. Dermatologica 1977;15:39–44.

145. Goette KD, Robinson JW. Atypical cellular blue nevus. J Assoc Milit Dermatol 1980.

146. Massi G. Melanocytic nevi simulant of melanoma with medicolegal relevance. Virchows Arch 2007; 451:623–47.

147. Rodriguez HA, Ackerman LV. Cellular blue nevus. Clinicopathological study of forty-five cases. Cancer 1968;21:393–405.

148. Epstein JI, Erlandson RA, Rosen RP. Nodal blue nevi. A study of three cases. Am J Surg Pathol 1984;8:907–15.

149. Masci P, Ciardi A, Di Tondo U. Blue nevus of the lymph node capsule. J Dermatol Surg Oncol 1984;10:596–8.

150. Antony FC, Sanclemente G, Shaikh H, et al. Pigment synthesizing melanoma (so-called animal type melanoma): a clinicopathological study of 14 cases of a poorly known distinctive variant of melanoma. Histopathology 2006;48:754–62.

151. Zembowicz A, Carney JA, Mihm MC. Pigmented epithelioid melanocytoma: a low grade melanocytic tumor with metastatic potential indistinguishable from animal-type melanoma and epithelioid blue nevus. Am J Surg Pathol 2004;28: 31–40.

152. Crowson AN, Magro CM, Mihm MC. Malignant melanoma with prominent pigment synthesis: "animal type" melanoma – a clinical and histological study of six cases with a consideration of other melanocytic neoplasms with prominent pigment synthesis. Hum Pathol 1999;30:543–50.

153. Vezzoni GM, Martini L, Ricci C. A case of animal-type melanoma (or pigmented epithelioid melanocytoma?): an open prognosis. J Dermatol Surg Oncol 2008;34:105–10.

154. Howard B, Ragsdale B, Lundquist K. Pigmented epithelioid melanocytoma: two case reports. Dermatol Online J 2005;11:1.

155. Ward JR, Brady SP, Tada H, et al. Pigmented epithelioid melanocytoma. Int J Dermatol 2006;45: 1403–5.

156. White S, Chen S. What is "pigmented epithelioid melanocytoma". Am J Surg Pathol 2005;29:1118–9.

157. Cecchi R, Rapicano V. Pigment synthesizing (animal type) melanoma with satellite metastasis. Eur J Dermatol 2007;17:335–6.

158. Tuthill RJ, Clark WH, Levene A. Pilar neurocristic hamartoma: its relationship to blue nevus and equine melanotic disease. Arch Dermatol 1982; 118:592–6.

159. Pathy AL, Helm TN, Elston D, et al. Malignant melanoma arising in a blue nevus with features of pilar neurocristic hamartoma. J Cutan Pathol 1993;20: 459–64.

160. Seab JA, Graham JH, Helwig EB. Deep penetrating nevus. Am J Surg Pathol 1989;13:39–44.

161. Barnhill RL, Mihm MC, Magro CM. Plexiform spindle cell naevus: a distinctive variant of plexiform melanocytic naevus. Histopathology 1991; 18:243–7.

162. Cooper PH. Deep penetrating (plexiform spindle cell) nevus. A frequent participant in combined nevus. J Cutan Pathol 1992;19:172–80.

163. Mehregan DA, Mehregan AH. Deep penetrating nevus. Arch Dermatol 1993;129:328–31.

164. Robson A, Morley-Quante M, Hempel H, et al. Deep penetrating naevus: clinicopathological study of 31 cases with further delineation of histological features allowing distinction from other pigmented benign melanocytic lesions and melanoma. Histopathology 2003;43:529–37.

165. Mehregan DR, Mehregan DA, Mehregan AH. Proliferating cell nuclear antigen staining in deep-penetrating nevi. J Am Acad Dermatol 1995;33:685–7.

166. Roesch A, Wittschier S, Becker B, et al. Loss of dipeptidyl peptidase IV immunostaining discriminates malignant melanomas from deep penetrating nevi. Mod Pathol 2006;19: 1378–85.

167. Roesch A, Becker B, Bentink S, et al. Ataxia telangiectasia-mutated gene is a possible biomarker for discrimination of infiltrative deep penetrating nevi and metastatic vertical growth phase melanoma. Cancer Epidemiol Biomarkers Prev 2007;16: 2486–90.

168. Graham J. Malignant deep penetrating nevus [abstract]. J Cutan Pathol 1996;23:76.

The Spitz Nevus: Review and Update

Valerie B. Lyon, MD[a,b,*]

KEYWORDS

- Spitz nevus • Atypical Spitz nevus
- Spindle and epithelioid cell nevus • Skin neoplasm
- Borderline melanoma • Spitz tumor
- Childhood melanoma • Juvenile melanoma

The Spitz nevus is a melanocytic lesion that has melanoma-like features on light microscopic examination but in typical form is distinguishable from melanoma, and usually exhibits benign behavior. There are also Spitz-like melanomas with microscopic features of Spitz lesions but otherwise distinctly malignant microscopy. Finally, borderline Spitz lesions have features of Spitz lesions and features of melanoma, and are recognized as of uncertain biologic potential and possible melanoma. These more rare borderline lesions are the most controversial regarding diagnosis and treatment. However, even Spitz nevi with typical histology have on very rare occasions unexpectedly led to metastasis and death.[1–3] Thus, even though Spitz lesions are easily recognized as distinct, they can defy current light microscopic diagnosis principles that are traditionally used to distinguish those malignant versus nonmalignant. There are many unanswered questions about the biologic nature of Spitz nevi. The diagnosis, prognosis, management, and even nomenclature of these lesions is controversial.

Despite improvements in diagnosis and combined experience over the past century since the Spitz lesion was first described,[4] this area remains one of the most controversial in pathology. To date investigations searching to more accurately diagnose and effectively treat these lesions have included limited numbers of cases and suffer from cohort bias. Multiple diagnostic and management strategies have been proposed and are individually utilized. Recently described investigational techniques seem promising. At this point, multicenter studies are needed to collectively determine whether they can be relied on to more accurately predict prognosis and therefore improve management.

EPIDEMIOLOGY

Spitz nevi are common in children but relatively uncommon in adults. Spitz nevi account for approximately 1% of excised nevi in children.[5] Many different names have been used for Spitz nevi since the original description of juvenile melanoma (**Box 1**), in an attempt to assign probable behavior. The names reflect a spectrum from benign to malignant, based on light microscopic analysis. Melanoma is probably best reserved in the name for Spitz lesions when referring to frank melanoma that has Spitz features ("spitzoid melanoma") or in Spitz lesions with features of Spitz and melanoma where biologic behavior is not predictable ("borderline melanoma"). The term "nevus" connotes benign behavior and is probably best reserved for lesions on the benign end of the spectrum or when atypical features are present if used with a qualifying description ("Spitz nevus with atypical features"). The term lesion is more neutral and can more broadly encompass all "Spitz lesions." Urso[6] and Piepkorn[7] suggest use of the term Spitz "tumor" to distinguish all Spitz lesions as separate entities from nevus and

a Department of Dermatology, Medical College of Wisconsin, Children's Hospital of Wisconsin, Milwaukee, WI, USA
b Department of Pediatrics, Medical College of Wisconsin, Children's Hospital of Wisconsin, Milwaukee, WI, USA
* Department of Dermatology, Medical College of Wisconsin, Children's Hospital of Wisconsin, Milwaukee, WI.
E-mail address: vlyon@mcw.edu

Clin Plastic Surg 37 (2010) 21–33
doi:10.1016/j.cps.2009.08.003
0094-1298/09/$ – see front matter

Box 1
Spitz nevus synonyms

Spitz nevus synonyms

  Juvenile melanoma

  Spindled and epithelioid cell nevus

  Pigmented spindle cell nevus of Reed

  Nevus of large spindleoid or epithelioid cells

Synonyms for Spitz that are neutral

  Spitz lesion

  Spitz tumor

  Spitzoid lesion; spitzoid tumor; spitzoid melanocytoma; spitzoid neoplasm

Atypical or borderline Spitz synonyms

  Atypical Spitz nevus

  Melanocytic tumor of uncertain potential (MELTUMP); melanocytic lesion of uncertain malignant potential (MUMP); Spitz tumor if uncertain potential (STUMP)

  Borderline melanoma

melanoma therby emphasizing separate diagnostic and biologic paths.[6,8] Individual names are used inconsistently between various investigators, and thus attention should be paid to the individual author's application of the terminology.

HISTORY

The Spitz nevus has been recognized in the literature since the early twentieth century, when Darier and Civatte[4] described a fast-growing red nodule on the cheek of a young boy and reported that they were unable to decide by light microscopy whether it was a melanoma or not. The pathology of the lesion they described, which would later be termed a Spitz nevus, was indistinguishable in their viewpoint from melanoma. Similar lesions would normally have been reported as malignant melanoma at this time; however, some researchers such as Darier and Civatte were beginning to recognize that these growths could exhibit benign clinical behavior. Still, the only criterion for distinguishing these lesions from melanoma was age of the patient. In 1948, Sophie Spitz[9] described in detail the light microscopic features of a group of these lesions, which she termed juvenile melanoma, and the diagnosis became widely recognized as distinct. Spitz compared the pathology of juvenile melanoma in individuals 18 months to 12 years old to melanoma in children 14 to 19 years old and to melanocytic

nevi in children. She described common features of these juvenile melanoma lesions, and emphasized the presence of giant cells as a distinguishing feature from postpubertal melanoma.

Spitz believed that these juvenile melanomas were unable to metastasize until adulthood because of a hormonal effect. The indicated treatment for juvenile melanoma in these years was removal before adulthood to prevent malignant degeneration. There were 2 problems with this assumption that she would later recognize: (1) a 12-year-old girl included in the original Spitz description died of metastasis,[2] and (2) benign Spitz lesions were found in adults as well. Both these factors implied that age was not the only factor in determining benign verses malignant behavior.

Allen and Spitz[10] later described a refined description of pathologic criteria for distinguishing Spitz nevi from melanoma in 1953. Arthur Allen, Sophie Spitz's husband,[11] eventually reviewed the pathology of the 12-year-old in the original description who died from melanoma and determined that the pathology was, in fact, not consistent with the diagnosis of juvenile melanoma.[2] Thus, the difficulty in pathologic diagnosis of Spitz nevi was apparent as early as the first description. Although more refined criteria for diagnosis of Spitz nevus are available today, the biologic potential remains unpredictable in a subset of lesions with atypical features that resemble melanoma.

CLINICAL PRESENTATION

Spitz nevi occur most often in children or young adults[12] but can occur at any age. Nearly half to two-thirds of Spitz nevi occur in individuals younger than 20 years.[13] Spitz nevi become less common with increasing age, and they are more likely to be diagnosed as melanoma with increasing age of the patient. Congenital Spitz nevi have been reported.[14,15] The lesions are more common in Caucasians with fair skin type and are slightly more frequently found in females.[5,16]

Spitz nevi commonly present on the face, head, neck, or lower extremities, but can occur anywhere on the body. In one study, Spitz nevi in children were more commonly on the head and neck whereas Spitz nevi in adults were more commonly located on the extremities (consistent with the observation in children that melanocytic nevi are found in greater frequency on the head and neck). The lesions are frequently solitary, but multiple and agminated (multiple grouped) lesions can occur. Grouped lesions may coalesce on a base of macular hyperpigmentation. Spitz nevi most often occur de novo but uncommonly can occur in association with an existing melanocytic nevus, usually either a congenital nevus or common melanocytic nevus.

The stereotypical Spitz nevus is a pink papule on the cheek of a child (**Fig. 1**). Spitz nevi are most commonly pink or flesh-colored owing to their relative paucity of melanin; however, red, brown, black, or brown/black lesions can occur (**Fig. 2**). The brown/black variant is also termed pigmented spindle cell nevus of Reed, and has been reported as a separate diagnostic entity, although most investigators consider it within the Spitz nevus spectrum.

Spitz nevi are usually flat-topped or dome-shaped papules that are symmetric and well circumscribed. The lesions are usually small (less than 6 mm) but can be larger (1 cm diameter or more). Lesions are generally round, but can be oval or rectangular. Telangiectasia may be associated with the lesion (**Fig. 3**). The surface can be ulcerated or scabbed (**Fig. 4**). More unusual clinical appearances such as halo phenomenon, polypoid shape, or pedunculated lesions can occur.

Spitz nevi are generally asymptomatic but growth can occur over a period of months. Eruptive Spitz nevi have also been described.[17-20] The lesions can uncommonly bleed, itch, or be reported as painful.

DIFFERENTIAL DIAGNOSIS

The Spitz nevus is commonly misdiagnosed based on clinical impression (**Box 2**). Red lesions are commonly misdiagnosed as pyogenic granuloma, especially if rapid growth, ulceration, or bleeding is found. Light brown lesions may mimic dermatofibroma and brown/black lesions can be mistaken for atypical nevi. Flesh-colored lesions

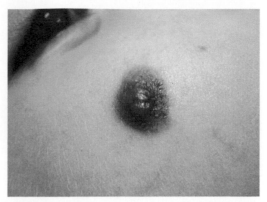

Fig. 2. Spitz nevus presenting as a brown/black nodule on the cheek.

may be misdiagnosed as a cyst, wart, or amelanotic melanoma. Spitz nevi presenting as a pink papule on the face in young children can be mistaken as a juvenile xanthogranuloma, a common skin lesion in young children. Misdiagnosis of angioma or hemangioma of infancy may also be made; however, clinical distinction should be possible given Spitz nevi have a firmer consistency, are more well demarcated than a hemangioma of infancy, and have a history of onset after the neonatal period.

DIAGNOSIS

The diagnosis of Spitz nevus can be suspected based on clinical presentation, and is confirmed by pathologic examination. As previously mentionid, lesions are, however, frequently misdiagnosed as either pyogenic granuloma or amelanotic melanoma, and the diagnosis is made retrospectively after light microscopic evaluation. If Spitz nevus is suspected, excisional biopsy is preferred in order to examine the entire specimen including the architectural details.

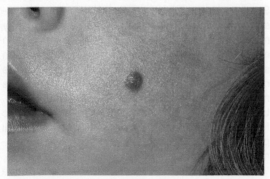

Fig. 1. Spitz nevus presenting as a pink papule on the cheek.

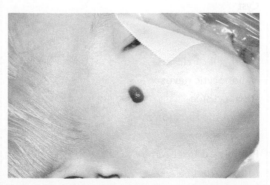

Fig. 3. Spitz nevus presenting as a red nodule. Note rectangular shape and radiating telangiectasia.

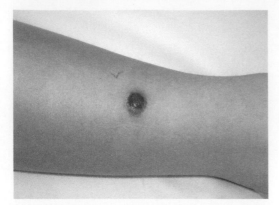

Fig. 4. Spitz nevus on the leg. Note ulcerated surface.

Full-thickness removal around the periphery of the lesion and through the dermis down to the mid or deep subcutaneous fat is ideal. Shave or partial excision may obscure pathologic features key to distinction from atypical nevi or melanoma. However, each case should be considered individually for its particular circumstances when biopsy technique is considered to avoid overtreatment, especially in very young children.

DERMOSCOPIC FEATURES

Dermoscopy (also known as dermatoscopy, epiluminescence microscopy, and skin surface microscopy) is a form of in vivo microscopy. Although recently described, it is now a routinely utilized diagnostic tool. Skin surface microscopy allows visualization of structures that are not

---

Box 2
Differential diagnosis of Spitz nevus

Pyogenic granuloma (lobular capillary hemangioma)

Hemangioma of infancy

Juvenile xanthogranuloma

Cyst

Wart

Melanoma

Basal cell carcinoma

Melanocytic nevus

Histiocytoma

Metastatic carcinoma

Pseudolymphoma

Primary adnexal tumor

Mastocytoma

Angioma

---

visible with the naked eye. The technique is especially useful for pigmented lesions and amelanotic lesions, and can improve diagnosis or delineate microscopic change in a lesion over time. Terminology used to describe dermoscopic features has been widely described. Several different methods of interpretation of the reflective pattern have been suggested, all combining overall features of symmetry observed within the lesion with detailed diagnostic criteria present or absent in the lesion for a given diagnostic entity.[21] Diagnostic accuracy improves with use of dermoscopy.[22]

The pigmented spindle cell nevus of Reed, a pigmented subset of Spitz nevus, has been well characterized on dermoscopy. Three main patterns have been described: (1) starburst, (2) globular, and (3) atypical. The globular and starburst patterns both consist of a central area surrounded by a prominent regular pigment network on the periphery. The starburst pattern is characterized by regularly spaced pigment globules that appear to stream outward toward the periphery of the lesion. Change from globular to starburst (stellate) pattern has been described over the course of evolution of a lesion, and thus these patterns may represent different stages of the lesion.[23,24] The central area of pigmentation can have a retiform pattern, or the pattern can be a reverse one characterized by dark holes with light network pattern intervening.

The dermoscopic pattern in nonpigmented Spitz nevi is characterized by the presence of dotted vessels regularly distributed throughout the nevus, and is often associated with network depigmentation. Other nonspecific patterns can be seen as well. The dermoscopic features of nonpigmented Spitz nevi are shared by melanoma, and dermoscopy cannot be used to distinguish these lesions.[25,26]

Use of dermoscopy can increase the accuracy of diagnosis of Spitz nevus based on globular or starburst subtype pigment patterns.[22] However, Spitz nevi showing an atypical pattern on dermoscopy or a multicomponent pattern are frequently misdiagnosed as other melanocytic nevi, skin neoplasms, or even nonmelanocytic lesions such as inflammatory conditions.[21,26] A final diagnosis of atypical Spitz nevi based on histopathology is made more than half of the time in these lesions. Unfortunately, a lack of distinctive dermoscopic features is found in approximately one-third of all pigmented Spitz nevi and in the most nonpigmented Spitz nevi.

Confocal microscopy (in vivo reflectance confocal microscopy) has been attempted as a way to improve the diagnosis of Spitz lesions without removal of the lesion, and has been able to identify characteristic features such as the presence of spindle cells and lateral shape demarcation of the lesion, but is not able to determine the presence of other characteristic features.[20,27,28] Confocal microscopy does not reach the vertical depth of the lesion that is required for accurate diagnosis.

PATHOLOGY

Spitz nevi are most commonly compound, but can be junctional or intradermal.[29–32] The hallmark of the pathology of Spitz nevus is the presence of large or spindle melanocytes, usually arranged in nests. The nests are composed of an admixture of spindle and epithelioid cells, although frequently spindle cells predominate. A striking feature is the uniformity of the cells horizontally from side to side. In deeper lesions, the cells also characteristically decrease in size from top to bottom within the lesion. Diagnosis requires a constellation of findings and is not based on any single finding (**Box 3**).

Spitz nevi resemble common nevi in their architectural features, are small and symmetric, and are well circumscribed. The intraepidermal component does not usually extend beyond the dermal component, and is arranged in nests that do not become confluent or vary a great deal in size and shape among each other. Nests in Spitz nevi are vertically arranged and regularly spaced, and can have clefting artifact above the nests at the dermal-epidermal junction (**Fig. 5**). In melanoma this retraction artifact is rare. Although junctional activity is characteristic in Spitz lesions, infiltration of cells into the upper layers of the epidermis is usually not present. There may be an occasional single cell infiltration in the upper epidermis, but pagetoid spread as seen in melanoma is not a feature. Epidermal changes include acanthosis, hyperkeratosis, and hypergranulosis. Rete ridges are usually elongated owing to the vertical orientation of the nests.

Spindle cells of a Spitz nevus are cells with fusiform shape, abundant cytoplasm, and a centrally located nucleus that has a conspicuous nucleolus. These cells are often plump. The nuclear chromatin pattern is usually finely dispersed but may be slightly vesicular. The cells are generally arranged in a fascicular pattern grouped in vertically oriented nests. The overall size of the nests and the cells within them are variable, but tend to decrease in size toward the deeper layers of the lesion.

The epithelioid cells of a Spitz nevus are large with abundant cytoplasm and have large nuclei.

Box 3
Summary of pathologic features of Spitz nevus

Symmetric lesion

Spindle or epithelioid melanocytic proliferation

"Maturation" of cells with increasing depth

Orderly infiltration of Spitz cells into surrounding collagen

Sharp lateral demarcation of lesion

Minor features

    Lack of mitoses, especially atypical or deep mitoses

    Presence of Kamino bodies

    Lack of single cell upward spread

    Presence of junctional clefts

    Loss of cohesion between cells

    Epidermal hyperplasia

    Superficial distribution of pigmentation

    Perivascular or diffuse inflammatory infiltrate

Ancillary tests differentiating benign from malignant Spitz lesion

    Low AgNOR score

    HMB-45 staining less intense deeply

    Ki-67 staining index

    Fatty acid synthase staining

    Chromosome copy analysis not consistent with melanoma

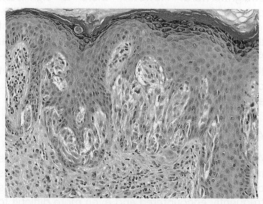

Fig. 5. High-power magnification of Spitz nevus showing vertically oriented nests of spindle and epithelioid cells in the dermal-epidermal junction extending down into the papillary dermis. The nests are fairly uniform (10 ×). (*Courtesy of* Annette Segura, MD, Department of Pathology, Children's Hospital of Wisconsin.)

These cells can be round, oval, polygonal, rhomboidal, or polyangular. The nuclei can be round, oval, irregularly shaped, or multilobulated. Multinucleated forms may be present. In some cases a minority of epithelioid cells can have cytoplasmic and or nuclear contours that are very irregular. The cells can be strikingly large or have a bizarre shape. Cytoplasm sometimes has a ground-glass appearance. Melanin is typically absent or not abundant, although melanin is prominent in melanophages in the pigmented spindle variant.

Within the dermis, the cells display maturation and the nests are replaced by a single cell infiltrating pattern into the base. Kamino bodies are pale eosinophilic globules (now known to be composed of basement membrane material) that stain positive with periodic acid Schiff and trichrome, and are commonly found in the dermal-epidermal junction of Spitz nevi.

Distinction of Spitz nevus from melanoma is made by a constellation of findings taken in the context of the clinical presentation. The symmetry of the lesion, absence of significant pleomorphism, deep mitoses or pagetoid spread, and lack of extension into surrounding structures are features recognized to suggest benign biology. In contrast, melanoma is typically a large lesion that is asymmetric and poorly demarcated. Nests are variable in size, shape, and orientation, and Kamino bodies are absent. In melanoma there is lack of maturation, mitoses are prominent and present in the depth of the lesion, and there is a lack of epidermal change. Cellular type is variable in melanoma, with various degrees of pigmentation.

The diagnosis of Spitz nevus with all the typical features in the setting of young children can be straightforward. However, there is significant potential for over- or underinterpretation of pathologic findings or absence of findings because of the baseline features that can mimic melanoma. As lesions become less characteristic, determination of benign Spitz nevi from those with malignant potential based on pathology can be problematic, even for experienced practitioners.

ATYPICAL SPITZ NEVUS PATHOLOGY

An atypical Spitz nevus is a Spitz lesion that has more atypia but not enough to render a diagnosis of melanoma. Spitz tumors with atypia are less frequently encountered and even more difficult to distinguish with certainty from melanoma. The number or degree of atypical features to qualify for the diagnosis of atypical Spitz nevus is not absolute. Atypia of architectural or cellular features can be found, and careful analysis of a range of features is required. Criteria for recognizing these

atypical Spitz lesions have been proposed[29,33] but are not uniformly practiced.

Atypical features can be either intraepidermal or intradermal.[29] The intraepidermal features are similar to those found in atypical common melanocytic nevi including variation in size, shape, orientation, and spacing of junctional nests, horizontal confluence and bridging of nests, diminished cellular cohesion of nests, and cytologic atypia of melanocytes. Atypical features recognized within the dermal component include increased cellularity, decreased cellular cohesion, asymmetry of the lesion, deep extension into the lowermost dermis or subcutis, cytologic atypia, presence of mitoses, lack of maturation of cells, disorderly infiltration of collagen, and presence of a mononuclear infiltrate (**Fig. 6**).[29] The presence and degrees of these features are weighed individually and collectively. Still, lack of consensus is the rule.[34]

A protocol for categorization of an atypical Spitz into a high-risk or low-risk lesion was proposed based on the size of the lesion, the presence of pathologic features (ulceration and mitotic activity), and the age of the patient.[33,35] A score is assigned based on presence or absence of these 4 features, and increasing scores are suggestive of malignancy. The diagnosis of Spitz lesions can also be divided into 3 categories[1] based on combined specific histologic criteria: (1) Spitz lesions without atypical features, (2) Spitz lesions with atypical features (regardless of the number or which features are present) including lesions with indeterminate biologic or malignant potential, and (3) melanoma. The rationale for this approach is to remove subjective, nonvalidated criteria for atypical lesions by lumping them together and separating them from the more easily distinguishable lesions on the opposite ends of the spectrum.

Misdiagnosis, either overdiagnosis of Spitz nevi as melanoma[36] or underdiagnosis of melanoma

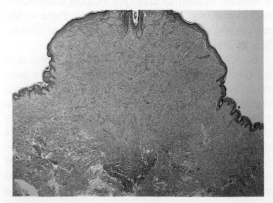

Fig. 6. Atypical Spitz lesion. At low-power magnification the lesion is large and asymmetric with variable nests and infiltration into the base (4 ×).

as Spitz nevi, is well documented.[37] The distinction of Spitz nevus from melanoma is one of the most important and challenging areas in pathology.[13,38–40] There is discordance of diagnosis of Spitz lesions of all types, even among expert practitioners.[41,42] The interobserver reliability in reading pathology of Spitz lesions is poor.[34] Most pathologists believe there is a spectrum of Spitz lesions from benign to malignant, but where they draw those lines can be different. Urso[6] writes that there is a core of 9 potential findings that may suggest malignancy, and that the presence of any one of the findings may represent sufficient conditions for diagnosis of malignancy. Potential significant findings relate the dermal growth pattern, extension of the tumor, location of mitoses, pleomorphism, presence of melanization deeply, asymmetry, cellular necrosis, epidermal melanocytes present below parakeratosis or epidermal ulceration, and presence of neoplastic cells in lymphatic vessels.[6]

In summary, for evaluation of Spitz nevus pathology, the symmetry of the lesion, the lateral and deep borders, the lateral and deep extension, the presence and proliferation of melanocytes within the epidermis, the nesting pattern, the cell type and cellularity, atypia of the cells, cohesion of the cells, the maturation of the cells, presence of ulceration, expansile nodules, Kamino bodies, deep mitoses, atypical mitoses, and mononuclear infiltrate should all be taken into account. The light microscopy of a Spitz lesion should be interpreted by an expert pathologist or dermatopathologist. The pathology report should reflect the degree of certainty of the resulting interpretation. Also, important clinical information should be recognized, such as the age of the patient and location of the lesion. For example, increasing age of the patient would suggest a diagnosis of melanoma over atypical Spitz nevus. Location that is uncommon for Spitz nevus, such as the back, would also suggest melanoma over Spitz nevus. There is no known clinical distinction of atypical Spitz lesions from Spitz nevi, but information known to be important in evaluating patients with melanocytic lesions includes history of change, symptoms, personal and family history of melanoma, skin phenotype, and personal history of predisposing condition.

PATHOLOGIC SUBTYPES OF SPITZ NEVUS
Desmoplastic Spitz Nevus

In lesions in which there is marked fibrosis in the dermis, the lesions can be termed desmoplastic Spitz nevus based on the presence of spindle or epithelioid cells. In desmoplastic Spitz lesions, junctional activity, nesting, and pigmentation are generally absent. When spindle or epithelioid cells are present within a paucicellular hyalinized collagenous stroma, the term hyalinizing Spitz nevus can be used. Rosette-like radial arrangement of cells of a Spitz nevus has been described.[43] Tubular arrangement of cells with centrally located empty spaces has also been reported in a series of cases.[44] Touton giant cell appearance of cells has also been described as have an angiomatoid, a myxoid and pagetoid, and plexiform variant of Spitz nevus.

Histologic variants also include combined lesions (blue nevus or deep penetrating nevus) and Spitz nevus with halo nevus features. The halo seems to be a particular feature of combined lesions.[45] When Spitz nevus is present within another lesion the term combined nevus is used. These lesions have spindle or epithelioid cells and features, but also have other cellular constituents. Spitz nodules are found within congenital nevi, and Spitz nevus may be seen in a lesion that also has histologic features of blue nevus or common melanocytic nevus.

Childhood Verses Adult Spitz Nevus

In general, Spitz lesions are much more common in children. Childhood Spitz nevi can exhibit less pigmentation than their adult counterpart, and not uncommonly display pagetoid proliferation. Purely epithelioid lesions are more common in children. Desmoplastic Spitz nevi are rare in children. The younger the age of the patient, the more likely the lesion is to be diagnosed as Spitz nevus; the older the age of the patient, the more likely the lesion is to be diagnosed as melanoma. It is important to be aware that there is no determined threshold age for malignancy. Melanoma in children is rare, but borderline Spitz lesions occur and some of these are melanomas. There are advocates for an age threshold for diagnosing malignant melanoma in Spitz lesions in children. This approach should be used with caution because it is not based on good evidence.

Differential diagnosis of the histologic findings in Spitz nevus

Melanoma and nonmelanoctyic lesions can be confused with Spitz nevi. Nonmelanocytic lesions that can have similar pathologic features include juvenile xanthogranuloma, cellular neurothekeoma, epithelioid cell histiocytoma, and reticulohistiocytoma. Hyalinizing Spitz nevi can be mistaken for metastatic carcinomas.

ANCILLARY TESTS

Spitz nevus cannot be diagnosed based on distinctive immunohistochemical markers. However, these stains are useful to distinguish pathologic findings from a nonmelanocytic lesion. The stains can be helpful as ancillary tests[46–56] to help determine malignant potential. Although there are differences in staining patterns between Spitz lesions and melanoma, there is often overlap. Sensitivity and specificity are not 100%.

Spitz lesions stain with melanocytic markers S100, Mart-1/Melan A, HMB-45 (gp100), tyrosinase, and microphthalmia transcription factor (Mitf), although expression may be low with the latter.[46,50,57,58] S100 and Mart-1 staining is diffuse, whereas HMB-45 and tyrosinase diminish toward the base of the lesion in Spitz nevus.[57,58] Immunohistochemical staining can also be helpful for detection of mitoses to determine relative mitotic rates. The rate of staining with proliferation markers is generally lower for Spitz lesions compared with melanoma. Ki-67/MIB-1 has been shown to correlate with risk stratification of Spitz tumors,[59] with a very low labeling index in normal nevi and a very high labeling index in melanoma, with intermediate grades of staining from typical to high-risk Spitz lesions. Ki-67/MIB-1[46,47,56] is a particularly helpful marker for distinguishing Spitz nevi from melanoma. Fatty acid synthase has also been shown to progressively increase in staining in a gradient from Spitz nevus to melanoma.[59] p53 does not seem to be expressed significantly in Spitz nevi, whereas there is higher expression in melanoma.[60,61] The pattern of staining in Spitz lesions within the tumor can also be significant because malignant lesions show increased proliferation at deeper levels. For instance, in one study Spitz nevi stain in the uppermost portion with HMB-45, compared with melanoma that stains throughout.[57] Others have found heterogeneous HMB-45 staining in Spitz nevi.[62]

Considerable overlap in the staining patterns for AgNOR, cyclin D1, c-myc, c-fos, telomerase, and Bcl-2 in Spitz lesions is observed, and these stains do not seem as useful.[52,63–67]

Spitz lesions have different nuclear features to melanoma lesions. Nuclear hyperchromatism, cellular pleomorphism, and mitotic activity can be quantified using image analysis cytometry and multivariate DNA cytometry. Image analysis cytometry revealed a difference in the amount of DNA content from the upper to the lower portion of Spitz nevi in comparison with melanoma, where there was no maturation found.[68] Differences in AgNOR number, size, and heterogeneity confirm the nuclear differences between Spitz nevi and melanoma.[69] A lesion is more likely to be a melanoma is the AgNOR is more than 2 per cell.[63] The use of multiple cytometric factors together (DNA microdensitometry, karyometry and AgNORs, and Ki-67/MIB-1) has been reported to improve the diagnosis of benign Spitz nevi from melanoma.[70] Telomerase activity is also much lower in Spitz nevi than in melanoma.[66]

MOLECULAR STUDIES

Abnormal DNA content has been detected in Spitz lesions. There seems to be heterogeneity of ploidy in various Spitz lesions.[71,72] However, at least some Spitz nevi seem to be diploid when compared with melanoma.[73] Recent studies show Spitz nevi generally to be devoid of chromosomal aberrations when measured by comparative genomic hybridization (CGH) and florescence in situ hybridization (FISH) studies.[74]

The exception of chromosomal normality found with CGH or FISH is the amplification of 11p in a subset of Spitz nevi.[75] (However, among the few oncogenes tested thus far, many Spitz nevi do not show mutations in oncogenes. A minority of Spitz nevi with 11p copy number increases also seem to have an HRAS mutation.)[75] These findings seem to occur in a subset of Spitz nevi with significant dermal and infiltrative involvement. The presence of HRAS mutation in the absence of other related oncogene mutations is different from the genetic signature of melanoma. These results have been interpreted by Maldonado and colleagues[76] as potentially conferring survival advantage of the Spitz lesion without conferring the ability to metastasize. On the other hand, BRAF mutation has also been found in a small subset of Spitz nevi, some with atypical features.[77] The significance of this finding is unknown because many types of nevi as well as a subset of melanoma lesions are found to have BRAF mutations.[78] Contrary to the aforementioned HRAS study findings, these investigators suggest that BRAF mutation may be a first event in melanocytic hyperplasia.

The use of whole genome CGH or FISH studies to detect chromosome number changes is potentially an exciting advance in the diagnosis of borderline Spitz lesions. The basis for this is a study in which researchers compared Spitz nevi and melanomas for chromosomal aberrations using these 2 methods.[74,79] The investigators found that whereas melanomas had frequent deletions of 9p, 10q, 6q, and 8p, and frequent gains of 7,8, 6p, and 1q, Spitz lesions were found to have no or very limited chromosomal gains or losses.

This test could potentially be used in patients with Spitz lesions that are borderline, to determine which patients should be offered further treatment. If chromosomal aberrations are found, especially if similar to melanoma, these patients may be offered sentinel lymph node biopsy, lymphadenectomy, or chemotherapy. Although these techniques are promising, they need to be validated by larger studies. The possibility that Spitz lesions metastasize based on different biologic mechanisms of malignancy (other than those of traditional melanoma) is a theory that has yet to be disproved. After all, as proponents of alternative pathways point out, traditional nevus-melanoma pathway mutations in BRAF or NRAS[80] have not been found in either Spitz nevi or spitzoid melanomas.[81–83]

TREATMENT OF SPITZ NEVUS

The majority of practitioners recommend biopsy of all Spitz nevi.[84] Most agree that Spitz nevi should be completely excised. Beyond surgical removal of the immediate lesion with 1- to 2-mm margin, there is no agreement regarding management. Wide 1-cm excisional margins in atypical Spitz lesions are recommended by some[1] and may be of particular relevance in atypical Spitz lesions. In children younger than 12 years with a starburst pattern of Spitz nevus on dermoscopy (indicating a diagnosis of pigmented spindle ell nevus of Reed), a proposal has been made for close clinical follow-up without necessary removal of these lesions if there are no complicating features or circumstances.[23] Treatment of spitzoid melanoma or melanoma with Spitz-like features is the same as that for malignant melanoma, with wide excision according to the depth of the lesion, and ancillary workup and nonsurgical treatment as deemed appropriate.

SENTINEL LYMPH NODE BIOPSY

Sentinel lymph node biopsy is the most important predictor of outcome in melanoma and as such, is one technique that has been used to gather more information regarding potential biologic behavior of borderline Spitz lesions.[85,86] An involved sentinel lymph node is defined as metastatic disease whereas a negative sentinel lymph nodes or node is somewhat reassuring. In cases of borderline Spitz lesions where the sentinel lymph node is positive, these patients may be offered lymphadenectomy, systemic therapy with interferon based on melanoma treatment protocols, or trial therapy to prevent further metastasis.

Kwon and colleagues[87] point out a frighteningly high rate of metastasis as an argument to question the validity of using sentinel node to determine metastasis. Nodal involvement can be defined in several ways, and is most commonly defined as presence of the same cell type as the original lesion within the parenchyma or the subcapsular sinus of the draining node(s), but stricter criteria would include replacement of a significant part of the node, mitoses, or necrosis. However, melanoma has been shown to metastasize to the capsule.[80] Still, benign nevi can be found in sentinel nodes as well, and therefore Kwon and colleagues[87] and others[80] question the usefulness and interpretation of the sentinel node biopsy.

In a series of patients (mean age 16 years) with borderline Spitz lesions indistinguishable from melanoma and more than 1-mm Breslow depth or borderline lesions with adverse features such as those with aberrant growth patterns, deep mitoses, or ulceration,[86] 44% of 18 patients had a positive sentinel lymph node. The mean Breslow depth of the original Spitz lesions in this series was 3.5 mm, and the predicted rate of sentinel node involvement for melanoma with the same depth would be expected to be approximately 40% to 50%. Thus the rate of sentinel node involvement was the same as that which would be expected in melanoma. There were no histologic or clinical predictors for a positive sentinel node In this series. All 8 patients with positive nodes underwent lymphadenectomy, 6 received interferon-α2b, and 2 received melanoma vaccine therapy. All these relatively young patients were alive at median 12 months follow-up. Sentinel node has been advocated for borderline Spitz lesions in multiple small studies and for other borderline melanocytic lesions.[88]

In summary, controversy remains concerning the significance of the presence of lymph node metastasis as an indication for broader-reaching metastasis.[89,90] Follow-up of patients found to have lymph node metastasis has not yet been long enough to determine relative outcomes, although outcomes so far for these borderline lesions seem favorable. Critics of sentinel node validity caution against overdiagnosis of malignancy in a lesion that has not been proven to be malignant. Some investigators believe Spitz lesions may metastasize to lymph nodes but are unable to metastasize further. Other possibilities to explain the limited experience so far are that treatment for these lesions was beneficial or that metastasis does not parallel the melanoma path. Additional evidence for lymph node metastasis as malignancy includes a case in which karyotyping performed on a lymph node metastasis in a child with a borderline Spitz lesion revealed deletion of chromos 6, consistent with diagnosis of melanoma.[90] Reports of atypical Spitz lesions that have metastasized[33,34,91] are interpreted by many as further proof of malignant potential. Yet critics argue that these lesions were misdiagnosed.[92]

EVOLUTION OF THE SPITZ NEVUS

Spitz nevi are usually clonal proliferations that are thought to be relatively stable. The different locations within the skin (ie, junctional, compound, dermal) may correspond to maturation of the lesion from a single cell to a collection of cells, and finally a larger growth.[93] At least some investigators[79] believe that the desmoplastic form of Spitz nevus may represent a later stage in evolution of the Spitz nevus where there is an increase in fibrosis without junctional activity or nesting. Some Spitz nevi have involuted over time. The presence of HRAS mutation in a subtype of Spitz lesion in the absence of other oncogenic mutations has been interpreted[75] as evidence for inability of at least this subset of Spitz lesion to metastasize, assuming activation of a senescence type stop of proliferation in these nevi.

PROGNOSIS

Spitz nevi with typical features on presentation and biopsy usually are associated with a favorable prognosis. These lesions that seem typical can rarely lead to metastasis and death.[34] Thus all biopsies of Spitz nevi should seek confirmatory consultation. Although benign Spitz features on biopsy are reassuring, they must of course be taken in the context of the other circumstances of the patient, including symptoms of recent change, pain, bleeding, or pruritus; location, age, personal and family history, skin phenotype, and other melanoma risk factors. Children have Spitz nevi more frequently, and it is notable that melanoma does not present with typical features of ABCD (Asymmetry, Border irregularity, Color variegation, Diameter >6 mm) criteria; instead clinical symptoms[94] seem paramount. In general, one can probably be cautiously optimistic with regard to the prognosis in the case of typical Spitz nevi in the setting of low-risk clinical features.

Spitz nevi with atypical features and Spitz nevi with borderline features require confirmatory consultation by a second expert dermatopathologist. There are 2 views regarding prognosis with this category of lesion. The first is that these lesions are a continuum from benign to malignant, and the second is that Spitz lesions are recognizable as distinct from melanoma and are not capable of metastatic behavior. If the Spitz lesion is a continuum from benign to malignant, criteria for grading atypical Spitz lesions should be achievable. In children a grading system for light microscopy has been proposed[33] based on a series of 30 cases with follow-up of at least 3 years. A limited selection of parameters was identified as potentially noteworthy, and 5 histologic criteria were determined to be significant. Atypical Spitz lesions are graded either 0 or 1 based on the absence or presence of the following criteria: age greater than 10 years, size greater than 10 mm, ulceration, mitotic rate greater than $6/mm^2$, and extension of the lesion into the fat. The higher the total score, the greater the risk for metastasis was felt to be. This system remains to be validated in a large series of patients and represents objective criteria for grading low-, medium-, or high-risk atypical Spitz lesions in children to more accurately diagnose and predict outcomes.

SUMMARY

The Spitz lesion can usually be determined to be benign or malignant, based on expert pathology examination with light microscopy when typical features are found. Benign lesions are commonly referred to as Spitz nevi and malignant lesions as melanoma. Atypical lesions are much more difficult to separate into benign lesions or lesions with malignant biologic behavior. Review by an expert pathologist of these atypical Spitz lesions is mandatory, and often subsequent expert consultation is required as well. In some borderline lesions, differentiating with certainty benign from malignant based on current techniques is not possible. Recent advances in ancillary testing and cytogenetic studies are promising. These new studies need to continue to be applied to a wide range of Spitz lesions in a large number of cases.

Future research studies should better delineate the nature of Spitz lesions. Analysis should confirm or dispute what seems to be a pathologic continuum of Spitz lesions on a spectrum from benign to malignant, and should help identify new diagnostic features or delineate existing light microscopic features that best differentiate benign versus malignant lesions. Patients with these lesions need to be followed in collective, multi-center, long-term studies to correlate the clinical behavior with the results of the diagnostic tests and treatment rendered in order to be able to eventually predict prognosis more accurately and to achieve the ultimate goal of improved treatment recommendations.

REFERENCES

1. Barnhill RL. The spitzoid lesion: the importance of atypical variants and risk assessment. Am J Dermatopathol 2006;28(1):75–83.
2. Spatz A, Barnhill RL. The Spitz tumor 50 years later: revisiting a landmark contribution and unresolved controversy. J Am Acad Dermatol 1999;40(2 Pt 1):223–8.
3. Kernen JA, Ackerman LV. Spindle cell nevi and epithelioid cell nevi (so-called juvenile melanomas) in children and adults: a clinicopathological study of 27 cases. Cancer 1960;13:612–25.
4. Darier J, Civatte J. Naevus ou Naevo-carcinome chez un n ourisson. Bull Soc Fr Dermatol Syphiligr 1910;21:61–3.
5. Casso EM, Grin-Jorgensen CM, Grant-Kels JM. Spitz nevi [see comment]. J Am Acad Dermatol 1992;27(6 Pt 1):901–13.
6. Urso C. A new perspective for Spitz tumors? Am J Dermatopathol 2005;27(4):364–6.
7. Piepkorn M. The Spitz nevus is melanoma. Am J Dermatopathol 2005;27(4):367–9.
8. Urso C. Melanocytic lesions, Spitz tumors, and Don Ferrante's logic. Am J Dermatopathol 2007;29(5):491–4.
9. Spitz S. Melanomas of childhood. 1948. CA Cancer J Clin 1991;41(1):40–51.
10. Allen AC, Spitz S. Malignant melanoma; a clinicopathological analysis of the criteria for diagnosis and prognosis. Cancer 1953;6(1):1–45.
11. Allen AC. Juvenile melanomas of children and adults and melanocarcinomas of children. Arch Dermatol 1960;82:325–35.
12. Herreid PA, Shapiro PE. Age distribution of Spitz nevus vs malignant melanoma. Arch Dermatol 1996;132(3):352–3.
13. Weedon D, Little JH. Spindle and epithelioid cell nevi in children and adults. A review of 211 cases of the Spitz nevus. Cancer 1977;40(1):217–25.
14. Harris MN, Hurwitz RM, Buckel LJ, et al. Congenital Spitz nevus. Dermatol Surg 2000;26(10):931–5.
15. Zaenglein AL, Heintz P, Kamino H, et al. Congenital Spitz nevus clinically mimicking melanoma. J Am Acad Dermatol 2002;47(3):441–4.
16. Bader JL, Li FP, Olmstead PM, et al. Childhood malignant melanoma. Incidence and etiology. Am J Pediatr Hematol Oncol 1985;7(4):341–5.
17. Fass J, Grimwood RE, Kraus E, et al. Adult onset of eruptive widespread Spitz's nevi. J Am Acad Dermatol 2002;46(5 Suppl):S142–3.
18. Levy RM, Ming ME, Shapiro M, et al. Eruptive disseminated Spitz nevi. J Am Acad Dermatol 2007;57(3):519–23.
19. Onsun N, Saracoglu S, Demirkesen C, et al. Eruptive widespread Spitz nevi: can pregnancy be a stimulating factor? J Am Acad Dermatol 1999;40(5 Pt 2):866–7.
20. Pellacani G, Longo C, Ferrara G, et al. Spitz nevi: In vivo confocal microscopic features, dermatoscopic aspects, histopathologic correlates, and diagnostic significance. J Am Acad Dermatol 2009;60(2):236–47.
21. Ferrara G, Argenziano G, Soyer HP, et al. The spectrum of Spitz nevi: a clinicopathologic study of 83 cases. Arch Dermatol 2005;141(11):1381–7.
22. Kittler H, Pehamberger H, Wolff K, et al. Diagnostic accuracy of dermoscopy. Lancet Oncol 2002;3(3):159–65.
23. Nino M, Brunetti B, Delfino S, et al. Spitz nevus: follow-up study of 8 cases of childhood starburst type and proposal for management. Dermatology 2009;218(1):48–51.
24. Piccolo D, Ferrari A, Peris K. Sequential dermoscopic evolution of pigmented Spitz nevus in childhood. J Am Acad Dermatol 2003;49(3):556–8.
25. Zalaudek I, Manzo M, Ferrara G, et al. New classification of melanocytic nevi based on dermoscopy. Expert Rev Dermatol 2008;3(4):477–89.
26. Pellacani G, Cesinaro AM, Seidenari S. Morphological features of Spitz naevus as observed by digital videomicroscopy. Acta Derm Venereol 2000;80(2):117–21.
27. Pellacani G, Guitera P, Longo C, et al. The impact of in vivo reflectance confocal microscopy for the diagnostic accuracy of melanoma and equivocal melanocytic lesions. J Invest Dermatol 2007;127(12):2759–65.
28. Pellacani G, Cesinaro AM, Seidenari S. Reflectance-mode confocal microscopy of pigmented skin lesions–improvement in melanoma diagnostic specificity. J Am Acad Dermatol 2005;53(6):979–85.
29. Barnhill R. Tumors of melanocytes. In: Barnhill RL, Crowson AN, Busam KJ, et al, editors. Textbook of dermatopathology. New York: McGraw-Hill; 1998. p. 550–8.
30. Weedon D. Lentigines, nevi and melanomas. In: Weedon D, Strutton G, editors. Skin pathology, vol.1 2nd edition. New York: Churchill Livingstone; 2002. p. 811–4.
31. McKee PH. Melanocytic nevi. In: Mckee PH, Calonje E, Granter SR, editors. Pathology of skin, vol. 2. 3rd edition. Philadelphia: Elsevier Mosby; 2005. p. 1268–75.
32. Paniago-Pereira C, Maize JC, Ackerman AB. Nevus of large spindle and/or epithelioid cells (Spitz's nevus). Arch Dermatol 1978;114(12):1811–23.
33. Spatz A, Calonje E, Handfield-Jones S, et al. Spitz tumors in children: a grading system for risk stratification. Arch Dermatol 1999;135(3):282–5.
34. Barnhill RL, Argenyi ZB, From L, et al. Atypical Spitz nevi/tumors: lack of consensus for diagnosis, discrimination from melanoma, and prediction of outcome. Hum Pathol 1999;30(5):513–20.

35. Barnhill RL, Flotte TJ, Fleischli M, et al. Cutaneous melanoma and atypical Spitz tumors in childhood. Cancer 1995;76(10):1833–45.

36. Orchard DC, Dowling JP, Kelly JW. Spitz naevi misdiagnosed histologically as melanoma: prevalence and clinical profile. Australas J Dermatol 1997;38(1):12–4.

37. Handfield-Jones SE, Smith NP. Malignant melanoma in childhood. Br J Dermatol 1996;134(4):607–16.

38. Mooi WJ. Spitz nevus and its histologic simulators. Adv Anat Pathol 2002;9(4):209–21.

39. Binder SW, Asnong C, Paul E, et al. The histology and differential diagnosis of Spitz nevus. Semin Diagn Pathol 1993;10(1):36–46.

40. Crotty KA, Scolyer RA, Li L, et al. Spitz naevus versus Spitzoid melanoma: when and how can they be distinguished? [see comment]. Pathology 2002;34(1):6–12.

41. Farmer ER, Gonin R, Hanna MP. Discordance in the histopathologic diagnosis of melanoma and melanocytic nevi between expert pathologists [see comment]. Hum Pathol 1996;27(6):528–31.

42. Ackerman AB. Discordance among expert pathologists in diagnosis of melanocytic neoplasms. Hum Pathol 1996;27(11):1115–6.

43. Kantrow S, Kalemeris GC, Prieto V. Spitz nevus with rosette-like structures: a new histologic variant. J Cutan Pathol 2008;35(5):510–2.

44. Burg G, Kempf W, Hochli M, et al. 'Tubular' epithelioid cell nevus: a new variant of Spitz's nevus. J Cutan Pathol 1998;25(9):475–8.

45. Harvell JD, Meehan SA, LeBoit PE. Spitz's nevi with halo reaction: a histopathologic study of 17 cases. J Cutan Pathol 1997;24(10):611–9.

46. Li LX, Crotty KA, McCarthy SW, et al. A zonal comparison of MIB1-Ki67 immunoreactivity in benign and malignant melanocytic lesions. Am J Dermatopathol 2000;22(6):489–95.

47. Bergman R, Malkin L, Sabo E, et al. MIB-1 monoclonal antibody to determine proliferative activity of Ki-67 antigen as an adjunct to the histopathologic differential diagnosis of Spitz nevi. J Am Acad Dermatol 2001;44(3):500–4.

48. Kapur P, Rakheja D, Roy LC, et al. Fatty acid synthase expression in cutaneous melanocytic neoplasms. Mod Pathol 2005;18(8):1107–12.

49. McNutt NS, Urmacher C, Hakimian J, et al. Nevoid malignant melanoma: morphologic patterns and immunohistochemical reactivity. J Cutan Pathol 1995;22(6):502–17.

50. Kanter-Lewensohn L, Hedblad MA, Wejde J, et al. Immunohistochemical markers for distinguishing Spitz nevi from malignant melanomas. Mod Pathol 1997;10(9):917–20.

51. Niemann TH, Argenyi ZB. Immunohistochemical study of Spitz nevi and malignant melanoma with use of antibody to proliferating cell nuclear antigen. Am J Dermatopathol 1993;15(5):441–5.

52. Tu P, Miyauchi S, Miki Y. Proliferative activities in Spitz nevus compared with melanocytic nevus and malignant melanoma using expression of PCNA/cyclin and mitotic rate. Am J Dermatopathol 1993;15(4):311–4.

53. Deeds J, Cronin F, Duncan LM. Patterns of melastatin mRNA expression in melanocytic tumors. Hum Pathol 2000;31(11):1346–56.

54. Duncan LM, Deeds J, Cronin FE, et al. Melastatin expression and prognosis in cutaneous malignant melanoma. J Clin Oncol 2001;19(2):568–76.

55. Ribe A, McNutt NS. S100A6 protein expression is different in Spitz nevi and melanomas. Mod Pathol 2003;16(5):505–11.

56. Harvell JD, Bastian BC, LeBoit PE. Persistent (recurrent) Spitz nevi: a histopathologic, immunohistochemical, and molecular pathologic study of 22 cases. Am J Surg Pathol 2002;26(5):654–61.

57. Bergman R, Dromi R, Trau H, et al. The pattern of HMB-45 antibody staining in compound Spitz nevi. Am J Dermatopathol 1995;17(6):542–6.

58. Rode J, Williams RA, Jarvis LR, et al. S100 protein, neurone specific enolase, and nuclear DNA content in Spitz naevus. J Pathol 1990;161(1):41–5.

59. Kapur P, Selim MA, Roy LC, et al. Spitz nevi and atypical Spitz nevi/tumors: a histologic and immunohistochemical analysis. Mod Pathol 2005;18(2):197–204.

60. Kaleem Z, Lind AC, Humphrey PA, et al. Concurrent Ki-67 and p53 immunolabeling in cutaneous melanocytic neoplasms: an adjunct for recognition of the vertical growth phase in malignant melanomas? Mod Pathol 2000;13(3):217–22.

61. Bergman R, Shemer A, Levy R, et al. Immunohistochemical study of p53 protein expression in Spitz nevus as compared with other melanocytic lesions. Am J Dermatopathol 1995;17(6):547–50.

62. Palazzo J, Duray PH. Typical, dysplastic, congenital, and Spitz nevi: a comparative immunohistochemical study. Hum Pathol 1989;20(4):341–6.

63. Howat AJ, Wright AL, Cotton DW, et al. AgNORs in benign, dysplastic, and malignant melanocytic skin lesions. Am J Dermatopathol 1990;12(2):156–61.

64. Bergman R, Kerner H, Manov L, et al. C-fos protein expression in Spitz nevi, common melanocytic nevi, and malignant melanomas. Am J Dermatopathol 1998;20(3):262–5.

65. Bergman R, Lurie M, Kerner H, et al. Mode of c-myc protein expression in Spitz nevi, common melanocytic nevi and malignant melanomas. J Cutan Pathol 1997;24(4):219–22.

66. Guttman-Yassky E, Bergman R, Manov L, et al. Human telomerase RNA component expression in Spitz nevi, common melanocytic nevi, and malignant melanomas. J Cutan Pathol 2002;29(6):341–6.

67. Nagasaka T, Lai R, Medeiros LJ, et al. Cyclin D1 overexpression in Spitz nevi: an immunohistochemical study. Am J Dermatopathol 1999;21(2):115–20.

68. LeBoit PE, Van Fletcher H. A comparative study of Spitz nevus and nodular malignant melanoma using image analysis cytometry. J Invest Dermatol 1987; 88(6):753–7.

69. Birck A, thor Straten P, Li L, et al. Analysis of T cell receptor AV and BV chain gene expression by infiltrating lymphocytes in Spitz naevi and in halo naevi. Melanoma Res 1997;7(1):49–57.

70. Li LX, Crotty KA, Scolyer RA, et al. Use of multiple cytometric markers improves discrimination between benign and malignant melanocytic lesions: a study of DNA microdensitometry, karyometry, argyrophilic staining of nucleolar organizer regions and MIB1-Ki67 immunoreactivity. Melanoma Res 2003;13(6):581–6.

71. Skowronek J, Warchol JB, Karas Z, et al. Significance of DNA ploidy measurements in Spitz nevi. Pol J Pathol 2000;51(1):45–50.

72. De Wit PE, Kerstens HM, Poddighe PJ, et al. DNA in situ hybridization as a diagnostic tool in the discrimination of melanoma and Spitz naevus. J Pathol 1994;173(3):227–33.

73. Vogt T, Stolz W, Glassl A, et al. Multivariate DNA cytometry discriminates between Spitz nevi and malignant melanomas because large polymorphic nuclei in Spitz nevi are not aneuploid. Am J Dermatopathol 1996;18(2):142–50.

74. Bastian BC, Wesselmann U, Pinkel D, et al. Molecular cytogenetic analysis of Spitz nevi shows clear differences to melanoma. J Invest Dermatol 1999; 113(6):1065–9.

75. Bastian BC, LeBoit PE, Pinkel D. Mutations and copy number increase of HRAS in Spitz nevi with distinctive histopathological features. Am J Pathol 2000; 157(3):967–72.

76. Maldonado JL, Timmerman L, Fridlyand J, et al. Mechanisms of cell-cycle arrest in Spitz nevi with constitutive activation of the MAP-kinase pathway. Am J Pathol 2004;164(5):1783–7.

77. Fullen DR, Poynter JN, Lowe L, et al. BRAF and NRAS mutations in spitzoid melanocytic lesions. Mod Pathol 2006;19(10):1324–32.

78. Thomas NE. BRAF somatic mutations in malignant melanoma and melanocytic naevi. Melanoma Res 2006;16(2):97–103.

79. Bastian BC, LeBoit PE, Hamm H, et al. Chromosomal gains and losses in primary cutaneous melanomas detected by comparative genomic hybridization. Cancer Res 1998;58(10):2170–5.

80. Busam KJ, Pulitzer M. Sentinel lymph node biopsy for patients with diagnostically controversial Spitzoid melanocytic tumors? Adv Anat Pathol 2008;15(5): 253–62.

81. Palmedo G, Hantschke M, Rutten A, et al. The T1796A mutation of the BRAF gene is absent in Spitz nevi. J Cutan Pathol 2004;31(3):266–70.

82. Gill M, Cohen J, Renwick N, et al. Genetic similarities between Spitz nevus and Spitzoid melanoma in children. Cancer 2004;101(11):2636–40.

83. Gill M, Renwick N, Silvers DN, et al. Lack of BRAF mutations in Spitz nevi. J Invest Dermatol 2004; 122(5):1325–6.

84. Gelbard SN, Tripp JM, Marghoob AA, et al. Management of Spitz nevi: a survey of dermatologists in the United States. J Am Acad Dermatol 2002;47(2): 224–30.

85. Lohmann CM, Coit DG, Brady MS, et al. Sentinel lymph node biopsy in patients with diagnostically controversial spitzoid melanocytic tumors. Am J Surg Pathol 2002;26(1):47–55.

86. Su LD, Fullen DR, Sondak VK, et al. Sentinel lymph node biopsy for patients with problematic spitzoid melanocytic lesions: a report on 18 patients. Cancer 2003;97(2):499–507.

87. Kwon EJ, Winfield HL, Rosenberg AS. The controversy and dilemma of using sentinel lymph node biopsy for diagnostically difficult melanocytic proliferations. J Cutan Pathol 2008;35(11):1075–7.

88. Kelley SW, Cockerell CJ. Sentinel lymph node biopsy as an adjunct to management of histologically difficult to diagnose melanocytic lesions: a proposal. J Am Acad Dermatol 2000;42(3):527–30.

89. Mooi WJ. Histopathology of Spitz naevi and "Spitzoid" melanomas. Curr Top Pathol 2001;94:65–77.

90. Smith NM, Evans MJ, Pearce A, et al. Cytogenetics of an atypical Spitz nevus metastatic to a single lymph node. Pediatr Pathol Lab Med 1998;18(1): 115–22.

91. Ghorbani Z, Dowlati Y, Mehregan AH. Amelanotic spitzoid melanoma in the burn scar of a child. Pediatr Dermatol 1996;13(4):285–7.

92. Shapiro PE. Spitz nevi. J Am Acad Dermatol 1993; 29(4):667–8.

93. LeBoit P. Spitz nevus: a look back and a look ahead. Adv Dermatol 2000;16:81–109.

94. Saenz NC, Saenz-Badillos J, Busam K, et al. Childhood melanoma survival. Cancer 1999;85(3): 750–4.

Lentigo Maligna: Diagnosis and Treatment

Mark W. Bosbous, MD[a],*, William W. Dzwierzynski, MD, FACS[a],
Marcelle Neuburg, MD[b]

KEYWORDS

- Melanoma in situ • Lentigo maligna
- Lentigo maligna melanoma • Diagnosis • Treatment

Lentigo maligna (LM) is a lesion of the dermal epidermal junction, which, if untreated, harbors the risk of dermal invasion progressing to invasive LM melanoma (LMM). In fact, multiple studies have shown that approximately 16% of lesions designated as LM (melanoma in situ) on biopsy actually harbor areas of early invasive melanoma (LMM).[1] A well-described condition, LMM has been estimated to comprise 4% to 15% of invasive melanomas.[2–4] Both the in situ and invasive lesions have a propensity for developing on the head and neck and together represent the most common melanocytic malignancy of that body region. A condition more common in the elderly and fair- skinned population related to chronic sun exposure and damage, LM/LMM is a problem on the rise. Incidence rates continue to increase, and although the number of cases increases significantly with age, lesions also have been diagnosed in the second and third decades of life.[5–7] As people live longer and lead more active lives, the incidence of LM/LMM will continue to rise. Coupled with this rise in incidence, the literature reflects renewed scrutiny of available treatment methods and the development of new therapeutic approaches to this disease. The histologic characteristics of LM/LMM, more specifically the diffuse nature of melanocytic overgrowth, make these lesions difficult to treat, with recurrence rates ranging from 2% to 50%.[8–10]

The current nomenclature for early melanoma of the skin can be confusing. The term lentigo maligna has been used by some to describe a proliferation of atypical melanocytes at the dermal–epidermal junction, which is not great enough in number or extent to constitute a melanoma in situ. Others, including the authors, assert that LM is melanoma in situ and should be regarded and treated as early melanoma. Moreover, the term lentigo maligna melanoma has been used to describe a melanoma arising from within an LM (melanoma in situ) as opposed to using the term to properly describe an advanced invasive LM (melanoma in situ). For the purposes of this article, LM is melanoma in situ, and LMM is an advanced invasive lesion that acts as any other cutaneous melanoma and should be evaluated and treated as such.

This article provides an overview of this disease and a critical examination of the data evaluating various treatment methods. In doing so, the authors hope to further the discussion of these treatment methods and aid in clinical decision making to provide patients optimal care while keeping in mind the critical issues of preserving both function and cosmesis in the head and neck region.

EPIDEMIOLOGY AND PATIENT DEMOGRAPHICS

Originally described by Hutchinson in 1912[11] and further defined by Dubrueilh[12,13] LM and LMM

[a] Department of Plastic Surgery, Medical College of Wisconsin, 8700 Watertown Plank Road, Milwaukee, WI 53226, USA
[b] Department of Dermatology, Medical College of Wisconsin, 9200 West Wisconsin Avenue, Milwaukee, WI 53226, USA
* Corresponding author.
E-mail address: mbosbous@mcw.edu (M.W. Bosbous).

Clin Plastic Surg 37 (2010) 35–46
doi:10.1016/j.cps.2009.08.006

are diseases that typically present in the sixth and seventh decades of life.[14] Although the average age of presentation for other subtypes of malignant melanoma has been estimated to be in the 45- to 57-year range,[15,16] the average age of presentation for LM and LMM falls slightly higher, in the 66- to 72-year range.[15–17] Because of varying degrees of sun exposure to the population, the incidence of LM/LMM varies from country to country and region to region. The overall annual incidence of LM/LMM in Australia at one point was estimated to be 1.3 cases per 100,000 population,[18] compared with the United States, where the incidence was estimated at 0.8 and 0.6 cases per 100,000 population for males and females, respectively, based on SEER (Surveillance, Epidemiology and End Results) data.[6] More recently, groups such as Swetter and colleagues[16] further examined SEER data looking at LM/LMM for a specific region and confirmed that in an area of high sun exposure such as southern California, the incidence of LM/LMM is on the rise overall and in specific patient populations related to sex and age. As indicated from the incidence data, there are slight differences in LM/LMM in relation to the sexes. Although the head and neck region has been documented to be the dominant site of presentation, the likelihood of developing LM/LMM at specific locations on the head and neck has been shown to differ between the sexes. Although the distribution of lesions on the cheek and nose remains equal between the sexes, males have a 3.1 times increased risk of development of ear lesions, and females are at 2.5 times increased risk of a lesion developing on the forehead.[19,20]

CLINICAL PRESENTATION/DIAGNOSIS

LM and LMM in many ways continue to present a clinical conundrum. Although the original description by Hutchison[11] describes a tan-colored lesion, hence the term Hutchison's melanotic freckle, savvy clinicians are aware of the vast differences in presentation that are associated with this disease. The typical presentation is that of a tan colored macule located on chronically sun-damaged skin on the head and neck of middle-aged and elderly patients (**Fig. 1**). Lesions, however, can vary in location, size, and color, ranging in spectrum from tan to black with or without variegation. In some cases, LM/LMM may present as a pink patch with little to no pigmentation, so-called amelanotic LM/LMM.[21,22] Clinicians also must keep in mind that previous treatments may alter the appearance of the lesions. Imiquimod, a treatment that will be discussed in more detail later, has been shown in

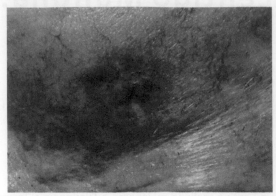

Fig. 1. Lentigo maligna (melanoma in situ) of the left cheek in an 84-yr-old man. Note the lesion's ill defined borders and variations in color. Areas of scarring are evident from previous treatment with cryotherapy. (*Courtesy of* Marcelle Neuburg, MD, Milwaukee, WI.)

some instances to remove visible pigment while having no effect on the histologic findings.[23] Similarly, treatment with cryotherapy may result in areas of depigmentation. Many of the these factors can lead to delays in diagnosis, which may be up to four times longer that other forms of cutaneous malignant melanomas.[20] Overall, a high clinical suspicion remains the best strategy in diagnosis.

Most patients will present to clinicians with a changing lesion on the head and neck, which, in many instances will be in high-stakes areas around the eyes, nose, mouth, and ears. It is not uncommon for patients to note a change in a lesion that has been present for years. The noted change in the lesion may be related to a number of characteristics but often is related to size, as the natural course of LM is to expand in a centrifugal fashion before progressing to LMM by invading vertically into the dermis. There is no exact time frame for dermal invasion of LM. These lesions generally are considered slow-growing. However, in recent histologic evaluations of staged excision lesions, 16% were found to have unexpected foci of invasion.[1] The risk of invasion also has been thought to be related to the size of the lesion, as in some case series, larger lesions have been the ones to frequently harbor invasive nests.[4,5]

The ill-defined nature of LM/LMM on presentation may generate a wide differential diagnosis including but not limited to dysplastic nevus, pigmented basal cell carcinoma, squamous cell carcinoma, seborrheic keratosis–lenticular form, actinic keratosis, and lentigo simplex. Clinical evaluation can be aided by tools such as the Wood's lamp, which can help highlight features such as subclinical pigmentation. Other forms of advanced imaging also can aid in diagnosis, including dermatoscopy,[24,25] epiluminescence microscopy,[25] and confocal laser microscopy.[26] These imaging modalities continue to evolve and remain outside the scope of plastic surgery practice. For plastic surgeons, high clinical suspicion, thorough physical examination, and a low threshold for excisional biopsy remain the tenets for clinical evaluation of these lesions. Excisional biopsy should continue to be the gold standard, as it eliminates sampling error and if done properly should prevent transection of the lesions at the deep margin, if invasion is present and further staging required. These lesions, however, are often quite large and approximate critical facial structures. In such cases, an incisional biopsy of the darkest or most raised portion of the lesion is the preferred approach.

HISTOLOGY

The histologic hallmark in diagnosing LM is the presence of an increased number of atypical melanocytes at the basal layer of the epidermis in small nests or single cells, usually with extension into the periadnexal structures (**Fig. 2**).[4,27] Melanocytic atypia can be characterized in various ways, including but not limited to the presence of

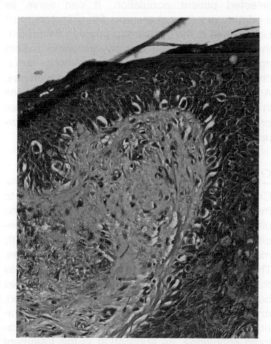

Fig. 2. Histology slide of lentigo maligna (melanoma in situ). Note the atypical melanocytic proliferation at the level of the basal epidermis with extension down the hair follicle. Additionally, there is effacement of the rete ridges and solar elastosis typically seen in heavily sun damaged skin. (*Courtesy of* Matthew Fleming, MD, Milwaukee, WI.)

dendritic melanocyte processes, multinucleated melanocytes, or cytoplasmic retraction artifact.[28,29] Other observed histologic markers that can aid in the diagnosis include effacement of rete ridges, atrophy of the epidermis, underlying solar elastosis, and the presence of an inflammatory dermal infiltrate.[4,29] These additional criteria are intimately related to the typical presence of solar damage to the skin in and around the area of the lesions.

Despite the many histologic markers, the diagnosis of lentigo maligna does not remain without significant problems. The most significant of these problems remains the fact that LM develops in areas of significant solar damage, which in essence muddies the water surrounding these lesions. These transition areas between the lesion itself and the surrounding solar damaged skin can lead to inadequate excisions and recurrent disease depending on the method of excision and how the histology is processed and evaluated. Several immunohistochemical stains have been employed in some studies to aid in diagnosis. The most commonly used are HMB45 and MART-1.

A second problem lies in the categorization of LM as melanoma in situ. Although the criteria for diagnosing LM are widely accepted, some pathologists will make a differentiation between lentigo maligna as a melanoma precursor and a true melanoma in situ based on the number of atypical melanocytes and their pattern of arrangement within the basal epidermis.[29–31] It is therefore imperative that plastic surgeons work closely with pathologists and have a knowledge of their methods of diagnosis and interpretation to understand the histologic diagnosis. The current standard nomenclature uses the term lentigo maligna to refer to malignant melanoma in situ occurring on the head/neck of elderly individuals in the setting of chronic actinic damage. LMM is an invasive melanoma that occurs within a lesion of LM. LM is a precursor to LMM.

TREATMENT

Treatment of LM and LMM has evolved over the years. Although surgical excision remains the gold standard, the methods by which excision is undertaken have changed significantly. Various methods are used, including direct excision with margins, Mohs micrographic surgery, and staged excision. Recurrence rates reported using these various methods range from 0.5% to 33% depending on technique.[4,32–34] Other less-invasive treatment methods including topical and physical nonspecific destructive modalities also have been introduced but ultimately have proven less effective, with recurrence rates ranging from 20% to 100%.[4,34] Many of these less-invasive therapies also lack long-term follow-up and have not stood the test of time.

The continuing dilemma that faces clinicians treating LM is balancing the morbidity of the various treatment methods with the risk of recurrence of these lesions. It has been shown that LM/LMM has higher rates of recurrence than other forms of cutaneous malignant melanoma.[35] This dilemma is particularly difficult in a predominantly elderly population, as some patients are not suitable to undergo excision procedures. Another consideration is that the location of these lesions tends to be on the head and neck in functionally and cosmetically sensitive areas that may not lend themselves to straightforward excisions and repairs/reconstructions.

As the treatment of LM/LMM continues to evolve, it is important to remember that various specialties including plastic surgery, dermatology, ophthalmology and otolaryngology treat this disease. Although most LM/LMM cases can be treated successfully by a single clinician performing both excision and defect repair, a team approach may be necessary to achieve optimal outcomes depending on lesion size and location. The remainder of this article will examine the various surgical and nonsurgical treatments of LM and LMM, focusing on the techniques and efficacy of the treatments and their practical applications in relation to plastic surgery practice.

NONSURGICAL THERAPY
Radiotherapy

Radiotherapy for LM first was described in the European literature by Miescher in the mid 1950s.[36,37] Widely accepted and used for primary treatment of LM and adjuvant treatment of LMM in Europe, this treatment modality has been speculated to be at least as effective as surgical excision.[38] Published recurrence rates have been found to be between 0% and 13%, with multiple studies having follow-up of 2 years or greater.[10,39,40]

Despite the use of radiotherapy as a primary treatment abroad, it for the most part has remained a secondary option to surgical excision within the United States. Typically, radiotherapy has been reserved for patients who have significant medical comorbidities, are unable to undergo surgical treatment, or have lesions in functionally or cosmetically sensitive areas that are not favorable for surgical excision. Treatments often are given once or twice a week and can provide

adequate local control without the inconvenience of needing daily therapy. Within the United States, regimens historically have used high voltage schedules of between 100 kV and 280 kV, delivering at depths of 5 to 6 mm depending on lesion size.[41,42] This method has proven successful, as it provides high tissue penetration and good field coverage but also exposes the patient to greater adverse effect risk secondary to exposure of underlying structures. In an effort to decrease morbidity, European centers have employed lower voltage regimens using 10 kV to 50 kV, applying at depths of around 1 mm.[20,39] Although this strategy intends to target these epidermal lesions more specifically, these soft x-ray regimens may run the risk of being too specific in the face of the diffuse nature of LM/LMM. In addition, the extension down follicular structures characteristic of LM/LMM suggests that 1 mm treatment depth might be insufficient. Close follow-up of patients treated with radiotherapy monitoring for both recurrence and treatment adverse effects is essential.

Despite the variable outcomes, radiotherapy remains another effective tool in the treatment of LM/LMM when surgical intervention is not possible or preferable. In the appropriately selected patient population, it can serve as a primary or adjuvant therapy. Many factors must be weighed in the decision to proceed with radiotherapy over surgical therapy, including patient age, comorbidities, goals of treatment, lesion characteristics/location, and patient preference. A team approach including input from colleagues in radiation oncology is imperative to ensure proper patient selection and appropriate follow-up care.

Cryotherapy

Cryotherapy employs the use of liquid nitrogen to freeze lesions, causing direct thermal injury and ultimately destruction. Cryotherapy is a nonspecific destructive modality. Melanocytes are slightly more sensitive to cold injury than keratinocytes. Thus, it is possible to use cryotherapy in a way that allows regrowth of damaged keratinocytes but largely destroys melanocytes. For this reason, cryotherapy often leads to hypo- or depigmentation of treated areas. Used for various dermatologic conditions, its application in the treatment of LM remains controversial. Several protocols have been investigated with varying characteristics. In general, lesions are treated with two to three freeze–thaw cycles of between 15 and 60 seconds of liquid nitrogen application covering an area 0.5 to 1 cm beyond the visible clinical margins. Reported recurrence rates have been highly variable. Early studies reported recurrence rates of 6.6% at 3 years,[7] while more recent studies have noted a recurrence rate of 34.3% at 5 years[10] and of 0% with an average follow-up of just over 6 years.[43] Varying recurrence rates may be attributed to differences in protocols and patient selection. High recurrence rates likely are related to the lack of histologic margin control and poor depth of penetration, leaving behind tumor nests near deeper epidermal appendages.

Because of the lack of consistency and definitive controlled studies within the literature regarding the efficacy of this modality, cryotherapy is not recommended as a preferred treatment for LM. Further investigation is necessary to develop proven protocols with long-term follow-up to ensure optimal patient care. Although this modality eventually may offer plastic surgeons an efficient, office-based treatment that can be provided under local anesthesia, several concerns remain. Among these concerns are excessive postoperative pain (like a burn), the need for postoperative wound care in a mostly elderly patient population, and poor aesthetic results, including development of keloids, hypertrophic scars, and loss of pigment.

Laser Therapy

The use of laser therapy within the practice of plastic surgery has expanded over the years. Many cosmetic and dermatologic problems are treated successfully with the use of lasers. This growing success, however, has not translated into the development of an effective laser-based treatment of LM. Throughout the literature, case reports and anecdotal evidence are present regarding the treatment of LM with laser therapy. Early reports used argon[44] laser treatments, and as technology progressed, various other laser therapies have been attempted including carbon dioxide,[45] Q-switched Nd:YAG,[46] and Q-switched ruby[47] laser therapy. More recently, attempts have been made using combination therapy such as Q-switched ruby and alexandrite lasers.[48] Despite the many attempts, no ideal treatment has been identified, as recurrences have been seen with each of the various laser therapies used. Most published reports have placed recurrence rates around the 40% to 50% mark.[49]

In light of the poor response rates to treatment and a body of evidence that lacks prospective controlled trials with long-term follow-up, laser therapy for LM cannot be recommended at this time. Perhaps as laser technology continues to move forward and knowledge of the histopathological basis of LM progresses, an effective laser based treatment will be identified.

Immunomodulation

Immune response modulators are a relatively new treatment for LM that has had promising early results. Already used to treat other conditions including basal cell carcinoma, squamous cell carcinoma, genital warts, actinic keratoses, and other forms of malignant melanoma, these agents are delivered either topically or via intralesional injection. The two commonly used immunomodulators are topical 5% imiquimod and injectable interferon alpha. Several small series and case reports have demonstrated early efficacy of intralesional interferon alpha[48,50]; however, more recent attention has been given to topical imiquimod.

Topical 5% imiquimod showed particularly promising early results in the literature as a solitary treatment agent and as preadjuvant therapy before surgical excision. As a primary treatment modality, several studies have shown impressive clinical and histologic response rates. In a study in 2003, Naylor and colleagues[51] showed a 93% clinical and histologic clearance rate after 4 weeks of treatment, with 80% of patients having no recurrence at 1 year follow-up. Several other small series have shown similar results, with combined response rates in the literature estimated to be 81% for clinical clearance and 85% for histologic clearance.[52] These early reports suggesting efficacy of imiquimod suffer from inadequate follow-up and reliance on clinical clearance as an indicator of histologic clearance. More recent studies have cast doubt on the reliability of the earlier reports. Among the other concerns remains the issue that some patients are complete nonresponders to therapy or respond clinically but not histologically to treatment. In a series reported by Fleming and colleagues[23] in 2004, one patient had complete clinical response with resolution of the lesion's pigmentation; however, histologically, there was no response to treatment. This scenario could prove extremely dangerous, as clinicians could mistake loss of pigmentation with resolution while the lesion itself remains intact. In another report by Cotter and colleagues in 2007, patients underwent staged surgical excision for histologic evaluation of margins after imiquimod therapy. After a full treatment course, 25% of patients were found to have residual disease, with one patient having invasive disease.[53] Reported recurrence is also present within the literature[52] and must remain a concern, as follow-up in published studies is relatively short.

Aside from questions relating to efficacy, treatment with imiquimod does have associated morbidity and adverse effects. Patients typically develop a striking inflammatory response to treatment with superficial crusting, which can be disconcerting and create an environment for infection. Patients also are required to continue treatment for 4 to 6 weeks or more depending on response.

The efficacy of treatment of LM with imiquimod remains unproven and represents an off-label use of this drug. Early results have been encouraging, but long-term follow-up of treated patients is necessary before this therapy can be recommended for use.

SURGICAL THERAPY

Surgical excision remains the gold standard for treating LM. Over the years, several different surgical techniques have been developed and applied to the treatment of LM. These include standard excision with margins, Mohs micrographic surgery, and staged excision procedures. The trend to develop improved techniques can be attributed to efforts to better control the clinically ill-defined margins of the disease while maximizing tissue sparing, as many of these lesions occur in cosmetically sensitive areas. For plastic surgeons, some of these techniques remain outside the scope of practice, as they require specialized training in Mohs micrographic surgery and dermatopathology. There are, however, several techniques that plastic surgeons can adopt easily with assistance from their institution's pathologist. These have proven superior to traditional wide local excision methods.

Traditional Surgical Excision

Traditional surgical excision refers to excision of LM and LMM with set surgical margins beyond the clinically defined lesion. The specimens then are sent to the pathologist, where a standard bread-loafing technique is used to analyze what amounts to less than 1% of the margins. This result then is extrapolated to the remaining surgical margin. In 1992, the National Institute of Health Consensus Conference on melanoma recommended 5 mm margins for the excision of malignant melanoma in situ, including LM.[54] The use of 5 mm margins for LM has been criticized as being inadequate, and critics argue that the published guidelines were based on excisional data for MMIS on the trunk and extremities rather than the head and neck. In response to these criticisms, the National Cancer Comprehensive Network published new guidelines stating that

margins beyond 5 mm may be necessary to fully clear LM lesions.[55] Statements such as this are based on recurrence rates for standard wide excision, which range from 8% to 20% in the literature.[56,57] Zitelli and colleagues used Mohs surgical technique to evaluate adequacy of 5 mm surgical margin for LM. Looking at 231 cases, these authors found that 0.6 cm resulted in clear margins in 75% of patients, and 1.5 cm cleared margins in 97%.[58,59] Using similar methods, Robinson and colleagues[60] found margins of greater than 6mm were required in 13 of 16 cases (81%). Zalla and colleagues[61] used Mohs surgery with immunostains to confirm surgical margins and found that 50% of LM lesions were cleared with margins of 6 mm or less, and that 71% of LMM lesions were cleared with margins of 10 mm or less. Similarly, Cohen and colleagues reported a mean margin of 13 mm to clear LM; Bricca and colleagues reported a 9 mm margin needed to clear 97% of LM cases, and Agarwal-Antal and colleagues found that 58% of 93 lesions of LM required margins greater than 5 mm.[1,62] In addition, multiple studies have shown that a significant number (5% to 22%) of LM lesions are found on postoperative examination to be LMM.[1,61]

Taken together, these studies provide an objective consensus that the recommended set surgical margins most plastic surgeons use for traditional surgical excision are inadequate, no matter what method of margin assessment is used. The explanation for this is likely multifactorial. As mentioned, bread-loafing, the standard method of assessing surgical margins, only examines a tiny fraction of the actual margin. Clinical margins of LM and LMM are notoriously difficult to assess, even with the addition of Wood's lamp illumination. These lesions often occur in a setting of severe sun damage with underlying dispigmentation, thus making it difficult to distinguish between tumor and the typical poikilodermatous changes of chronically sun-damaged skin. This may be complicated further by the fact that previous treatment with liquid nitrogen may cause loss of pigment, further obscuring clinical boundaries. Lastly, the phenomenon of subclinical extension and the finding of amelanotic LM make clinical examination a poor predictor of histologic extent.

There is little doubt that because of the known tendency of LM to have significant subclinical extension, traditional resection with 5 mm margins and standard pathologic evaluation are inadequate. Multiple techniques have been developed or adapted to the treatment of LM in an effort to address theses issues. They represent a second generation of treatment that offers better margin evaluation, leading to decreased recurrence rates and the ability in some cases to resect less tissue. If traditional resection is to be undertaken, the plastic surgeon should consider excision with margins beyond what traditionally is recommended with close follow-up. Once again, many of these second-generation techniques can be practiced easily by plastic surgeons with support from their institutional pathologists.

Mohs Micrographic Surgery

Mohs micrographic surgery for LM remains outside of the practice of plastic surgery. It is imperative, however, that plastic surgeons be educated on the variety of second-generation LM treatments available. Although plastics surgeons do not provide Mohs micrographic surgery, at many institutions, they are involved intimately with the reconstructive procedures following Mohs. The technique of Mohs surgery refers to the removal of lesions in a staged fashion with serial examination of histologic margins by the Mohs surgeon using horizontally oriented frozen sections. This technique is intended to maximize tissue sparing while providing complete, meticulous margin control. Key to the process is the excision of the specimen margins at 45° angles and preparation of the specimens in a horizontal en face fashion. This allows for optimal view of the histologic margins. This specimen preparation is done in a fresh-frozen section manner with staining. Along with the use of traditional Mohs surgery, various modified Mohs procedures have been used to treat LM/LMM.

The use of Mohs in the treatment of melanomas and melanocytic lesions such as LM has been evaluated in the literature and remains a subject of controversy. The main issue in the use of this technique revolves around the quality of frozen sections in comparison with traditional paraffin-embedded permanent section tissue preparations when examining melanocytic atypia. Vast differences in the literature exist, as some groups have reported frozen section to have 100% sensitivity and 90% specificity[63] in the detection of melanoma, while others have reported a sensitivity of 59% and specificity of 81% for detection of marginal melanocytic atypia.[64] Also, previous studies have shown that there may be considerable intraobserver differences in differentiating LM from the melanocytic atypia seen in chronically solar-damaged skin.[65] The possibility of the quality of frozen sections compounding these differences remains real.

Despite its potential problems, traditional Mohs micrographic surgery has been used with success for treating LM and LMM. There are few studies within the literature examining traditional Mohs techniques for the excision of LM. Local recurrence rates for Mohs treatment have been reported to be in the 0% to 33% range over an average follow-up ranging from 29 months to 10 years[17,19,33,59,66] (Table 1) with the majority of studies having rates less than 3%. Although this is a significant improvement of traditional excision, many Mohs surgeons remain uncomfortable with margin assessment based on frozen section. Immunostains have been used by some Mohs surgeons to attempt to increase the accuracy of frozen section histology. Examples of immunostains that have been used include MART-1/Melan-A, and HMB 45. These techniques may enhance diagnosis, as one study has shown a recurrence rate of 0.5% at 38 months.[67] There remains concern, however, for overestimation of marginal involvement, as these stains have been shown to prominently stain sun-damaged skin.[68] They also add considerable time and expense to the performance of Mohs surgery.

Another strategy that has been used to minimize frozen section inaccuracy is overnight rush permanent sections, so-called slow Mohs. In some cases, the specimens are sent immediately without being evaluated using frozen section by the Mohs surgeon,[69] while in other cases, the specimens are sent only if unable to be cleared

Table 1
Local recurrence rates after Mohs' micrographic surgery

Study	Recurrence Rate	Average Follow-up
Walling et al (2007)[33]	33% (6/18)	117 months
Temple and Arlette (2006)[17]	3% (6/202)	29.8 months
Bricca et al (2005)[66]	0% (0/331)[a]	58 months
Beinert et al (2003)[19]	0% (0/92)	33 months
Zitelli et al (2005)[59]	0.5% (1/184)	59 months

[a] 1 distant recurrence over follow-up period (1/331), 0.3%.

by initial frozen section evaluation.[62] This can lengthen the procedure to at least a 2-day process but then reduces the possibility of frozen section error. Recurrence rates for these procedures range from 0.02% to 2.8%, with average follow-up ranging from 22 months to 5 years.[62,70,71]

Traditional Mohs micrographic surgery with or without the use of adjuncts such as immunostaining and rush permanent sections is a reliable treatment for LM. The use of various adjuncts needs to be investigated further to delineate their efficacy long term. In general, the use of Mohs surgery as a treatment for LM and LMM is experiencing a downward trend, as it has been superceded by alternative methods.

Staged Excision Procedures

Staged excision procedures are powerful tools at the disposal of plastic surgeons for treating LM and LMM. Requiring no additional training or specialized laboratory facility as in Mohs surgery, these techniques can be performed easily in an efficient manner with emphasis on achieving complete margin control. Originating from the Mohs procedure with the addition of rush permanent section, these procedures typically incorporate multiple excisional biopsies in a patterned fashion with overnight permanent sections. Completed over several visits, positive margins then can be re-excised and sent again for permanent histology and reconstruction performed once the lesion has been cleared.

Several techniques have been developed and published incorporating various excisional patterns and pathologic processing methods. Depending on the technique, the original lesion is excised with the initial margin specimens or left in place until the margins are cleared. If the central lesion is left intact, the surrounding biopsy sights can be closed so the patient is not left with open wounds between stages. Despite their differences, the principles remain the same, with the key to success lying in good communication between surgeon and pathologist regarding specimen collection, marking, and pathology.

One of the more popular techniques used is the square procedure. Originally described by Johnson and colleagues[34] in 1997, this technique involves using a double-bladed scalpel to excise a 2 mm strip of tissue in a square pattern starting at 5 mm from the original lesion. The square is removed in four strips, oriented and sent for rush overnight permanent sections, and analyzed in en face sections of the surgical margin in a vertical orientation. Positive areas are mapped, and repeat excisions of 2 mm strips are performed as dictated by the margin assessment results. Closure of the initial square remains the surgeon's choice. Alternative techniques to the square procedure include those described by Mahoney and colleagues,[72] Bub and colleagues,[73] Hazan and colleagues,[57] and Huilgol and colleagues.[74] These techniques differ in not only excision procedure but also pathologic evaluation methods. Mahoney describes a surgical excision that involves 2 mm strip biopsies harvested at 5 mm around the lesion circumferentially. The original lesion is left intact until the margins are cleared. The excision is planned out in various geometric shapes including triangles, rectangles, and pentagons to aid in orientation and reconstruction. Bub takes a different approach excising the original lesion, taking care to include a 2 to 3mm rim of normal-appearing skin. This entire specimen then is oriented and sent to pathology, where 1 mm radial sections are taken for permanent histologic evaluation. Hazan describes a different approach, in which the biopsies are excised in a circular four-quadrant pattern with 5 to 7 mm margins around the initial lesion. The biopsies then are oriented, and the remainder of the lesion is removed as an en bloc disk and sent labeled "tumor debulking." The original lesion then is examined in 3 mm bread-loaf sections, while the radial biopsies are sectioned at 2 mm. Finally, Huilgol excises lesions en bloc with

Table 2
Local recurrence rates after staged excision

Study	Recurrence Rate	Average Follow-up
Walling et al (2007)[33]	7.3% (3/41)	96 months
Johnson et al (1997)[34]	0% (0/35)	Not reported
Mahoney et al (2005)[72]	0% (0/11)	4.7 months
Bub et al (2004)[73]	4.8% (3/62)	57 months
Huilgol et al (2004)[74]	2.5% (4/161)	38 months

a 5 mm margin. After orienting the specimen, it is sent to pathology, where it is examined in 1 to 2 mm bread-loaf sections.

Although there are differences amongs the techniques, staged procedures have had excellent results, with local recurrence rates ranging from 0% to 7.3%,[33,34,72] with follow up ranging from 4.7 to 96 months (**Table 2**). Recently, staged excision were compared with Mohs micrographic surgery by Walling and colleagues,[33] with results favoring the use of staged excision due to a marked difference in recurrence rates between the two procedures. Other studies have demonstrated staged procedures can allow the surgeon to ensure margin control and minimize patient morbidity associated with wound care.[75] By leaving the initial lesion intact until margins are clear, the surgeon can perform the bulk of excision and reconstruction in the same setting. In addition, the geometric patterns that are the basis for some of the staged excision procedures can aid in reconstruction, lending themselves to the design of various local flaps.

Staged excision is the method of choice at the authors' institution, and it is performed as a team with excision by dermatology, histologic evaluation by pathology, and reconstruction by plastic surgery. The procedure is protocol driven such that the involvement of dermatology is not essential, meaning that this or similar techniques can be performed easily by plastic surgeons. Briefly, all suspicious lesions are biopsied to confirm the diagnosis of LM or LMM. Biopsies of smaller lesions are excisional with narrow margins, whereas biopsies of larger lesions are typically incisional at the darkest or most raised area of the lesion. Patients then are scheduled for surgery over 3 consecutive days. On the first day, the clinical lesion is excised with 0.5 to 1.0 cm margins beyond the clinically apparent lesion or scar. The wider margin is chosen for multiply recurrent lesions or lesions of LMM. The surgical wound is covered with a moist dressing, and the patient is discharged with scheduled return the following morning. The excised specimen and the patient are marked with a suture at the 12:00 position, and the surgical specimen is submitted to the hospital pathology laboratory on a saline-soaked gauze. The laboratory technicians follow a set protocol for grossing and cutting the tissue, with direct oversight by an attending pathologist familiar with the procedure. Thin strips are removed from the periphery of the specimen, maintaining orientation with colored stains. The strips are processed en face with rush overnight permanent sections. The remaining central portion of the surgical specimen is processed with standard bread-loafing, allowing for the assessment/confirmation of tumor depth. The pathologist reports positive margins based on a 12:00 reference point. These results are reported via phone to the surgeon the following morning, and the process is repeated using 5 mm margins at each area reported as positive for tumor cells. The surgical specimens and the patient again are marked carefully with reference sutures. On the third day, the patient undergoes further excision as needed followed by plastic reconstruction.

Staged excision of LM and LMM carries the advantages of Mohs surgery (complete margin control and maximal tissue conservation) without the requirement for specialized training, personnel, or laboratory facilities. Although further 5- to 10-year follow-up studies are necessary to confirm some of the earlier reports, staged excision is an efficient, reliable method for treating LM and LMM that can be incorporated into the practice of plastic surgery.

SUMMARY

The treatment of LM and LMM is a difficult problem that crosses specialty lines. As these lesions tend to occur most often in the head and neck, function and cosmesis are of paramount concern. Issues confounding the diagnosis and treatment of the disease include the diffuse nature of the lesions and confusing nomenclature, which can lead clinicians away from the reality that LM is melanoma in situ. Various treatment options are available depending on patient preference and goals of therapy. Despite an array of data examining surgical and nonsurgical treatments, excision remains the treatment of choice. Optimal margin control with the least tissue excision and patient morbidity remains the goals of surgical therapy. Several methods have proven effective in achieving these goals, including Mohs micrographic surgery and staged excision procedures. Typically, plastic surgeons have used wide local excision with 5 mm margins to treat LM. After careful review of the literature, one can say this method is prone to local recurrence. Moving forward, one needs to re-examine the recommended margins for wide local excision of LM and begin to incorporate into practice current excisional techniques that offer better marginal control of these lesions. Despite plastic surgical involvement in the reconstructive aspects of Mohs micrographic surgery, only staged excision allows for the total care of the patient by the plastic surgeon. Protocol-driven staged excision procedures can be adopted easily into plastic surgery practice, moving the specialty away from inadequate treatment by wide local excision with 5 mm margins. The possibility for reliable nonsurgical treatment options in the future exists. These methods may prove effective and offer better functional and cosmetic results in the head and neck region. But as the face of treatment of LM changes, the role of the plastic surgeon remains the same, to provide quality care to patients ensuring optimal oncologic, functional, and cosmetic results.

REFERENCES

1. Agarwal-Antal N, Bowen GM, Gerwela JW. Histologic evaluation of lentigo maligna with permanent sections: implications regarding current guidelines. J Am Acad Dermatol 2002;47:743–8.
2. Clark WH Jr, Elder DE, Van Horn M. The biologic forms of malignant melanoma. Hum Pathol 1986; 17:443–50.
3. Langley RGB, Flotte TJ, Sober AJ. Clinical characteristics. In: Balch CMHA, Sober AJ, Soong S, editors. Cutaneous melanoma. St. Louis (MO): Quality Medical Publishing Incorporated; 1998. p. 81–101.
4. McKenna JK, Florell SR, Goldman GD, et al. Lentigo maligna/lentigo maligna melanoma: current state of diagnosis and treatment. Dermatol Surg 2006;32: 493–504.
5. Cohen LM. Lentigo maligna and lentigo maligna melanoma. J Am Acad Dermatol 1995;33:923–36.
6. Newell GR, Sider JG, Bergfelt L, et al. Incidence of cutaneous melanoma in the United States by histology with special reference to the face. Cancer Res 1988;48:5036–41.
7. Kuflik EG, Gage AA. Cryosurgery for lentigo maligna. J Am Acad Dermatol 1994;31(1):75–8.
8. Pitman GH, Kopf AW, Bart RS, et al. Treatment of lentigo maligna and lentigo maligna melanoma. J Dermatol Surg Oncol 1979;5:727–37.
9. Bartoli C, Bono A, Clemente C, et al. Clinical diagnosis and therapy of cutaneous melanoma in situ. Cancer 1996;77:882–92.
10. Zalaudek I, Horn M, Richtg E, et al. Local recurrence in melanoma in situ: influence of sex, age, site of involvement, and therapeutic modalities. Br J Dermatol 2003;148:703–8.
11. Hutchinson J. On tissue dotage. Arch Surg (London) 1892;3:315–32.
12. Dubreuilh MW. Lentigo malin de vieillards. Ann Dermatol Syphiligr 1894;3:1092–9.
13. Dubreuilh MW. De la melanose circonscrite precancereuse. Ann Dermatol Syphil 1912;5:129–51, 205–30.
14. Nestle FO, Kerl H. Melanoma. In: Bolognia JL, Jorizzo JL, Rapini RP, editors. 1st edition, Dermatology, volume 2. Philadelphia: Mosby; 2003. p. 1789–815.
15. Cox NH, Aitchison TC, Sirel JM, et al. Comparison between lentigo maligna melanoma and other histogenic types of malignant melanoma of the head and neck. Br J Cancer 1996;73:940–4.
16. Swetter SM, Boldrick JC, Jung SY, et al. Increasing Incidence of lentigo maligna melanoma subtypes: northern California and national trends 1990–2000. J Invest Dermatol 2005;125:685–91.
17. Temple CL, Arlette JP. Mohs micrographic surgery in the treatment of lentigo maligna and melanoma. J Surg Oncol 2006;94:287–92.
18. Holman CD, Mulroney CD, Armstrong BK. Epidemiology of preinvasive and invasive malignant melanoma in western Australia. Int J Cancer 1980;25:317–23.
19. Bienert TN, Trotter MJ, Arlette JP. Treatment of cutaneous melanoma of the face by Mohs micrographic surgery. J Cutan Med Surg 2003;7:25–30.
20. Arlette JP, Trotter MJ, Trotter T, et al. Management of lentigo maligna and lentigo maligna melanoma: seminars in surgical oncology. J Surg Oncol 2004; 86:179–86.
21. Su WP, Bradely RR. Amelanoic lentigo maligna. Arch Dermatol 1980;116(1):82–3.
22. Rahbari H, Nabai H, Mehregan A, et al. Amelanotic lentigo maligna melanoma: a diagnostic conundrum—presentation of four new cases. Cancer 1998;77(10):2052–7.
23. Fleming CJ, Bryden AM, Evans A, et al. A pilot study of treatment of lentigo maligna with 5% imiquimod cream. Br J Dermatol 2004;151:485–8.
24. Cognetta AB Jr, Stolz W, Katz B, et al. Dermatoscopy of lentigo maligna. Dermatol Clin 2001; 19(2):307–18.
25. Stante M, Giorgi V, Stanganelli I, et al. Dermoscopy for early detection of facial lentigo maligna. Br J Dermatol 2005;152:361–4.
26. Chen CS, Elias M, Busam K, et al. Multimodal in vivo optical imaging, including confocal microscopy, facilitates presurgical margin mapping for clinically complex lentigo maligna melanoma. Br J Dermatol 2005;153(5):1031–6.
27. Clark WH Jr, Mihm MC Jr. Lentigo maligna and lentigo maligna melanoma. Am J Pathol 1969;55:39.
28. Weyers W, Bonczkowitz M, Weyers I, et al. Melanoma in situ versus melanocytic hyperplasia in sun damaged skin. Am J Dermatopathol 1996;18:560–6.
29. Farrahi F, Egbert BM, Swetter M. Histologic similarities between lentigo maligna and dysplastic nevus: importance of clinicopathalogic distinction. J Cutan Pathol 2005;32(6):405–12. Erratum in: J Cutan Pathol 2005;32(7):521.
30. Barnhill RL, Mihm MC Jr. The histopathology of cutaneous malignant melanoma. Semin Diagn Pathol 1993;10:47–75.
31. Flotte TJ, Mihm MC. Lentigo maligna and malignant melanoma in situ, lentigo maligna type. Hum Pathol 1999;30:533–6.

32. Malhotra R, Chen C, Huilgol S, et al. Mapped serial excision for periocular lentigo maligna and lentigo maligna melanoma. Ophthalmology 2003;110:2011–8.

33. Walling HW, Scupham RK, Bean AK, et al. Staged Excision versus Mohs micrographic surgery for lentigo maligna and lentigo maligna melanoma. J Am Acad Dermatol 2007;57(4):659–64.

34. Johnson TM, Headington JT, Baker SR, et al. Usefulness of the staged excision for lentigo maligna and lentigo maligna melanoma: the square procedure. J Am Acad Dermatol 1997;37:758–64.

35. Wildemore JK, Schuchter L, Mick R, et al. Locally recurrent malignant melanoma—characteristics and outcomes: a single-institution study. Ann Plast Surg 2002;55:611–5.

36. Miescher G. Uber Melanotische Precancerose [Melanotic Precancerosis]. Oncologia 1954;7:92–4 [in German].

37. Miecher G. Die Behandlung der Malingnen Melanome der Haut mit EinschluB der Melanotischen Pracancerose [The treatment of malignant melanoma of the skin including the melanotic precancerous stage]. Strahlentherapie 1960;46:25–35 [in German].

38. Wilson L. Radiation therapy. In: Bolognia JL, Jorizzo JL, Rapini RP, editors. 1st edition, Dermatology, volume 2. Philidelphia: Mosby; 2003. p. 2185–95.

39. Schmid-Wendtner MH, Brunner B, Konz B, et al. Fractionated radiotherapy of lentigo maligna and lentigo maligna melanoma in 64 patients. J Am Acad Dermatol 2000;43(3):477–82.

40. Farshad A, Burg G, Panizzon R. A retrospective study of 150 patients with lentigo maligna and lentigo maligna melanoma and the efficacy of radiotherapy using Grenz or soft x-rays. Br J Dermatol 2002;143:843–5.

41. Harwood AR. Conventional radiotherapy in the treatment of lentigo maligna and lentigo maligna melanoma. J Am Acad Dermatol 1982;6:310–6.

42. Tsang RW, Liu FF, Wells W, et al. Lentigo maligna of the head and neck. Arch Dermatol 1994;130: 1008–12.

43. Machado de Moreas A, Pavarin LB, Herreros F, et al. Cryosurgical treatment of lentigo maligna. JDDG 2007;5:477–81.

44. Arndt KA. New pigmented macule appearing four years after argon laser treatment of lentigo maligna. J Am Acad Dermatol 1986;14:1092.

45. Kopera D. Treatment of lentigo maligna with carbon dioxide laser. Arch Dermatol 1995;131(6):735–6.

46. Orten SS, Waner M, Dinehart SM. Q switched neodymium; yttrium-aluminum-garnet laser treatment of lentigo maligna. Otolaryngol Head Neck Surg 1999;120:296–302.

47. Kauvar ANB, Geronemus RG. Treatment of lentigo maligna with the Q-switched ruby laser. Lasers Surg Med 1995;7:48.

48. Cornejo P, Vanaclocha F, Polimon I. Intralesional interferon treatment of lentigo maligna. Arch Dermatol 2000;136:428–30.

49. Iyer S, Goldman MP. Treatment of lentigo maligna with combination laser therapy: recurrence at 8 months after initial resolution. J Cosmet Laser Ther 2003;5:49–52.

50. Carucci JA, Leffell DJ. Intralesional interferon for treatment of recurrent lentigo maligna for the eyelid in a patient with primary melanosis. Arch Dermatol 2000;136:1415–6.

51. Naylor MF, Crowson N, Kuwahara R, et al. Treatment of lentigo maligna with topical imiquimod. Br J Dermatol 2003;149(Suppl 66):66–9.

52. van Meurs T, van Doorn R, Kirtschig G. Recurrence of lentigo maligna after initial complete response to treatment with 5% imiquimod cream. Dermatol Surg 2007;33(5):623–7.

53. Cotter MA, McKenna JK, Bowen GM. Treatment of lentigo maligna with imiquimod before staged excision. Dermatol Surg 2007;34(2):147–51.

54. National Institutes of Health Consensus Development Conference Statement on diagnosis and treatment of early melanoma. Am J Dermatopathol 1993; 15:34–43.

55. NCCN clinical practice guidelines in oncology: melanoma V.2.2008. Available at: http://www.nccn.org/prefessionals/physician_gls/PDF/melanoma.pdf. Accessed August 5, 2008.

56. Osborne JE, Hutchison PE. A follow-up study to investigate the efficacy of initial treatment of lentigo maligna with surgical excision. Br J Plast Surg 2002;55:611–5.

57. Hazan C, Dusza S, Delgado R, et al. Staged excision for lentigo maligna and lentigo maligna melanoma: a retrospective analysis of 117 cases. J Am Acad Dermatol 2008;58(1):142–8.

58. Zitelli JA, Brwon CD, Hanusa BH. Surgical margins for excision of primary cutaneous melanoma. J Am Acad Dermatol 1997;37:422–9.

59. Zitelli JA, Brown C, Hanusa BH. Mohs micrographic surgery for the treatment of primary cutaneous melanoma. J Am Acad Dermatol 1997;37:236–45.

60. Robinson JK. Margin control for lentigo maligna. J Am Acad Dermatol 1994;31:79–85.

61. Zalla MJ, Lim KK, Dicaudo DJ, et al. Mohs micrographic excision of melanoma using immunostains. Dermatol Surg 2000;26:771–84.

62. Cohen LM, McCall MW, Hodge SJ, et al. Successful treatment of lentigo maligna and lentigo maligna melanoma with Mohs micrographic surgery aided by rush permanent section. Cancer 1994;73(12):2964–70.

63. Zitelli JA, Mow RL, Abell E. The reliability of frozen sections in the evaluation of surgical margins for melanoma. J Am Acad Dermatol 1991;24:102–6.

64. Barlow RJ, White CR, Swanson NA. Mohs micrographic surgery using frozen section alone may be

unsuitable for detecting single atypical melanocytes at the margins of melanoma in situ. Br J Dermatol 2002;146:290–4.

65. Florell SR, Boucher KM, Leachman SA. Histopathologic recognition of involved margins of lentigo maligna excised by staged excision: an interobserver comparison study. Arch Dermatol 2003;139: 595–604.

66. Bricca GM, Brodland DJ, Ren D. Cutaneous head and neck melanoma treated with Mohs micrographic surgery. J Am Acad Dermatol 2005;52: 92–100.

67. Bhardwaj SS, Tope WD, Lee PK. Mohs micrographic surgery for lentigo maligna and lentigo maligna melanoma using Mel-5 immunostaining: University of Minnesota experience. Dermatol Surg 2006;32: 690–7.

68. Shabrawi-Caelen LE, Kerl H, Cerroni L. Melan-A: not a helpful marker in distinction between melanoma in situ on sun damaged skin and actinic keratosis. Am J Dermatopathol 2004;26:364–6.

69. Stonecipher MR, Leshin B, Patrick J, et al. Management of lentigo maligna and lentigo maligna melanoma with paraffin-embedded tangential sections: utility of immunoperoxidase staining and supplemental vertical sections. J Am Acad Dermatol 1994;29(4):589–94.

70. Cohen LM, McCall MW, Zax RH. Mohs micrographic surgery for lentigo maligna and lentigo maligna melanoma: a follow-up study. Dermatol Surg 1998;24:673–7.

71. Clayton BD, Leshin B, Hitchcock MG, et al. Utility of rush paraffin-embedded tangential sections in the management of cutaneous neoplasms. Dermatol Surg 2000;26:671–8.

72. Mahoney MH, Josephy M, Temple CLF. The perimeter technique for lentigo maligna: an alternative to Mohs micrographic surgery. J Surg Oncol 2005;91:120–5.

73. Bub JL, Berg D, Slee A, et al. Management of lentigo maligna and lentigo maligna melanoma with staged excision: a 5-year follow up. Arch Dermatol 2004; 140:552–8.

74. Huilgol SC, Selva D, Chen C, et al. Surgical margins for lentigo maligna and lentigo maligna melanoma: the technique of mapped serial excision. Arch Dermatol 2004;140:1087–92.

75. Jejurikar SS, Borschel GH, Johnson TM, et al. Immediate, optimal reconstruction of facial lentigo maligna and melanoma following total peripheral margin control. Plastic and Reconstructive Surgery 2007;120(5):1249–55.

Epidemiology, Staging (New System), and Prognosis of Cutaneous Melanoma

Younghoon R. Cho, MD, PhD[a],*, Melissa P. Chiang, MD, JD[b]

KEYWORDS
- Melanoma • Epidemiology • Staging • Risk factors
- Prognosis • TNM

The incidence of malignant melanoma is rising steadily and rapidly in the United States. Melanoma is now the sixth and seventh most common new cancer among men and women respectively.[1] An estimated 62,480 new cases of cutaneous melanoma will be diagnosed in 2008, a 13% increase compared with 2004 (55,100 new diagnoses). In addition, there will be an estimated 54,020 new cases of melanoma in situ in 2008. From 1975 to 2005, data from the National Cancer Institute Surveillance Epidemiology and End Results (SEER)[2] show that the incidence of melanoma nearly tripled (**Fig. 1**). One in 55 men and women in the United States will be diagnosed with cutaneous melanoma.

Prevalence is also increasing. In 2005, 723,416 men and women alive in the United States had a history of melanoma of the skin—349,414 men and 374,002 women.[2]

The mortality rate for melanoma increased by about 20% from the 1970s to 1990, but has largely stabilized from the 1990s onwards (**Fig. 2**). In 2008, an estimated 8,420 people will die from melanoma compared with 7,910 in 2004. Currently, one person in the United States dies from melanoma every hour.

INCIDENCE AND MORTALITY BY AGE, SEX, AND RACE

Based on the SEER data for 2001 to 2005, the median age at diagnosis for melanoma of the skin was 59 and the median age at death was 68. Additional breakdown in incidence and mortality by age group is shown in **Table 1**.

The age-adjusted incidence and death rates for melanoma were 19.4 and 2.7 per 100,000 per year respectively between the years 2001 and 2005. This data is further divided by sex and race in **Table 2**. Melanoma is several times more common in whites compared with more deeply pigmented ethnic groups. Men are approximately 1.5 times more likely to develop melanoma than are women, and more than twice as many die of melanoma compared with women (see **Table 2**). In men, the most common area for melanoma development is the back. In women, melanoma most commonly arises on the arms and legs.[3]

RISK FACTORS

Risk factors can be divided into environmental factors and host factors. The main environmental risk is ultraviolet radiation (UVR). The increasing incidence of melanoma may be partially due to the depletion of the ozone layer, which allows more UVR to penetrate the atmosphere. In addition, many people use tanning beds, which emit high amounts of UVR.

A history of sunburns confers twice the risk of developing melanoma compared with no prior history of sunburns Those with a childhood history of sunburns are at an even higher risk.[4] Patients

[a] Department of Plastic Surgery, Medical College of Wisconsin, Milwaukee, 8700 Watertown Plank Road, Milwaukee, WI 53226, USA
[b] Department of Dermatology, Medical College of Wisconsin, Milwaukee, 8700 Watertown Plank Road, Milwaukee, WI 53226, USA
* Corresponding author.
E-mail address: ycho@mcw.edu (Y.R. Cho).

Clin Plastic Surg 37 (2010) 47–53
doi:10.1016/j.cps.2009.07.001
0094-1298/09/$ – see front matter © 2010 Elsevier Inc. All rights reserved.

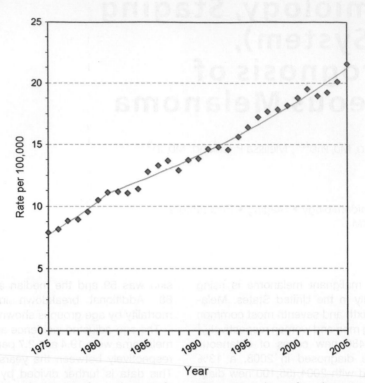

Fig. 1. Age-adjusted incidence rates for melanoma from 1975 to 2005. (*Data from* http://seer.cancer.gov/SEER 9 areas [San Francisco, Connecticut, Detroit, Hawaii, Iowa, New Mexico, Seattle, Utah and Atlanta]. *Data from* National Cancer Institute. Surveillance, Epidemiology and End Results (SEER). Available at: http://www.seer. cancer.gov.)

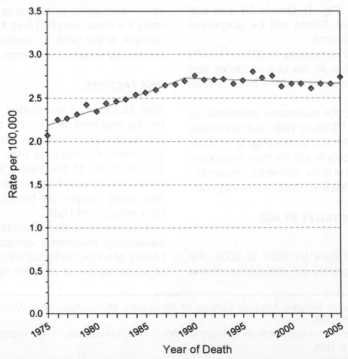

Fig. 2. Age-adjusted mortality rates for melanoma from1975 to 2005. Modified from a graph generated on SEER Web site using United States' Mortality Files, National Center for Health Statistics, CDC. (*Data from* National Cancer Institute. Surveillance, Epidemiology and End Results (SEER). Available at: http://www.seer.cancer.gov.)

Table 1
Incidence and death for melanoma by age

Age	Incidence (%)	Deaths (%)
<20	0.9	0.1
20–34	8.1	2.9
35–44	12.9	7.2
45–54	18.9	15.0
55–64	19.5	18.8
65–74	17.8%	21.3
75–84	16.4	23.6
>85	5.5	11.0

Data from National Cancer Institute. Surveillance, Epidemiology and End Results (SEER). Available at: http://www.seer.cancer.gov.

with a history of more than 10 severe painful sunburns increase their risk for developing melanoma in the upper extremity by up to 6.8-fold; 2.4-fold in the head or neck; 2.1-fold in the lower extremity; and 1.7-fold in the trunk, shoulder, hip, back, or abdomen.[5] Tanning bed exposure may lead to a higher risk of melanoma with one meta-analysis showing a 1.25 odds ratio (CI 95%) in patients with prior exposure compared with those with no prior exposure.[6] Interestingly, the use of sunscreen as a UVR-protective device has not been shown to reduce the risk of melanoma. This may be explained by the results of several studies that show that those using sunscreen are more likely to spend more time in the sun and hence increase their total UVR exposure.[7]

Certain phenotypic characteristics such as red hair, skin type, sun sensitivity, and freckles are associated with an increased risk of developing melanoma.[8] Skin type is determined by the quantity and type of melanin. Melanin, produced by the melanocyte, is the skin's natural protectant against ultraviolet damage. Melanin absorbs UVR and possesses potent antioxidant properties that can neutralize free radicals produced by the radiation. There are two types of melanin produced in the skin: eumelanin and pheomelanin. The ratio of eumelanin to pheomelanin is controlled by the melanocortin 1 receptor, which, when functioning well, leads to an increased amount of eumelanin production. Eumelanin is responsible for gray, black, yellow, and brown colors found in hair and skin and confers greater UVR protection. Pheomelanin produces more pink and red colors and is the primary form of melanin in people with red hair. People with red hair have diminished melanocortin 1 receptor function—an independent risk factor for developing melanoma.[9]

Family history and the presence of melanocytic nevi are also strong risk factors for melanoma. Patients with a first-degree relative with melanoma have a twofold higher risk of developing melanoma compared with patients with no family history of melanoma.[5] The risk of developing melanoma increases with the number of moles. Having more than ten moles greater than three millimeters on the arm can increase the risk of melanoma development by up to 4.7-fold on the trunk, shoulder, hip, back, or abdomen; 3.5-fold on the head or neck; 2.5-fold on the upper extremity; and 2-fold on the lower extremity.[5] Sunscreen (sun protection factor 30) usage has been shown to decrease the number of acquired nevi that develop in children.[10]

Evidence suggests that the presence of dysplastic nevi confer an independent risk factor

Table 2
Incidence and death rates for melanoma by age and sex between 2001 and 2005

Race or Ethnicity	Incidence Rates by Race		Death Rates by Race	
	Male (per 100,000)	Female (per 100,000)	Male (per 100,000)	Female (per 100,000)
All races	24.6	15.6	3.9	1.7
White	28.5	18.5	4.4	2.0
Black	1.1	0.9	0.5	0.4
Asian or Pacific Islander	1.6	1.3	0.5	0.3
American Indian or Alaska Native	3.9	2.6	1.5	0.7
Hispanic	4.8	4.9	0.9	0.6

Data from National Cancer Institute. Surveillance, Epidemiology and End Results (SEER). Available at: http://www.seer.cancer.gov.

for melanoma. A recent meta-analysis concluded that subjects with five or more dysplastic nevi had six times the risk of developing melanoma compared with subjects with no atypical nevi.[11]

The Spitz nevus sometimes causes diagnostic confusion with melanoma. Most Spitz nevi are found in children. However, there are spitzoid melanomas, and these are usually found in adults, that share microscopic features of Spitz nevi, but are malignant, with the potential to metastasize. Lyon provides detailed discussion in this issue.

Larger nevi are associated with a greater risk of melanoma. In particular, giant congenital melanocytic nevi (>20 cm) have a substantial risk of malignant transformation. The estimated lifetime of risk of melanoma in these patients has been reported to be between 5% and 40%.[12] Their melanomas tend to occur within the first 3 to 5 years of life (50% of occurrences by 3 years of life, 60% by childhood, 70% by puberty).[13]

Women with a history of breast cancer may have a slightly higher chance of developing melanoma (standardized incidence ratio = 1.41, CI 0.91–2.09).[14] This has fueled speculation that hormonal factors can influence the development of melanoma. Interestingly, a pooled-analysis study showed a reduced risk (odds ratio 0.33) of melanoma among women with higher parity (>5) with an early age at first birth (<20 years) compared with women with a later age at first birth (>25 years) and lower parity.[15]

The overall risk of melanoma increases when multiple risk factors including family history, increased number of nevi, history of severe sunburn, freckling on the upper back, light hair color are present. Having one or two risk factors can increase the risk of melanoma by two- to fourfold, and more than three risk factors can increase the risk by more than twentyfold.[5]

STAGING

The 2002 American Joint Committee on Cancer (AJCC) tumor-nodes-metastasis (TNM) staging classification (**Fig. 3**) incorporates Breslow depth, Clark's level, ulceration and pathologic microstaging attributes.[16] The AJCC Melanoma Staging Committee studied a cohort of 17,600 melanomas from major melanoma centers in the United States, Europe, and Australia. This staging system parallels staging for other cancers: patients with localized melanoma are characterized as stages I or II, those with regional metastases are considered stage III, and those with distant metastases are stage IV. In the previous staging system, melanomas greater than 4.0 mm were characterized as stage III regardless of nodal involvement. In addition, the previous system did not incorporate the presence of ulceration or pathologic information obtained after lymphatic mapping.

Approximately 81% of cutaneous melanomas are locally confined; 12% are diagnosed after the

	Tis	T1 (< 1.0 mm)		T2 (1.01–2.0 mm)		T3 (2.01–4.0 mm)		T4 (> 4.0 mm)	
		a no ulceration and level II/III	**b** ulceration or level IV/V	**a** without ulceration	**b** with ulceration	**a** without ulceration	**b** with ulceration	**a** without ulceration	**b** with ulceration
N0	0	IA (95%, 88%)	IB (91%, 83%)	IB (89%, 79%)	IIA (77%, 64%)	IIA (79%, 64%)	IIB (63%, 51%)	IIB (67%, 54%)	IIC (45%, 32%)
N1a (1 node, micrometastisis)		IIIA (70%, 63%)	IIIB (53%, 38%)	IIIA (70%, 63%)	IIIB (53%, 38%)	IIIA (70%, 63%)	IIIB (53%, 38%)	IIIA (70%, 63%)	IIIB (53%, 38%)
N1b (1 node, macrometastisis)		IIIB (59%, 48%)	IIIC (29%, 24%)	IIIB (59%, 48%)	IIIC (29%, 24%)	IIIB (59%, 48%)	IIIC (29%, 24%)	IIIB (59%, 48%)	IIIC (29%, 24%)
N2a (2-3 nodes, micrometastisis)		IIIA (63%, 57%)	IIIB (50%, 36%)	IIIA (63%, 57%)	IIIB (50%, 36%)	IIIA (63%, 57%)	IIIB (50%, 36%)	IIIA (63%, 57%)	IIIB (50%, 36%)
N2b (2-3 nodes, macrometastisis)		IIIB (46%, 39%)	IIIC (24%,15%)	IIIB (46%, 39%)	IIIC (24%,15%)	IIIB (46%, 39%)	IIIC (24%, 15%)	IIIB (46%, 39%)	IIIC (24%, 15%)
N2c (in transit met(s) / satellites (s)) without metastatic nodes		IIIB (46%, 39%)							
N3 (> 4 nodes, in transit met(s) / satellites with metastatic node(s))		IIIC (27%, 18%)							
M1a (distant skin, subcutaneous, or nodal metastases, normal LDH)		IV (19%, 16%)							
M1b (lung metastases, normal LDH)		IV (7%, 3%)							
M1c (any other visceral with normal LDH or distant metastases and ↑LDH)		IV (10%, 6%)							

Fig. 3. Integrated TNM staging with five- and ten-year survival data. The T classifications are outlined on the top rows; the N and M classifications are outlined on the far-left column. The melanoma stage is determined by the intersection between the T category and the N and M categories. The 5- and 10-year survival rates are listed in that order in parentheses for each stage.

cancer has spread regionally; 4% are diagnosed with distant metastasis and for the remaining 4% the staging information is unknown.[2]

TNM

The TNM classification is widely used to characterize a variety of cancers. In general, T describes the size of the tumor, N describes involvement of regional lymph nodes, and M describes distant metastasis. The T in melanoma uses Breslow depth,[17] the presence or absence of ulceration, and Clark's level[18] to characterize the primary tumor.

Breslow depth is measured in millimeters and is characterized by the following depths: less than 1.0 mm (T1), 1.01 to 2.0 mm (T2), 2.01 to 4.0 mm (T3), and greater than 4.0 mm (T4). The presence or absence of ulceration is based on microscopic examination of the tumor. The pathologist must differentiate between ulceration and traumatic disruption of the epidermis (eg, excoriation). Traumatic disruption is characterized by hemorrhage, brightly eosinophilic fibrin exudation, and a characteristic disruption of the architecture of the specimen. In contrast, specimens with ulceration will have a partial or total absence of the epidermal layer overlying the tumor. Ulceration is important since it signifies a greater risk for metastases such that the survival rates for patients with a given T category with ulceration are nearly equivalent to patients of the next T category without ulceration, provided that nodal status does not exceed N2b (see **Fig. 3**). The incidence of ulceration increases with tumor thickness with a 6% incidence of ulceration for tumors less than 1 mm, 23% for tumor thickness 1.1 to 2.0 mm, 47% for 2.1 to 4.0 mm, and 63% for tumors greater than 4 mm in thickness.[19] In the absence of nodal or distant metastases, tumor thickness (odds ratio 1.56) and ulceration (odds ratio 1.9) remain the most significant predictors of survival outcome.[19]

Clark's level describes the depth of invasion and is useful for prognostic differentiation for T1 lesions. Level I is limited to the epidermis (tumor in situ); Level II reaches the underlying papillary dermis; Level III fills the papillary dermis; Level IV involves the reticular dermis; and Level V reaches the subcutaneous fat. Tumors that have a Breslow depth of less than 1 mm and have a Clark's level of II or III without ulceration remain T1a melanomas. In contrast, melanomas that are ulcerated or Clark's level IV or V are reclassified as T1b melanomas.

To obtain accurate Breslow or Clark's measurements, the biopsy sample must include the deepest portion of the tumor. Inadequate specimens can result from superficial shave or curettage biopsies and are categorized as Tx. The same Tx designation is also used when a regional or distant metastasis is discovered with an unknown primary melanoma. When multiple primaries are present, the melanoma with the worst features is used to determine the T-category.

REGIONAL AND DISTANT METASTASES

The N category incorporates the status of regional lymph nodes. Stages I and II do not include any nodal or metastatic involvement. For Stage III melanomas, the number of nodal metastases is the most significant predictor of outcomes. A single nodal metastasis is classified as N1. N2 signifies that two or three nodes are involved, or that in-transit metastases or satellite lesions are present in the absence of regional nodal involvement. Satellite lesions are defined as discontinuous foci of tumor that reside within 5 cm from the primary tumor. In-transit metastases are lesions of discontinuous foci that reside more than 5 cm from the primary tumor. These discontinuous foci of melanoma are considered intralymphatic metastases and signify a poorer prognosis.[20] The N3 classification has four or more metastatic nodes, matted nodes, or the presence of in-transit metastases or satellite lesions in addition to regional nodal involvement. The level of tumor burden within the nodes is also of prognostic importance. Microscopic tumor burden refers to metastatic spread to nodes that is not clinically detectable. Macroscopic tumor burden refers to clinically or radiographically detectable nodes that have pathologic confirmation of metastatic deposits. Patients with macroscopic nodal spread have worse outcomes than patients with microscopic tumor burden within the same T classification (see **Fig. 3**). The presence of ulceration upstages a melanoma and confers a poorer prognosis when the melanoma is locally confined (no in-transit metastases or satellite lesions) and there are less than four nodes.

The sentinel node refers to the first lymph node in a nodal basin to which a cancer would travel. The presence or absence of melanoma in the sentinel node correlates closely to the presence or absence of melanoma in the remainder of the nodal basin. The role of sentinel node biopsy in the treatment of melanoma has reduced the need for complete surgical resection of regional nodal basins and has become an important tool in the staging of melanoma. The indications for sentinel node are discussed more thoroughly in this issue by Stadelmann; and the pathologic considerations are discussed by Shidham.

Distant metastases can occur in skin and subcutaneous tissues, distant lymph node basins (M1a), lung (M1b), and other visceral sites (M1c). Any distant metastatic spread is characterized as Stage IV with lung and other visceral site metastases having a worse prognosis compared with distant metastatic spread to skin, subcutaneous tissues, or lymph nodes.

Fig. 3 gives the 5- and 10-year survival outcomes for each TNM stage.[16] Stage IIa melanomas can serve as an illustration. Locally confined T2b tumors (1.01–2.0 mm with ulceration) have 5- and 10-year survivals of 77% and 64% respectively. Similarly, T3a tumors (2.01–4.0 mm without ulceration) have 5- and 10-year survivals of 79% and 64%. Note that the survival rates are similar between T2b tumors, which are shallower and ulcerated, and T3a tumors, which are thicker without ulceration.

UNKNOWN PRIMARY

Patients with an unidentifiable primary tumor location account for approximately 2% to 6% of all patients with melanoma. One study showed a 5-year survival of 83% in patients with cutaneous or subcutaneous in-transit metastases; 50% in patients with a lymph node metastasis, and a median survival of 6 months for patients with disseminated disease.[21]

DIAGNOSTIC BIOPSY

Biopsy is mandatory for the evaluation of a concerning pigmented lesion. Whether the type of biopsy can influence melanoma prognosis is controversial. One study examined head and neck melanomas to evaluate differences in survival in patients who underwent an excisional biopsy (79 patients), incisional biopsy (48 patients), or another procedure (shave, needle biopsy, cauterization, or cryotherapy; 32 patients) before definitive surgical treatment. They found 31.3%, 25%, and 8.9% death rates for incisional, other biopsy types, and excisional biopsies respectively. A similar trend was found when comparing the development of distant metastases: 31.3% for incisional biopsy; 28.1% for other biopsy type, and 10.1% for excisional biopsy. These results suggest that for head and neck melanoma, the type of biopsy may influence clinical outcome.[22] A separate study, which included biopsies from all anatomic locations, found no statistical difference in the development of distant metastases between incisional (265 patients) and

excisional (496 patients) biopsy.[23] A more comprehensive discussion on the work-up of melanoma is included in this issue by Lifchez and Kelamis. The histologic subtypes of melanoma are discussed in detail by Fleming.

TREATMENT

Surgery remains integral to the treatment of melanoma, particularly in the early stages. This issue addresses several different treatment protocols for melanoma. Surgical treatment for melanoma is discussed by Rees with special consideration of complete lymph node dissection in a separate article by Dzwierzynski. Treatment of melanoma of the head and neck is discussed separately by Larson and Larson. Surgical treatment of advanced melanoma is discussed by Hussussian. Bosbous and colleagues discuss the treatment of lentigo maligna using staged local excision. The role of radiation therapy for local and regional control is discussed by Shuff and colleagues, and the role of chemotherapy by Teisman. Advances in melanoma focusing on the genetics and biology of melanoma are discussed by Hornyak.

SUMMARY

Melanoma remains a disease that, when treated in advanced stages, portends a poor prognosis. Early diagnosis and treatment is paramount to improving clinical outcomes. A review of the epidemiology, staging, and prognosis has been presented. This can serve as an aid for clinicians to have meaningful discussions with their patients regarding different risk factors for melanoma, accurate staging for their disease process, and prognosis.

REFERENCES

1. Jemal A, Siegel R, Ward E, et al. Cancer statistics, 2008. CA Cancer J Clin 2008;58:71–96.
2. Surveillance E, and End Results (SEER), National Cancer Institute D, Surveillance Research Program. Available at: http://www.seer.cancer.gov. CSB. Accessed November 11, 2008.
3. Boyle P, Maisonneuve P, Dore JF. Epidemiology of malignant melanoma. Br Med Bull 1995;51:523–47.
4. Elwood J, Jopson J. Melanoma and sun exposure: an overview of published studies. Int J Cancer 1997;73:198–203.
5. Cho E, Rosner B, Colditz G. Risk factors for melanoma by body site for whites. Cancer Epidemiology, Biomarkers & Prevention 2005;14:1241–4.
6. Gallagher R, Spinelli J, Lee T. Tanning beds, sunlamps, and risk of cutaneous malignant

melanoma. Cancer epidemiology, Biomarkers & Prevention 2005;14:562–6.

7. Autier P, Dore J, Reis A, et al. Sunscreen use and intentional exposure to ultraviolet A and B radiation: a double blind randomized trial using personal dosimeters. Br J Cancer 2000;83:1243–8.

8. Veierod M, Weiderpass E, Thorn M, et al. A prospective study of pigmentation, sun exposure, and risk of cutaneous malignant melanoma in women. J Natl Cancer Inst 2003;95:1530–8.

9. Rees J. The genetics of sun sensitivity in humans. Am J Hum Genet 2004;75:739–51.

10. Gallagher R, Rivers J, Lee T, et al. Broad-spectrum sunscreen use and the development of new nevi in white children: a randomized controlled trial. JAMA 2000;283:2955–60.

11. Gandini S, Sera F, Cattaruzza M, et al. Meta-analysis of risk factors for cutaneous melanoma: I. Common and atypical naevi. Eur J Cancer 2005;41:28–44.

12. Tannous Z, Mihm M, Duncan ASL. Congenital melanocytic nevi: clinical and histopathologic features, risk of melanoma, and clinical management. J Am Acad Dermatol 2005;52:197–203.

13. Watt AJ, Kotsis SV, Chung KC. Risk of melanoma arising in large congenital melanocytic nevi: a systematic review. Plast Reconstr Surg 2004;113:1968–74.

14. Levi F, Te VC, Randimbison L, et al. Cancer risk in women with previous breast cancer. Ann Oncol 2003;14.71–3.

15. Karagas M, Zens M, Stukel T, et al. Pregnancy history and incidence of melanoma in women: a pooled analysis. Cancer Causes Control 2006;17:11–9.

16. Balch C, Buzaid A, Soong S, et al. Final version of the American Joint Committee on Cancer staging system for cutaneous melanoma. J Clin Oncol 2001;19:3635–48.

17. Breslow A. Thickness, cross-sectional areas and depth of invasion in the prognosis of cutaneous melanoma. Ann Surg 1970;172:902–8.

18. Clark WJ, From L, Berardino E, et al. The histogenesis and biologic behavior of primary human malignant melanomas of the skin. Cancer Res 1969;29:705–27.

19. Balch C, Soong S-J, Gershenwald J, et al. Prognostic factors analysis of 17,600 melanoma patients: validation of the American Joint Committee on Cancer melanoma staging system. J Clin Oncol 2001;19:3622–44.

20. Rao U, Ibrahim J, Flaherty L, et al. Implications of microscopic satellites of the primary and extracapsular lymph node spread in patients with high-risk melanoma: pathologic corollary of Eastern Cooperative Oncology Group Trial E1690. J Clin Oncol 2002;20:2053–7.

21. Schlagenhauff B, Stroebel W, Ellwanger U, et al. Metastatic melanoma of unknown primary origin shows prognostic similarities to regional metastatic melanoma: recommendation for initial staging examinations. Cancer 1997;80:60–5.

22. Austin J, Byers R, Brown W, et al. Influence of biopsy on the prognosis of cutaneous melanoma of the head and neck. Head Neck 1996;18:107–17.

23. Bong J, Herd R, Hunter J. Incisional biopsy and melanoma prognosis. J Am Acad Dermatol 2002;46:690–4.

Melanoma: Workup and Surveillance

Scott D. Lifchez, MD[a],*, J. Alex Kelamis, MD[b]

KEYWORDS

- Melanoma • Staging • Surveillance • Sentinel lymph node
- Recurrence

Initial evaluation of the patient suspected of having a melanoma consists of a thorough physical examination. If a suspicious lesion is identified, palpation of the nearby regional lymph node basins should be performed to assess for clinical adenopathy. For lesions on an extremity, the ipsilateral axillary (upper extremity) or inguinal (lower extremity) should be examined. For lesions in the head and neck, the parotid and cervical nodes should be evaluated. For lesions on the trunk, bilateral axillary and inguinal nodal basins should be examined, as multiple studies have demonstrated that the first draining node for a cutaneous area is not necessarily the closest nodal basin by distance, and multiple nodal basins may drain a cutaneous area.[1,2]

The American Joint Committee on Cancer (AJCC) groups primary tumor (T) staging based on thickness of the tumor and ulceration.[3] Surveillance recommendations by the AJCC by stage are as follows:

Stage 0—patient education, follow-up with primary doctor annually as part of any patient's annual physical examination

Stage 1—patient education; baseline chest radiograph; baseline complete blood cell count (CBC), liver function test (LF),T and lactate dehydrogenase (LDH); history and physical examination every 6 to 12 months for 3 years, then annually thereafter; further imaging studies or laboratory studies as indicated

Stage 2A—patient education; baseline CBC, LFT, and LDH and then annually for life; baseline chest radiograph; history, physical examination and chest radiograph every 6 to 12 months for 3 years, then annually; further imaging and laboratory testing as indicated

Stage 2B/C—patient education; baseline CBC, LFT, and LDH and then every 6 months for 5 years, then annually for life; baseline chest radiograph and then every 6 to 12 months for 3 years then annually; history and physical examination every 6 months for 5 years then annually; baseline computed tomography (CT) chest/abdomen/pelvis; further imaging and laboratory testing as indicated

Stage 3—patient education; baseline CBC, LFT, LDH, with surveillance labs every 6 months for 5 years, then annually for life; baseline chest radiograph, then every 6 months for 5 years, then annually; history and physical examination every 6 months for 5 years then annually thereafter; baseline CT chest/abdomen/pelvis; Further imaging and laboratory testing as indicated

Stage 4—individualized

For ulcerated lesions, the measured distance from the base of the ulcer to the deepest point of invasion is recorded as the thickness of the lesion; one should not construct an imaginary line to represent the superficial limit of the lesion before ulceration or alter the actual measured thickness in any manner. Lesions without ulceration and

[a] Division of Plastic Surgery, Johns Hopkins Bayview Medical Center, Johns Hopkins University School of Medicine, 4940 Eastern Avenue, Suite A520, Baltimore, MD 21224, USA
[b] Division of Plastic Surgery, Johns Hopkins Outpatient Center, Johns Hopkins University, 601 North Caroline Street, Room 8150, Baltimore, MD 21287, USA
* Corresponding author.
E-mail address: slifche1@jhmi.edu (S.D. Lifchez).

Clin Plastic Surg 37 (2010) 55–63
doi:10.1016/j.cps.2009.08.004
0094-1298/09/$ – see front matter © 2010 Elsevier Inc. All rights reserved.

less than or equal to 1.0 mm thick are characterized further by Clark's level[4]; such lesions that abut the junction of the papillary and reticular dermis but have not violated the reticular dermis are classified as T1A. Invasion into the reticular dermis or ulceration for lesions less than or equal to 1.0 mm changes the classification to T1B. Lesions 1.01 to 2.0 mm, 2.01 to 4.0 mm, and greater than 4.0 mm are placed into T2, T3, and T4 groups, respectively. For T2 to T4 lesions, the presence of ulceration changes the T classification to subgroup b (eg, a 1.5 mm ulcerated lesion would be characterized as T2B), whereas nonulcerated lesions are in subgroup A. Clark's level has no impact on T staging for lesions greater than 1.0 mm thick.

In the AJCC system, patients then are staged based on initial tumor, nodal status, and metastatic disease.[3] Patients are staged both clinically at the initiation of treatment, and later pathologically, based on microscopic evaluation of sentinel lymph node(s) or completion lymph node dissection specimens. Clinical stage 3 disease groups all patients with nodal disease together, whereas pathologic staging stratifies stage 3 patients based on the number of positive nodes and whether these nodes are clinically identifiable as involved or only by microscopic Hematoxylin and Eosin (H&E) assessment.[5] Patients with fewer nodes that are only identifiable by microscopic assessment have better survival than those with more positive nodes or clinically identifiable lymph node disease.[6] Patients with distant metastases, those with skin, subcutaneous, or distant lymph node disease (M1) were noted to have better survival with those with lung (M2) or other visceral sites of disease (M3). Elevation of serum LDH was noted to be a poor prognostic indicator regardless of location of the metastasis, and patients with this finding also are included in the M3 group.[5] A complete discussion of the AJCC staging of melanoma is beyond the scope of this article.

EVALUATION OF THE PRIMARY LESION

Initial pathologic assessment of the primary lesion is performed by full-thickness biopsy. It is imperative that any lesion suspicious for melanoma be biopsied in a full-thickness fashion. Shave biopsies that demonstrate melanoma often have positive deep margins, and it may not be possible to obtain a proper full-thickness biopsy once shave biopsy has been performed. Staging for these patients, assuming node and metastases assessment is negative, becomes impossible because of an inability to obtain accurate assessment of the lesion's thickness. This problem is completely avoidable by obtaining a full-thickness initial biopsy. For patients with localized melanoma, tumor thickness and ulceration were the two most powerful predictors of outcome.[6]

Whenever possible, excisional biopsy is ideal for evaluating pigmented lesions. If the lesion is negative for melanoma, treatment is complete. If positive for melanoma, width of the re-excision depends on depth of the lesion. In cosmetically sensitive areas, or areas where primary closure of an excisional biopsy would not be possible, incisional biopsy is an appropriate alternative. For any such initial biopsy, the surgeon should plan the incision with local geography (relaxed skin tension lines, facial aesthetic subunits) and possible future treatments in mind.

Patients with no evidence of distant disease by history or clinical examination and in situ or T1a disease require close clinical follow-up, but most authors do not advocate further intervention. Multiple studies have demonstrated no benefit to serologic or radiographic evaluation in these patients.[7,8] Patients should be re-examined at least annually for the rest of their lives. Multiple studies[9–11] have advocated sentinel node biopsy for T1A lesions if the lesion has certain characteristics on light microscopy.

SENTINEL LYMPH NODE BIOPSY

Sentinel lymph node (SLN) biopsy is generally advocated for patients with clinical stage 1B or 2 disease. Further evaluation for patients with palpable adenopathy or distant disease will be discussed later. SLN identification is performed in the standard manner with radiolabeled tracer before surgery and a colored lymphatic tracer intraoperatively. Multiple studies have demonstrated near 100% ability to identify one or more SLNs.[12,13] Because up to 80% of patients with stage 1B or 2 disease do not have positive SLN, these patients can be spared the morbidity of lymph node dissection that would not be expected to provide them any benefit. Zogakis and colleagues reported disease-free survival and overall survival of 88% and 93% respectively in 773 patients with negative SLN biopsies. The subset of patients with thick, ulcerated primary lesions in the head and neck did notably poorer than the overall group.[14]

Patients who have at least one SLN typically then undergo completion lymph node dissection for therapeutic benefit. Interestingly, a large, multi-institutional series failed to demonstrate any detriment to recurrence risk or survival in patients with positive SLN biopsy who did not undergo completion dissection.[15] In addition, several authors caution against the risk of false-positive SLN biopsy if the immunohistochemical staining results are not well correlated with the H&E assessment, or if the results are not evaluated in the context of the clinical picture.[16,17]

The clinical utility of SLN biopsy in patients with melanomas greater than or equal to 4 mm thick but no clinical adenopathy or distant disease (stages 2B and C) is somewhat controversial. Multiple studies, however, have demonstrated value of SLN assessment for prognosis and directing further treatment.[18-20]

POSITIVE SLN BIOPSY AND CLINICAL ADENOPATHY

Patients with positive SLN biopsy typically undergo completion dissection of the involved nodal basin(s). Patients with palpable lymph nodes, particularly if the primary melanoma is thin or nonulcerated, present a clinical dilemma, as the adenopathy may not be related to the melanoma. Multiple authors have advocated ultrasound-guided fine needle aspiration (FNA) to evaluate these nodes.[21-23] The presence of melanoma in these nodal aspirations mandates completion nodal dissection. Open biopsy of palpable nodes is also an option for patients with clinically palpable adenopathy to determine if completion node dissection is necessary. After nodal assessment is completed (either by SLN biopsy, or completion dissection, if performed), patients with stage 3 clinical disease will be placed into subgroups (A to C) based on the number of nodes or if macroscopic disease is present.

A major reason for the interest in reducing the frequency of completion lymph node dissection is the significant morbidity associated with the procedure. Completion lymph node dissection is performed much less frequently since the introduction of SLN evaluation for melanoma. Patients are at risk for several complications from this procedure, including wound problems and lymphedema. Sabel and colleagues[24] found that risk of lymphedema (42% vs 24%) and major wound problems (28% vs 14%) was notably higher for patients undergoing completion lymph node dissection for clinically palpable disease than for positive SLN, although no increased risk of nodal recurrence was identified for the clinically palpable group. Serpell and colleagues[25] noted a higher complication rate (71% vs 47%) for inguinal node dissection than for axillary node dissection. Roaten and colleagues reported a 19.5% overall complication rate for patients undergoing completion lymph node dissection, although 5.9% of their SLN biopsy patients had complications including

seroma and transient nerve injury. They correlated removal of two or more nodes and placement of a closed suction drain with increased complications in the sentinel lymph node biopsy group.[26]

IMAGING AND LABORATORY EVALUATION

Multiple studies have been evaluated for the evaluation of distant disease in melanoma patients. Chest radiograph has been evaluated by multiple studies as a screening tool for metastatic disease.[7,27,28] All of the previously mentioned studies demonstrated no survival benefit for chest radiograph evaluation in asymptomatic melanoma patients. These studies also demonstrated notably high incidences of false-positive findings (abnormal findings that did not represent metastatic melanoma). Further evaluation of these chest radiograph findings led to significant cost and heightened anxiety in the patients evaluated.

Other imaging modalities, including positron emission tomography (PET) and CT scanning also have been evaluated as staging tools for melanoma, both for distant metastases and for occult lymph node disease. Multiple studies have demonstrated poor sensitivity and high cost for these techniques as screening tools.[29,30]

Serologic evaluation also has been considered for melanoma patients to evaluate for occult distant disease and to detect recurrence. Nonspecific markers such as LDH[7] have been shown not to be of benefit in identifying occult distant disease. Melanoma-specific markers such as tyrosinase and Melanoma Antigen Recognized by T-cells-1[31-33] have shown promise in identifying occult disease and detecting disease progression. A large, prospective, multi-institutional study of molecular staging of melanoma with these markers, however, did not demonstrate any additional prognostic benefit to patients.[34] There are no established guidelines regarding which patients, what time points, and which markers should be used; these serologic markers remain purely investigational tools at this time.

Although melanoma patients presenting without symptoms to suggest distant disease should not undergo imaging or serologic workup routinely, those patients presenting with symptoms suggestive of distant disease should be worked up as appropriate for the organ system in question. In this patient population, distant disease may be identified by symptom-directed workup. These patients may be eligible for medical or surgical treatment of their distant disease, which may prolong their survival.[35]

POSTOPERATIVE SURVEILLANCE OF PATIENTS WITH CUTANEOUS MALIGNANT MELANOMA

Postoperative surveillance of patients who have been treated for melanoma is clearly important as evidenced by the frequent reoccurrence of primary melanomas or the development of additional primary melanomas. Early detection of melanoma and recurrence thereof is the most important factor in regards to overall prognosis.

Despite extensive research on the topic, there is little agreement as to what optimal surveillance is. Many questions remain as to how frequently patients should be examined, for how long they should be followed, and to what extent laboratory tests and imaging studies should be used. The specific staging of a melanoma patient also will impact the degree of surveillance needed to adequately follow a patient. Melanoma incidence is increasing; optimal surveillance can offer several advantages not only for patients, but also for the health care system.

IMPACT OF STAGING ON SURVEILLANCE

It generally is agreed upon that patients with a melanoma in situ have low risk with regards to local, regional, or distant spread. High-risk patients, however, are those who have been diagnosed with invasive melanoma (AJCC stage 1 or higher) or those with a sporadic or familial dysplastic nevus syndrome.[36] These are the patients in need of surveillance. Lifelong follow-up is needed for these patients, but there is no consensus on the frequency of follow-up or the methods of surveillance.

The most common sites of distant spread in patients with melanoma are: distant skin, subcutaneous tissue or lymph nodes (42% to 59%), lungs (18% to 36%), liver (14% to 20%), brain (12% to 20%), bone (11% to 17%) and gastrointestinal (GI) system (1% to 7%).[37] Christianson and Anderson reported that the overall 3-year survival rate in patients with AJCC stage 1 or 2 was 76% for those whose metastases were discovered early, as opposed to 38% for those whose metastases were discovered late. For stage 3 patients, the survival rate was 60% versus 18% for early versus late discovery of metastases, respectively. Most recurrences and metastases occur within the first 3 years.[38] Mooney and colleagues reported that most recurrences occur in the first 2 years and that most are local or regional and not systemic. They went on to suggest that systemic surveillance such as chest radiographs should not be used more frequently than every 6 months for the first 2 years for better cost-effectiveness. Further,

Mooney and colleagues[39] recommended that surveillance cease after 5 to 10 years if the patient remains disease-free. Recurrence after 10 years is infrequent (about 3%) and occurs with approximately equal frequency between local, regional, and distant involvement. Christianson and Anderson reported the median time intervals and ranges between initial visits and diagnosis of recurrences according to AJCC staging:

> Stage 1 had a median recurrence of 22 months (range of 2.0 to 60.5 months).
> Stage 2 had a median recurrence of 13.2 months (range of 2.0 to 71.0 months)
> Stage 3 had a median recurrence of 10.6 months (range 2.3 to 53.8 months).[38]

METHODS OF SURVEILLANCE

Poo-Hwu and colleagues[40] reported that 44% of recurrences were patient-detected, whereas 56% were detected by a physician. For recurrences detected by physicians, 57% were detected through the physical examination or patient history. This underscores the importance of patient education and clinician history and physical examination. Physical examination should pay particular attention to the site of melanoma removal and to the lymph nodes draining the area.

Garbe and colleagues[41] compared ultrasound and CT surveillance with physical examination for detecting recurrence in a prospective study on 2008 patients with invasive melanomas. Sonography of lymph nodes detected 13.7% of all recurrences (stage 1, 16.7%; stage 2, 22.4%; stage 3, 9.5%; stage 4, 20.0%). The authors reported recurrences detected by physical examination to be 47% (stage 1, 55.6%; stage 2, 51.0%; stage 3, 48.2%; stage 4, 13.3%). CT scans detected 23.7% of recurrences (stage 1, 5.6%; stage 2, 14.3%; stage 3, 27.7%; stage 4, 40.0%). Chest radiograph detected 5.5% of recurrences (stage 1, 11.1%; stage 2, 2.0%; stage 3, 5.1%; stage 4, 13.3%). Abdominal ultrasound detected 3.7% of recurrences (stage 1, 0%; stage 2, 2.0%; stage 3, 4.4%; stage 4, 6.7%). Lastly, blood tests detected 1.4% of recurrences (stage 1, 0%; stage 2, 2.0%; stage 3, 1.5%; stage 4, 0%). No imaging or laboratory study was superior or even equal to physical examination.

PATIENT HISTORY

Weiss and colleagues[42] performed a study with 261 patients who had melanomas over 1.69 mm in thickness. Of the 145 patients who had recurrence, 68% of the recurrences were discovered by the patient's interval history during routine follow-up. Although this number may seem high given that nearly 50% were detected by physical examination alone by the Garbe study, symptom changes reported by the patient will direct an effective physical examination. A complete interval history must be taken from the patient. Questions should be asked in regards to the surgical excision site and any changes in color, texture, size, or any changes in sensation, including paresthesias, numbness or pain. Patients also should be asked about any changes in the regional lymph nodes including pain, fullness, swelling, erythema, or other concerns. A complete review of systems should be performed with careful attention paid to the integument, lymph nodes, pulmonary, abdomen (especially liver and GI), brain, and skeletal systems.

PHYSICAL EXAMINATION

Physical examination is an indispensable tool for detecting primary melanomas and recurrences. Nearly 50% of melanoma recurrences are detected by the physical examination alone[41]; this is particularly true for the first 2 years after initial diagnosis of invasive melanoma. Over 50% of recurrences are local or regional and not distant.[39] Of recurrences that are distant, 42% to 59% are within the skin, subcutaneous tissue, or distant lymph nodes.[37] Therefore, for about half of melanoma patients, there appears to be a window of opportunity in which one can detect recurrences with only a thorough physical examination. Of all surveillance techniques, the physical examination will afford the earliest detection of recurrence in most patients. During the physical examination, the entire cutaneous surface should be inspected, with careful attention directed toward the scar of the surgical excision and to the lymph nodes draining that region.

IMAGING TESTS BY ORGAN SYSTEMS
Skin and Lymphatics

Most melanoma recurrences occur first within the skin, subcutaneous tissue, or regional lymph nodes.[37] There is little beyond a good history and physical examination that is needed to aid in the diagnosis of a recurrence within the integument. Several methods, however, deserve mentioning. Although photographic surveillance is used commonly in high-risk patients who have yet to be diagnosed with a melanoma, it is also useful in patients who have multiple nevi or skin lesions, patients who have had multiple excisions of melanomas, or patients with complex or extensive surgical excision scars. Photographic surveillance is simple, takes little time, is inexpensive, and can make documentation much easier and faster to review. Another method for skin surveillance is surface microscopy. This method entails the use of a microscope with high illumination to view a suspicious skin lesion. It is useful in differentiating high-risk skin lesions in need of biopsy or excision from low-risk skin lesions. It is not intended to be used for examination of every skin lesion in a high-risk patient. With proper use, it can increase the sensitivity and specificity of the physical examination. It is likely to be detrimental, however, for the untrained examiner. Although popular in Europe, this technique has yet to be used routinely in the United States.[43]

The use of ultrasound to examine lymph nodes is popular among European physicians and is particularly useful for patients with excess scarring or obesity, or in patients whose lymphatic beds are difficult to palpate because of anatomy.[37] Ultrasound is useful for local and regional surveillance, including the site of surgical resection, and regional lymph nodes at risk of recurrence. Ultrasound combined with FNA has a sensitivity of 95% and a specificity of 100% for detecting recurrent disease.[44] The use of ultrasound within the United States, however, is limited in terms of lymph node examination. In the United States, CT is used more commonly to image lymph nodes that are inaccessible because of scarring, obesity, or anatomy.[37]

Pulmonary

After the skin and lymphatics, the lungs are the most likely to be affected by metastases. Morton and colleagues enrolled 108 patients in a prospective study to evaluate the accuracy of surveillance chest radiographs to detect asymptomatic pulmonary metastases in patients who were AJCC stage 3A/B. Confirmation of pulmonary metastases was done through biopsy. The sensitivity and specificity of the surveillance chest radiographs were 48% and 78%, respectively.[45] The authors concluded that chest radiographs do not lead to earlier detection of pulmonary metastases, and few patients who are detected will be candidates for curative surgery. There was a high rate of false-positives, which may lead to increased expenses, surgical procedures (mediastinoscopy, thoracoscopy), and increased patient anxiety.

Given the relatively inexpensive cost of a chest radiograph, it is still used by many physicians.[45] Chest radiographs are not optimal for detection of metastases, but baseline and surveillance radiographs allow for interval changes to be detected.

Mooney and colleagues[39] recommend chest radiographs not be performed more often that every 6 months in the first 2 years and be discontinued after 10 years if patients are disease-free. Other authors have slightly different recommendations regarding chest radiographs. Christianson and Anderson advocate the following[38]:

Stage 1—baseline chest radiograph with further imaging based on history and physical examination findings

Stage 2—baseline chest radiograph followed by one every 6 to 12 months for 3 years, then annually

Stage 3—baseline chest radiograph followed by one every 3 to 6 months for 3 years, then every 6 months for 2 years, then annually

Stage 4—individualized

The authors recommended using stage 3 guidelines for stage 2B/C melanomas because of comparable 10-year survival rates.

CT scans are more sensitive than chest radiographs in detecting pulmonary metastases, but they are much less specific. This lack of specificity is because of the small benign nodules that often are picked up during a CT of the chest.[37] Thoracic CT scans, however, are useful and recommended in these situations: before pulmonary resection, in symptomatic patients, and as part of a research protocol.[46]

Abdomen and Pelvis

CT scans of the abdomen and pelvis rarely detect occult GI tract metastases. Surgery, however, may be an option when they are discovered. In one study, the mean survival was 27.2 months, with 5-year survival of 28.3% for patients with GI metastases who underwent complete resection. Those who did not undergo surgery had a mean survival of 2.9 months with a 0% 5-year survival.[47]

The use of CT, magnetic resonance imaging (MRI) or ultrasound of the liver or spleen has not been shown to offer any benefit for detecting occult metastases.[41] Even in patients with occult liver metastases, widespread disease is so common that these patients are extremely unlikely to have surgical options.

Skeletal

Screening for bone metastases in asymptomatic patients also has not been shown to be of any benefit. Once bone metastases occur, widespread disease is so common that skeletal screening is of no benefit.[48]

Brain

Occult brain metastases usually are not detected by CT or MRI for stage 1 to 3 melanoma. Brain imaging should be performed only when there appear to be neurologic signs or symptoms suggesting brain metastases.[38] MRI with gadolinium imaging is superior to CT scanning for detecting brain, spinal cord, and meninges metastases.[48]

LABORATORY TESTS

Laboratory tests are seldom ever the sole abnormality in initial recurrence. By the time these are abnormal, there are usually multiple other abnormalities detectable by history, physical examination, and imaging studies.[40] Laboratory tests, however, are inexpensive, easy to perform, and take little time or effort from the patients or physicians. Although many guidelines still call for routine laboratory tests, the physician should keep in mind that these tests should be interpreted in the context of all other data. It is useful to draw baseline laboratory tests upon initial diagnosis, when it is unlikely that distant metastases have not yet occurred. Laboratory tests that often are drawn as part of baseline surveillance, or continued surveillance, are CBC, LFT, and LDH. There have been few reports as to the utility of alkaline phosphatase in regards to surveillance. Based on the available literature, the authors make the following recommendations for laboratory surveillance of melanoma:

Stage 0—no laboratory baseline or surveillance

Stage 1—baseline CBC, LFT, LDH with further laboratory tests as indicated by history or physical examination

Stage 2A—baseline CBC, LFT, and LDH with surveillance labs annually for life

Stage 2B/C and stage 3—baseline CBC, LFT, LDH, with surveillance laboratory tests every 6 months for 5 years, then annually for life

Stage 4—individualized

SUMMARY RECOMMENDATIONS FOR SURVEILLANCE GUIDELINES

The overall prognosis of melanoma is improved by earlier detection of the primary tumor, and it follows that prognosis likely can be improved in patients with recurrence through earlier detection. Patient education is paramount for overall success in terms of recurrence detection. Patients need to be educated on the nature of their disease, what their specific staging means, and, most importantly, what they need to look for to detect any recurrence. If the surgical excision is located in a place not readily visible to the patient, such as the back, then a family member or significant other also can be educated for signs of recurrence or regional spread. The history and examination are also important for the early detection of recurrence. A thorough history should be elicited from the patient on each visit, and care should be taken during the physical examination with the use of photographic surveillance in appropriate patients.

The use of CT scans to image lymph nodes is common in patients with dense scar tissue overlying the lymph nodes, in patients who are obese, or in instances where anatomy is a limiting factor to physical examination. Although chest radiographs have not been shown to improve the overall outcome of patients with melanomas, they are inexpensive and easy to obtain; sensitivity is low, but there is a possibility that a patient may benefit. Those against the use of chest radiographs can argue that they lead to expensive tests and procedures and that they can be another drain to the health care system. There is no consensus on the use of surveillance chest radiographs. The use of thoracic CT scans should be reserved for those patients who are symptomatic. CT scans have a low specificity and therefore will have a high false-positive rate if used in routine surveillance.

CT scans of the GI tract can offer patients a chance at successful palliative treatment, which has been shown to prolong survival after complete resection. Occult metastases, however, are unlikely to be picked up by CT. This test should be reserved for patients complaining of symptoms suggestive of GI metastases or findings on physical examination.

CT, MRI, and ultrasound scans of the liver or spleen seldom detect occult metastases and have shown no benefit in outcome. Likewise, by the time metastases to the bone or brain have occurred, it is very likely that widespread involvement is present. Routine scanning of the liver, spleen, bone, brain, or spinal cord should not be performed. Imaging of these sites only should be done if indicated by symptoms or physical findings.

Baseline CT scans may be ordered as part of a workup for a patient with positive SLNs to rule out systemic involvement. Therefore, these can be used as a baseline given the patient has no distant metastases.

It is unlikely that there will ever be a formal consensus for surveillance based on prospective studies showing clear results. Instead, the physician should gain an understanding of the nature of melanomas, how the staging system affects prognosis, which organ systems to carefully monitor, and what techniques are available for patient surveillance.

REFERENCES

1. McHugh JB, Su L, Griffith KA, et al. Significance of multiple lymphatic basin drainage in truncal melanoma patients undergoing sentinel lymph node biopsy. Ann Surg Oncol 2006;13(9):1216–23.
2. Leong SP, Morita ER, Südmeyer M, et al. Heterogeneous patterns of lymphatic drainage to sentinel lymph nodes by primary melanoma from different anatomic sites. Clin Nucl Med 2005;30(3):150–8.
3. Balch CM, Buzaid AC, Soong SJ, et al. Final version of the American Joint Committee on Cancer staging system for cutaneous melanoma. J Clin Oncol 2001; 19(16):3635–48.
4. Clark WH Jr, From L, Bernardino EA, et al. The histogenesis and biologic behavior of primary human malignant melanomas of the skin. Cancer Res 1969;29(3):705–27.
5. Kim CJ, Reintgen DS, Balch CM. The new melanoma staging system. Cancer Control 2002;9(1):9–15.
6. Balch CM, Soong SJ, Gershenwald JE, et al. Prognostic factors analysis of 17,600 melanoma patients: validation of the American Joint Committee on Cancer melanoma staging system. J Clin Oncol 2001;19(16):3622–34.
7. Wang TS, Johnson TM, Cascade PN, et al. Evaluation of staging chest radiographs and serum lactate dehydrogenase for localized melanoma. J Am Acad Dermatol 2004;51(3):399–405.
8. Hofmann U, Szedlak M, Rittgen W, et al. Primary staging and follow-up in melanoma patients—monocenter evaluation of methods, costs, and patient survival. Br J Cancer 2002;87(2):151–7.
9. Gimotty PA, Elder DE, Fraker DL, et al. Identification of high-risk patients among those diagnosed with thin cutaneous melanomas. J Clin Oncol 2007; 25(9):1129–34.
10. Bedrosian I, Farjes MB, Guerry D 4th, et al. Incidence of sentinel node metastasis in patients with thin primary melanoma (< or = 1mm) with vertical growth phase. Ann Surg Oncol 2000;7(4):262–7.
11. Ranieri JM, Wagner JD, Wenck S, et al. The prognostic importance of sentinel lymph node biopsy in thin melanoma. Ann Surg Oncol 2006;13(7):927–32.
12. McMasters KM, Reintgen DS, Ross MI, et al. Sentinel lymph node biopsy for melanoma: controversy despite widespread agreement. J Clin Oncol 2001;19(11):2851–5.
13. Gershenwald JE, Thompson W, Mansfield PF, et al. Multi-institutional lymphatic mapping experience: the prognostic value of sentinel lymph node status

in 612 stage I or II melanoma patients. J Clin Oncol 1999;17(3):976–83.

14. Zogakis TG, Essner R, Wang HJ, et al. Natural history of melanoma in 773 patients with tumor-negative sentinel lymph nodes. Ann Surg Oncol 2007;14(5):1604–11.

15. Wong SL, Morton DL, Thompson JF, et al. Melanoma patients with positive sentinel lymph nodes who did not undergo completion lymphadenectomy: a multi-institutional study. Ann Surg Oncol 2006;13(6):809–16.

16. Brennick JB, Yan S. False-positive cells in sentinel lymph nodes. Semin Diagn Pathol 2008;25(2):116–9.

17. Thomas JM. Prognostic false-positivity of the sentinel node in melanoma. Nat Clin Pract Oncol 2008;5(1):18–23.

18. Gutzmer R, Satzger I, Thoms KM, et al. Sentinel lymph node status is the most important prognostic factor for thick (> or = 4mm) melanomas. J Dtsch Dermatol Ges 2008;6(3):198–203.

19. Cecchi R, Buralli L, Innocenti S, et al. Sentinel lymph node biopsy in patients with thick (=4mm) melanoma: a single-centre experience. J Eur Acad Dermatol Venereol 2007;21(6):758–61.

20. Jacobs IA, Chang CK, Salti GI. Role of sentinel lymph node biopsy in patients with thick (>4 mm) primary melanoma. Am Surg 2004;70(1):59–62.

21. Dalle S, Paulin C, Lapras V, et al. Fine-needle aspiration biopsy with ultrasound guidance in patients with malignant melanoma and palpable lymph nodes. Br J Dermatol 2006;155(3):552–6.

22. Jaffer S, Zakowski M. Fine-needle aspiration biopsy of axillary lymph nodes. Diagn Cytopathol 2002;26(2):69–74.

23. Voit C, Schoengen A, Schwürzer-Voit M, et al. The role of ultrasound in detection and management of regional disease in melanoma patients. Semin Oncol 2002;29(4):353–60.

24. Sabel MS, Griffith KA, Arora A, et al. Inguinal node dissection for melanoma in the era of sentinel lymph node biopsy. Surgery 2007;141(6):728–35.

25. Serpell JW, Carne PW, Bailey M. Radical lymph node dissection for melanoma. ANZ J Surg 2003;73(5):294–9.

26. Roaten JB, Pearlman N, Gonzalez R, et al. Identifying risk factors for complications following sentinel lymph node biopsy for melanoma. Arch Surg 2005;140(1):85–9.

27. Tsao H, Feldman M, Fullerton JE, et al. Early detection of asymptomatic pulmonary melanoma metastases by routine chest radiographs is not associated with improved survival. Arch Dermatol 2004;140(1):67–70.

28. Miranda EP, Gertner M, Wall J, et al. Routine imaging of asymptomatic patients with metastasis to sentinel lymph nodes rarely identifies systemic disease. Arch Surg 2004;139(8):831–6.

29. Veit-Haibach P, Vogt FM, Jablonka R, et al. Diagnostic accuracy of contrast-enhanced FDG-PET/CT in primary staging of cutaneous malignant melanoma. Eur J Nucl Med Mol Imaging 2009;36(6):910–8.

30. Singh B, Ezziddin S, Palmedo H, et al. Preoperative 18FDG-PET/CT imaging and sentinel node biopsy in the detection of regional lymph node metastases in malignant melanoma. Melanoma Res 2008;18(5):346–52.

31. Voit C, Kron M, Rademaker J, et al. Molecular staging in stage II and stage III melanoma patients and its effect on long-term survival. J Clin Oncol 2005;23(6):1218–27.

32. Koyanagi K, Kuo C, Nakagawa T, et al. Multimarker quantitative real-time PCR detection of circulating melanoma cells in peripheral blood: relation to disease stage in melanoma patients. Clin Chem 2005;51(6):981–8.

33. Max N, Willhauck M, Wolf K, et al. Reliability of PCR-based detection of occult tumour cells: lessons from real-time RT-PCR. Melanoma Res 2001;11(4):371–8.

34. Scoggins CR, Ross MI, Reintgen DS, et al. Prospective multi-institutional study of reverse transcriptase polymerase chain reaction for molecular staging of melanoma. J Clin Oncol 2006;24(18):2849–57.

35. Essner R, Lee JH, Wanek LA, et al. Contemporary surgical treatment of advanced-stage melanoma. Arch Surg 2004;139(9):961–6.

36. ESMO Guidelines Working Group, Jost L. Cutaneous malignant melanoma: European Society for Medical Oncology clinical recommendations for diagnosis, treatment and follow-up. Ann Oncol 2007;18(Suppl 2):ii71–3.

37. Huang CL, Provost N, Marghoob AA, et al. Laboratory tests and imaging studies in patients with cutaneous malignant melanoma. J Am Acad Dermatol 1998;39(3):451–63.

38. Christianson DF, Anderson CM. Close monitoring and lifetime follow-up are optimal for patients with a history of melanoma. Semin Oncol 2003;30(3):369–74.

39. Mooney MM, Mettlin C, Michalek AM, et al. Life-long screening of patients with intermediate thickness melanoma for asymptomatic pulmonary recurrences: a cost-effectiveness analysis. Cancer 1997;80(6):1052–64.

40. Poo-Hwu WJ, Ariyan S, Lamb L, et al. Follow-up recommendations for patients with American Joint Commission on Cancer stages I–III malignant melanoma. Cancer 1999;86:2252–8.

41. Garbe C, Paul A, Kohler-Spath H, et al. Prospective evaluations of a follow-up schedule in cutaneous melanoma patients: recommendations for an effective follow-up strategy. J Clin Oncol 2003;21:520–9.

42. Weiss M, Loprinzi CL, Creagan ET, et al. Utility of follow-up tests for detecting recurrent disease in patients with malignant melanomas. JAMA 1995; 274:1703–5.

43. Rhodes AR. Cutaneous melanoma and intervention strategies to reduce tumor-related mortality: what we know, what we don't know, and what we think we know that isn't so. Dermatol Ther 2006;19:50–69.

44. Choi EA, Gershenwald JE. Imaging studies in patients with melanomas. Surg Oncol Clin N Am 2007;16(2):403–30.

45. Morton RL, Craig JC, Thompson JF. The role of surveillance chest x-rays in the follow-up of high-risk melanoma patients. Ann Surg Oncol 2009;16:571–7.

46. Chalmers N, Best JJ. The significance of pulmonary nodules detected by CT but not by chest radiography in tumor staging. Clin Radiol 1991; 41:410–2.

47. Ricaniadis N, Konstadoulakis MM, Walsh D, et al. Gastrointestinal metastases from malignant melanoma. Surg Oncol 1995;4:105–11.

48. Meyers MO, Yeh JJ. Method of detection of initial recurrence of stage II/III cutaneous melanoma: analysis of the utility of follow-up staging. Ann Surg Oncol 2009;16(4):941–7.

Surgical Management of Primary Disease

Jeffrey H. Kozlow, MD, Riley S. Rees, MD*

KEYWORDS

- Melanoma • Surgery • Management
- Reconstruction • Sentinel node biopsy

Melanoma is a malignancy that plastic surgeons frequently manage. The current incidence of melanoma is estimated at more than 68,000 new cases per year in the United States.[1] Despite aggressive research into chemotherapy, radiation, immunomodulation, and other treatment modalities, surgery remains the cornerstone for treatment, and the best chance for cure and long-term survival.[2] Given the spectrum of disease and variety in location, multiple surgical specialties are involved in the care of a patient with melanoma. All patients with melanoma should be evaluated in multidisciplinary clinics with tumor boards so that appropriate surgical referrals can be based on patient characteristics, disease location, and experience of surgeons. The most important component of melanoma care includes patient education and early screening. Early detection leads to early surgical excision and, therefore, increased survival.[3]

PRIMARY SURGICAL CARE

All suspicious cutaneous lesions require biopsy for definitive pathologic diagnosis. In addition to evaluation lesions for changes based on the "ABCD" (Asymmetry, Border irregularity, Color variation, Diameter >6 mm) criteria, it is notable that approximately 5% of melanomas are not pigmented[3] and the "ABCD" criteria may not indicate the typical malignant lesions in younger patients. The recommended biopsy techniques are excisional biopsies with narrow margins (1–2 mm) for small lesions or incisional biopsy for larger lesions. Punch biopsies should be performed for larger pigmented lesions with multiple suspicious areas. The design of incisional and excisional biopsies should also take into account the location of the lesion, to allow for improved reconstructive and cosmetic outcomes if additional resection is needed. Shave biopsies of pigmented lesions are never recommended, given the importance of tumor depth for staging and treatment recommendations. Excisional biopsies well outside the tumor margin are also not recommended, because it can destroy the local lymphatic drainage pattern that is important for accurate sentinel lymph node biopsy. A poorly planned biopsy technique can not only make excision and reconstruction more difficult but may adversely effect treatment options for the patient. Recent studies have shown that in patients initially undergoing an incisional biopsy with greater than 50% of the primary lesion remaining who then later underwent a narrow margin microstaging procedure, an average increase in depth from 0.66 to 1.07 mm resulted, with 21% of patients upstaged and 10% more requiring sentinel lymph node biopsy.[4]

Surgical Excision Including Margins

Evolving treatment of primary melanoma has transitioned from radical surgical treatment to more appropriate excisional margins. This trend has been especially true for lesions of the head and neck where disfigurement is important to the patients. Early descriptions of the surgical treatment of melanoma recommended 5-cm margins around the primary lesion including fascia and muscle, regional lymphadenectomy, and sometimes all subcutaneous tissues in between.[5] The current practice of more reasonable margins has

Section of Plastic and Reconstructive Surgery, University of Michigan, 2130 Taubman Center, 1500 East Medical Center Drive, Ann Arbor, MI 48108, USA
* Corresponding author.
E-mail address: rreese@med.umich.edu (R.S. Rees).

Clin Plastic Surg 37 (2010) 65–71
doi:10.1016/j.cps.2009.07.006

not changed survival. In meta-analysis of randomized controlled trials comparing narrow and wide margins for resection, there was no difference in death, disease-free survival, or recurrence when narrow (1–2 cm) margins were used compared with wider (3–5 cm) margins.[6,7] In addition to equal oncologic outcomes, the smaller margin significantly decreased the need for split-thickness skin graft reconstruction or delayed reconstruction.[8] The data for margins of 1 cm on melanomas less than 1 mm in depth are supported, but it is unclear if a 1-cm margin for thicker melanoma is sufficient. **Table 1** shows the typical margins of resection used at the authors' institution for lesions not involving the head and neck. Studies comparing the risk of regional metastasis based on preservation versus inclusion of the fascia in the surgical resection surprisingly have shown no difference in outcome.[9,10] Therefore, current standards of case include dissection only down to the fascia unless the tumors have already evaded through the fascial layer.

Special care is required for lentigo maligna melanomas due to difficulties in determining lesion margins. The role of first determining lesion margins using boundary biopsy techniques (such as the 2-blade square technique described later) allows for fewer recurrences and more satisfactory reconstructions. Desmoplastic melanomas, which are locally more aggressive, require more extensive surgical margins of 3 to 5 cm.

Sentinel Lymph Node Biopsy/Completion Lymph Node Dissection

In all melanoma patients with lesions at a Breslow depth greater than 1 mm, consideration must be made for evaluation of the lymph node basins. It is well established that increasing depth of invasion is associated with increased risk of distant disease. Metastatic disease to regional lymph nodes has been demonstrated in even thin lesions.[11] At a minimum, all patients require physical examination of all lymph node basins including the cervical, axillary, epitrochlear, popliteal, and inguinal drainage basins, regardless of primary disease location. For patients with lesions greater than 1 mm in depth and clinically node-negative disease, lymphoscintigraphy with sentinel lymph node biopsy must be performed. The Multicenter Selective Lymphadenectomy Trial-I demonstrated the prognostic value of sentinel lymph node biopsy.[12] In addition, this study showed that for intermediate thickness melanomas (1.2–3.5 mm in depth), sentinel lymph node biopsy with completion lymphadenectomy in patients with a positive sentinel node improved overall survival.

In younger patients, consideration for sentinel node biopsy with lesions less than 1 mm may be warranted because there is suggestive evidence that they have a higher frequency of regional metastatic disease.[13,14] The only *potential* exception is for the severely medically compromised patient with a negative clinical examination who would not be a candidate for completion lymph node dissection due to significant surgical risk. Any patient with clinically positive lymph nodes should undergo fine-needle aspiration for confirmation of metastatic disease with subsequent lymph node dissection if testing is positive. Patients with inconclusive fine-needle aspirations should be evaluated for excisional lymph node biopsy. For patients with thin melanomas (<1.0 mm in depth), recommendations are currently being reviewed with attempts to identify pathologic characteristics that may predict high-risk thin lesions, including mitotic rate or primary tumor location.[15] The data remain controversial for lesions between 0.75 and 1.00 mm. Lesions less than 0.75 mm should not undergo sentinel node biopsy because it does not seem to be a predictor of outcome. It is still unclear as to what additional surgical care is needed for a small focus of micrometastatic disease in the sentinel lymph node;[16] however, the current standard of care is for completion lymph node dissection for any positive sentinel

Table 1
Recommended surgical margins for primary disease[a]

Tumor Thickness	Margin of Excision
Melanoma in situ	0.5 cm or pre-resection margin control
Less than 1.0 mm	1 cm
Greater than 1.0 mm	2 cm
Recurrent local disease	2 cm
In-transit disease	2 cm
Desmoplastic melanoma	3–5 cm

[a] Excludes lesions located on the head, neck, and digits.

lymph node biopsy. Future data from the Multicenter Selective Lymphadenectomy Trial-II should help address some of these issues.

Resection of Metastasis

Melanoma is one of the few malignancies for which surgical resection of metastasis has been shown to prolong survival in selected patients.[17] In addition to excision of recurrences at the primary site, in-transit disease, and lymph node drainage basins, surgical excision should be considered for distant disease if clinically isolated and appropriate. This approach is particularly true in the head and neck, where control of local disease will prolong the quality of survival. It is the authors' institutional practice to perform radical resection of recurrent disease when clinically feasible unless there is extensive distant metastasis. For extensive extremity in-transit disease that is not amenable to surgical resection, the patient should be evaluated for a limb perfusion or infusion technique.[2]

Reconstruction

After surgical excision with pathologically cleared margins, reconstruction can be performed in either an immediate or staged fashion, depending on location. For example, hand and ear melanomas may require immediate reconstruction to avoid infected critical structures such as tendons or auricular cartilage. Reconstruction should be aimed at closure of the defect without compromising the ability for surveillance. Melanoma is prone to local recurrence even after clear surgical margins. For superficial lesions on areas with increased tissue laxity, surgical excision in an elliptical fashion with layered closure is preferred. After identification of the lesion, the appropriate surgical margins are marked around the lesion. This mark is then turned into an elliptical incision using roughly a 3:1 length to width ratio designed parallel to the relaxed lines of tension. Alternatively, one can remove the lesion with the marked circular margin and then start to close the defect, with excision of any remaining standing cutaneous deformities. Both of these primary closure techniques are ideal from a reconstructive perspective and a future surveillance standpoint.

On the face and extremities, however, primary closure following excision may not always be possible due to a lack of soft tissue laxity or distortion of critical structures. Local skin flaps including the keystone, V-Y advancement, rotational, and rhomboid flaps, are popular techniques that allow closure of extremity defects without skin grafting. Larger areas, or when local reconstructive options are not available, can also be treated with split-thickness skin grafting. The role of bilaminar dermal regenerative templates (Integra) is an advance in the surgical treatment of melanoma. Using bilaminar dermal regenerative template on the resection defect allows the surgeon to clear the margins in high-risk lesions or provide a collagen base to cover defects, particularly lesions in the scalp. Extensive reconstruction including muscle flaps or free flap is generally not indicated except in rare circumstances.

SPECIAL AREAS
Scalp

Surgical management of melanoma on the scalp is challenging because reconstruction options are limited to skin grafts. Moreover, tumor recurrence, particularly in males, makes scalp flaps undesirable. Unlike in other areas of the body, the authors believe that surgical margins for scalp melanoma should include resection of the galea aponeurotica down through the pericranium. This action forces the surgeon to use skin substitutes such as Integra to populate the bone with fibroblasts so that delayed skin grafting can occur. The delay in reconstruction allows the pathologist to assess the surgical margin and determine if the sentinel node is positive, thus requiring regional lymphadenectomy.[18] Integra occasionally fails, and successful reconstruction requires bone burring and reapplication. It is important to counsel patients that melanoma of the scalp and neck have a high rate of mortality compared with other sites, when controlled for other prognostic factors.[19]

Face

Lentigo maligna (melanoma in situ) and lentigo maligna melanoma occur frequently on the face, and are challenging because clear surgical margins are hard to achieve. Margins frequently are positive for atypical junctional melanocytic hyperplasia, which is a precursor of melanoma. The surgical management of melanoma on the face is challenging because of the close proximity of multiple structures that are not easily sacrificed with the typical margins. The 2-blade "square" technique has been shown to allow for peripheral margin control before resection on the face.[20,21] For atypical junctional melanocytic hyperplasia or melanoma in situ, the 2-blade square technique for peripheral control allows for improved margin control and the ability to perform formal excision with immediate reconstruction. In this technique, parallel incisions are made around the lesion typically by a dermatologic cutaneous surgeon. The incisions are then closed while a pathologic review is conducted. Further resection is then performed if necessary until margins are negative. The patient then undergoes a secondary excision of the entire square with immediate reconstruction. Standard techniques for facial reconstruction are then used, including skin grafting, local tissue rearrangement, and local-regional flaps. At the authors' institution, the 2-blade square technique is most commonly employed for lesions on the nose, cheek, eyelid, and neck.

Ears

The ear is the site of primary melanoma in 7% to 20% of head and neck melanomas,[22] with approximately half occurring on the helix.[23] Surgical management previously included standard margins based on Breslow depth. However, initial narrower margins of surgical resection with staged reconstruction after negative pathology may be necessary.[22,23] Depth of excision should be down to and including the cartilage in most cases. Wedge excision leaves good surgical options for reconstruction. Wedge excision also allows for further excision if the margins are close. The authors have found management of auricular melanoma with this technique to be successful from both an oncologic and a reconstructive outcome. Atypical junctional melanocytic hyperplasia and melanoma in situ can be managed with preservation of the cartilage and temporary coverage. If final pathology reveals no invasive disease, then reconstruction using skin grafting or local flaps is performed. Previous recommendations for complete or partial auriculectomy are now reserved only for recurrent or extensive disease. Lymphatic drainage of the ear is often to the parotid basin. Positive sentinel lymph node requires regional lymphadenectomy in the area of drainage. Experience clearly is necessary to perform these procedures.[24] Most commonly, superficial parotidectomy and anterior neck dissections are required for positive sentinel nodes. The drainage occasionally is into the posterior neck, and level V nodes must be dissected.

Eyelid

Primary melanoma of the eyelids is seen in substantial volume only in large melanoma centers. Given the small, but important amount of soft tissue in the periocular region, recommended excisional margins tend to be smaller, with no clear decrease in survival benefit. Margins of 5 mm have been suggested for lesions with Breslow depth less than 1 mm.[25] However, lesions greater than 2 mm in depth likely require 10 mm

to decrease local recurrence.[25] After achieving local control, standard techniques for eyelid reconstruction are employed. Specialized oculoplastic surgeons may be involved in reconstruction, based on local referral patterns.

Hands

Melanomas on the hand occur in distinct anatomic locations: dorsal skin, palmar skin, digits, or subungal nail. For dorsal hand skin, surgical management requires resection down to the paratenon, and requires immediate reconstruction with skin grafts or flaps to prevent tendon exposure. Lesions of the palm are best treated by radical excision and skin grafting. Superficial lesions of the digit (Breslow depth less than 1 mm) can be treated with radical excision, and flap or skin graft reconstruction. In contrast, invasive lesions of the digit (Breslow depth greater than 1 mm) require amputation at one joint proximal to the melanoma along with sentinel lymph node biopsy. For the index finger, ray amputation should be discussed with the patient, given the improved functional outcome and ability for the middle finger to be used for pinching. Subungal melanoma is a unique problem because it is impossible to determine the Breslow depth without excisional biopsy. Moreover, the quality of the biopsy, due to the anatomy of the nail matrix, makes interpretation of the depth circumspect. In these cases, the authors favor amputation at the level of the distal interphalangeal joint.

Toes

Melanoma of the feet can be divided into lesions of the dorsal surface, plantar surface, or digits. Dorsal foot melanomas can either be skin grafted or closed linearly, depending on the laxity of the skin. Melanoma of the plantar surface of the foot represents a particular challenge. Skin grafts do not heal well in this area, particularly if the patient has diabetes. Application of Integra after resection of acrolentiginous lesion is a good solution, because it allows time to clear the margins and provides a collagen mat for a subsequent skin graft. Lesions of the digits are best treated with amputation; however, superficial lesions (<1.0 mm) can be treated with Integra and skin grafting to preserve the aesthetic appearance of a 5-digit foot. Postoperative ambulation may also be improved with preservation of the great toe treated with reconstruction rather than amputation.

Genitalia

Melanoma of the female genitalia is rare, occurring in 0.23% of all melanomas.[26] The most common site for primary disease is the vulva, with histology typically of a mucosal lentiginous type.[27] Staging specifically for vulva melanoma has not been clearly established. Current surgical recommendations are based on standard Breslow depth determined margins, with radical surgery including vulvectomy, used only in exceptional cases.[28] Early lesions that present with melanoma in situ usually can be treated with resection and skin grafts. Vaginal melanomas are advanced and typically have a nodular histologic type. Actual tumor size and not tumor thickness is the best predictor of long-term survival.[29]

Although rare, melanoma of the male genitalia is frequently located on the penis, with case reports existing for primary scrotal melanoma.[30,31] Although surgical standards for care have not been fully evaluated, it is the authors' practice to perform partial or total penectomy for invasive penile melanoma. Thin lesions can be managed with wide local excision and skin graft reconstruction. Scrotal melanoma is rarer, and managed with wide local excision and scrotal reconstruction as necessary. Sentinel lymph node biopsy is performed for all lesions with Breslow depth greater than 1 mm.

SPECIAL POPULATIONS
Children

Melanoma accounts for 1% to 3% of old childhood malignancies; however, in patients diagnosed with melanoma, approximately 50% have regional disease based on sentinel lymph node biopsy or clinical examination.[32] The compounding difficulty in children is the number of lesions with unknown biologic potential. The differentiation between Spitz nevi, Spitz tumors, and melanomas with Spitzoid features are difficult for pathologists and surgeons alike. Primary management includes local excision of primary disease and sentinel lymph node biopsy in patients thought to have Spitz tumors or melanoma with Spitzoid features when the lesions are greater than 1.0 mm in depth. Although the incidence is more limited, completion lymph node dissection is indicated for pediatric patients with positive sentinel lymph node biopsies.[32,33] Pediatric patients are more likely to present with amelanotic disease, which delays the diagnosis and subsequent treatment. Unlike the adult population, it is unclear whether a negative sentinel lymph node biopsy in children is a prognostic indicator for survival.[34]

It is unclear whether pediatric patients have an increased risk for discovery of a positive sentinel lymph node compared with adults with similar Breslow depth; however, disease-free survival and overall survival do not seem to differ for similar-staged disease, assuming true melanomas are separated from Spitz nevi and Spitz tumors. Sentinel lymph node biopsy in pediatric cases has been shown to be safe.[35,36] In addition, it can be used as an adjunct to diagnosis in lesions with difficult pathology, including Spitz nevus.[36,37] Adjuvant therapies for metastatic diseases are still being evaluated; however, current protocols include interferon α-2b,[38] which children tolerate better than adults.

Pregnancy

It was historically believed that pregnancy increased the risk and worsened the outcome for melanoma. However, multiple studies have now demonstrated no correlation between pregnancy and the development of melanoma, prognosis of a melanoma, or survival rates.[39,40] From a surgical perspective, the management of primary melanoma is no different in the pregnant woman than in any other patient. Wide local excisions can still be performed under local anesthesia. When necessary, general anesthesia can be used with fetal monitoring. General anesthesia is clearly indicated for melanomas greater than 1 mm in depth for which sentinel lymph node biopsy can still safely be performed. A recent study examining the radiation exposure to the uterus during lymphoscintigraphy revealed that the exposure to the uterus was less than the daily background dose.[41] Thus, the surgical oncologist should make no significant changes to standard protocol for the pregnant patient. For pregnant patients with stage IV disease, the use of systemic agents is more controversial, and should involve the local medical oncologist and obstetrician. For women who have already been treated for melanoma, these patients may be counseled that future pregnancies have not been shown to increase the risk of recurrence. However, women with high-risk lesions may benefit from waiting 2 to 3 years in case there is a recurrence that requires advanced therapies.[42] Hormone replacement therapies and oral contraceptives do not seem to increase the risk of recurrence in melanoma.[39]

Elderly

Melanoma is more common in the elderly male because of multiple factors including decreased melanoma awareness, decreased access to health care, vision changes resulting in decreased skin surveillance, and accumulative long-term sun exposure.[43] The management of melanoma in the elderly requires a balance between the overall risks of the melanoma compared with the secondary complications from treatment. However, age alone is not a contraindication for the surgical care of melanoma in the elderly population. Surgical excision of the primary lesion is performed based on the standard techniques, although patients with multiple medical comorbidities may be treated under intravenous sedation and local anesthesia instead of general anesthesia.

Sentinel lymph node biopsy should still be performed in most circumstances, and by itself does not seem to have increased the rate of complications in the elderly.[43] Although sentinel lymph node biopsy can be performed under local anesthesia, the potential for increased systemic stress to the patient may require that the anesthetist and surgeon consider general anesthesia as the safest alternative. This procedure under intravenous sedation is generally not well suited for head and neck or axillary sentinel nodes. However, some controversy exists in elderly, sick patients with multiple comorbidities and melanomas greater than 1.0 mm and no clinical lymphadenopathy. Are these patients better served by serial clinical examinations than by sentinel lymph node biopsy? The authors' institutional view at the University of Michigan Multidisciplinary tumor board is to treat elderly patients no differently than others. Otherwise, the appearance of clinically positive regional disease at a later time increases the complication with surgical removal.[44] A particular problem in the elderly patient is the presence of desmoplastic melanomas or melanoma in situ. Both of these lesions share the difficulty of clearing the surgical margin because of their local aggressive nature. Overall, the surgical treatment of melanoma for the elderly is the same as the surgical care for younger patients, with exceptions made only in patients with multiple high-risk medical comorbidities.

SUMMARY

Plastic surgeons will continue to have a leading role in the surgical management of melanoma. A thorough understanding of the surgical management of melanoma and a breadth of experience in operating on the head, neck, and extremities allows plastic surgeons to appropriately care for the melanoma patient. The continued development of surgical standards of care will ultimately lead to improved survival from melanoma.

REFERENCES

1. American Cancer Society. Available at: http://www.cancer.org/docroot/cri/content/cri_2_4_1x_what_are _the_key_statistics_for_melanoma_50.asp. Last revised 05/14/2009. Accessed June 15, 2009.
2. Demierre MF, Sabel MS, Margolin KA, et al. State of the science 60th anniversary review: 60 years of advances in cutaneous melanoma epidemiology, diagnosis, and treatment, as reported in the journal cancer. Cancer 2008;113(Suppl 7): 1728–43.
3. Thompson JF, Scolyer RA, Kefford RD. Cutaneous melanoma. Lancet 2005;365:687–701.
4. Karimipour DJ, Schwartz JL, Wang TS, et al. Microstaging accuracy after subtotal incisional biopsy of cutaneous melanoma. J Am Acad Dermatol 2005; 52(5):798–802.
5. Pringle JH. A method of operation in cases of melanocytic tumors of the skin. Edinburgh Med J 1908; 123:496–9.
6. Haigh PI, DiFronzo LA, McCready DR. Optimal excision margins for primary cutaneous melanoma: a systematic review and meta-analysis. Can J Surg 2003;46(6):419–26.
7. Lens MB, Nathan P, Bataille V. Excision margins for primary cutaneous melanoma updated pooled analysis of randomized controlled trials. Arch Surg 2007; 142(9):885–91.
8. Balch CM, Urist MM, Karakousis CP, et al. Efficacy of 2-cm surgical margins for intermediate-thickness melanomas (1-4 mm). Ann Surg 1993;218: 262–9.
9. Olsen G. The malignant melanoma of the skin. Acta Chir Scand Suppl 1966;365:1–222.
10. Kenady DE, Brown BW, McBride CM. Excision of underlying fascia with a primary malignant melanoma: effects on recurrence and survival rates. Surgery 1982;92:615–8.
11. Lowe JB, Hurst E, Moley JF. Sentinel lymph node biopsy in patients with thin melanoma. Arch Dermatol 2003;39(5):617–21.
12. Morton DL, Thompson JF, Cochran AJ, et al. Sentinel-node biopsy or nodal observation in melanoma. N Engl J Med 2006;355:1307–17.
13. Sondak VK, Taylor JM, Sabel MS, et al. Mitotic rate and younger age are predictors of sentinel lymph node positivity: lessons learned from the generation of a probabilistic mode. Ann Surg Oncol 2004;11: 247–58.
14. Thompson JF, Shaw HM. Should tumour mitotic rate and patient age, as well as tumour thickness, be used to select melanoma patients for sentinel node biopsy? Ann Surg Oncol 2004;11:233–5.
15. Paek SC, Griffith KA, Johnson TM, et al. The impact of factors beyond Breslow depth on predicting sentinel lymph node positivity in melanoma. Cancer 2007;109(1):100–8.
16. Frankel TL, Griffith KA, Lowe L, et al. Do micromorphometric features of metastatic deposits within sentinel nodes predict nonsentinel lymph node

involvement in melanoma? Ann Surg Oncol 2008; 15(9):2403–11 [Epub 2008 Jul 15].

17. Meyer T, Merkel S, Goehl J, et al. Surgical therapy for distant metastases of malignant melanoma. Cancer 2000;89(9):1983–91.

18. Wilensky JS, Rosenthal AH, Bradford CR, et al. The use of a bovine collagen construct for reconstruction of full-thickness scalp defects in the elderly patient with cutaneous malignancy. Ann Plast Surg 2005; 54(3):297–301.

19. Lachiewicz AM, Berwick M, Wiggins CL, et al. Survival differences between patients with scalp or neck melanoma and those with melanoma of other sites in the Surveillance, Epidemiology, and End Results (SEER) program. Arch Dermatol 2008; 144(4):515–21.

20. Hazan C, Dusza SW, Delgado R, et al. Staged excision for lentigo maligna and lentigo maligna melanoma: a retrospective analysis of 117 cases. J Am Acad Dermatol 2008;58(1):142–8.

21. Jejurikar SS, Borschel GH, Johnson TM, et al. Immediate, optimal reconstruction of facial lentigo maligna and melanoma following total peripheral margin control. Plast Reconstr Surg 2007;120(5): 1249–55.

22. Jahn V, Breuninger H, Garbe C, et al. Melanoma of the ear: prognostic factors and surgical strategies. Br J Dermatol 2006;154:310–8.

23. Ravin AG, Pickett N, Johnson JL, et al. Melanoma of the ear: treatment and survival probabilities based on 199 patients. Ann Plast Surg 2006; 57(1):70–6.

24. Ollila DW, Foshag LJ, Essner R, et al. Parotid region lymphatic mapping and sentinel lymphadenectomy for cutaneous melanoma. Ann Surg Oncol 1999;6: 150–4.

25. Esmaeli B, Youssef A, Naderi A. Margins of excision for cutaneous melanoma of the eyelid skin: the collaborative eyelid skin melanoma group report. Ophthal Plast Reconstr Surg 2003;19(2): 96–101.

26. Chang AE, Karnell LH, Menck HR. The National Cancer Data Base report on cutaneous and noncutaneous melanoma: a summary of 84.836 cases from the past decade. The American College of Surgeons Commission on Cancer and the American Cancer Society. Cancer 1998;83:1664–78.

27. Ragnarsson-Olding BK, Nilsson BR, Kanter-Lewensohn LR, et al. Malignant melanoma of the vulva in a nationwide, 25-year study of 219 Swedish females: predictors of survival. Cancer 1999;86: 1285–93.

28. Piura B. Management of primary melanoma of the female urogenital tract. Lancet Oncol 2008;9: 973–81.

29. Sugiyama VE, Chan JK, Kapp DS. Management of melanomas of the female genital tract. Curr Opin Oncol 2008;20(5):565–9.

30. Sánchez-Ortiz R, Huang SF, Tamboli P, et al. Melanoma of the penis, scrotum and male urethra: a 40-year single institution experience. J Urol 2005;173(6):1958–65.

31. Vasudeva P, Agrawal D, Goel A. Malignant melanoma of the scrotum. Urology 2008;71(6):1053–4.

32. Gow KW, Rapkin LB, Olson TA, et al. Sentinel lymph node biopsy in the pediatric population. J Pediatr Surg 2008;43(12):2193–8.

33. French JC, Rowe MR, Lee TJO, et al. Pediatric melanoma of the head and neck: a single institution experience. Laryngoscope 2006;116:2216–20.

34. Butter A, Hui T, Chapdelaine J, et al. Melanoma in children and the use of sentinel lymph node biopsy. J Pediatr Surg 2005;40:797–800.

35. Topar G, Zegler B. Assessment of value of the sentinel lymph node biopsy in melanoma in children and adolescents and applicability of subcutaneous infusion anesthesia. J Pediatr Surg 2007;42:1716–20.

36. Pacella SJ, Lowe L, Bradford C, et al. The utility of sentinel lymph node biopsy in head and neck melanoma in the pediatric population. Plast Reconstr Surg 2003;112(5):1257–65.

37. Downard CD, Rapkin LB, Gow KW. Melanoma in children and adolescents. Surg Oncol 2007;16: 215–20.

38. Shah NC, Gerstle JT, Stuart M, et al. Use of sentinel lymph node biopsy and high-dose interferon in pediatric patients with high-risk melanoma: the Hospital for Sick Children experience. J Pediatr Hematol Oncol 2006;28:496–500.

39. Katz VL, Farmer RM, Dotters D. Focus on primary care: from nevus to neoplasm: myths of melanoma in pregnancy. Obstet Gynecol Surv 2002;57(2): 112–9.

40. Silipo V, De Simone P, Mariani G, et al. Malignant melanoma and pregnancy. Melanoma Res 2006; 16(6):497–500.

41. Spanheimer PM, Graham MM, Sugg SL, et al. Measurement of uterine radiation exposure from lymphoscintigraphy indicates safety of sentinel lymph node biopsy during pregnancy. Ann Surg Oncol 2009;16(5):1143–7 [Epub 2009 Mar 7].

42. Driscoll MS, Grant-Kels JM. Nevi and melanoma in the pregnant woman. Clin Dermatol 2009;27: 116–21.

43. Testori A, Soteldo J, Sances D, et al. Cutaneous melanoma in the elderly. Melanoma Res 2009; 19(3):125–34.

44. Sabel MS, Griffith KA, Arora A, et al. Inguinal node dissection for melanoma in the era of sentinel lymph node biopsy. Surgery 2007;141(6):728–35.

Head and Neck Melanoma

David L. Larson, MD[a],*, Jeffrey D. Larson, MD[b]

KEYWORDS

- Malignant melanoma • Head and neck
- Sentinel lymph node • Staging • Lymphadenectomy
- Neck dissection • Treatment

Nearly 20% of malignant melanoma in the human body occurs in the head and neck.[1] Most studies divide the sites of origin of malignant melanoma in the head and neck into the following areas: the face, the scalp and neck, the external ear, and the eyelid or medial or lateral canthal area.[2] Sixty-five percent of malignant melanomas occur in the facial region. Given that the face represents only 3.5% of total body surface area, the face is overrepresented when compared with other sites in the head and neck.

Of the sites of origin in the head and neck, melanoma of the scalp and neck carries the highest mortality, with 10-year survival being only 60%.[3] Melanoma of the ear, face, and eyelid have 10-year survival rates of 70%, 80%, and 90%, respectively.

PATIENTS' WORKUP

Whether patients are being evaluated for the first time or seen in referral from a primary care physician, a thorough patients' workup begins with a complete history of exposure to risk factors and the lesion in question.[4] Patients should be assessed for sun exposure in early childhood, episodes of severe sunburn, or a personal and family history of cutaneous malignancy. Patients should also be questioned about the nature of the lesion, specifically whether there has been a recent change in the last few weeks or months, or if there are symptoms, such as bleeding, itching, pain, or ulceration.

Certain characteristics of skin lesions may indicate a process consistent with melanoma; the acronym "ABCDE" highlights some features of cutaneous lesions that have a high likelihood of being melanomas: Asymmetry, Border irregularity, Color variegation, Diameter greater than 6 mm, Evolution.[5]

When dealing with melanoma, a complete physical examination includes careful palpation of the nodal basins draining the area: the preauricular, parotid, postauricular, suboccipital, posterior cervical, anterior cervical, and supraclavicular nodal groups. If clinical lymphadenopathy is present, further imaging, such as a CT scan, MRI, ultrasound, or fine-needle biopsy may be indicated.

TYPES OF MELANOMA

The most common type of melanoma is superficial spreading, which represents 70% of the cases of melanoma diagnosed in the head and neck.[6]

Nodular melanoma represents 15% to 30% of all cases of melanoma and may easily be mistaken for hemangioma, blue nevi, pyogenic granuloma, or a pigmented basal cell carcinoma.

Lentigo maligna, also known as intraepidermal melanoma or melanoma-in situ, is a precursor to melanoma. Lentigo maligna disease represents a diagnostic dilemma as atypical junctional melanocytic hyperplasia, so adequate margins may be difficult.

Desmoplastic melanoma features abundant collagen and has features consistent with

a Department of Plastic Surgery, Medical College of Wisconsin, 8700 Watertown Plank Road, Milwaukee, WI 53122, USA
b Department of Surgery, Section of Plastic Surgery, University of Wisconsin, Madison, WI, USA
* Corresponding author.
E-mail address: dlarson@mcw.edu (D.L. Larson).

Clin Plastic Surg 37 (2010) 73–77
doi:10.1016/j.cps.2009.08.005

fibromas.[7] There is a high tendency for perineural spread in these lesions. Although this histologic variant represents a small percentage of melanomas throughout the human body (1%), it is over-represented in the head and neck, where 75% of all desmoplastic neurotropic melanomas are found. Furthermore, many of these lesions are amelanotic and thereby make diagnosis difficult.

Mucosal melanoma is a rare, distinct, and separate entity from cutaneous melanoma and should be considered as such. Similar to desmoplastic melanoma, it represents a small portion of overall melanoma subtypes, but nearly half of those diagnosed are found in the head and neck. The nasal cavity is the most common site, specifically the anterior septum, followed by the inferior and middle turbinates. The oral cavity is the second most common site, followed by the larynx.[8]

RISK FACTORS

Risk factors for melanoma of the head and neck are commonly associated with sun exposure, specifically intermittent sun exposure, fair complexion, elevated geographic latitude, and number of lifetime sunburns.[9] Although numerous studies have tried to identify particular patterns of sun exposure that may carry higher risk for developing melanoma, they have failed to display consistent definitions and are subject to recall bias.

Given its numerous deleterious effects on the skin, it is not surprising that sun exposure is a risk factor for developing melanoma.[10] Intermittent sun exposure or an increased number of lifetime sunburns predispose individuals to melanoma formation. Intermittent sun exposure tends to occur on unprotected skin, which penetrates to the melanocytes in the basal layer of the epidermis, whereas repeated exposure of thickened, darkly tanned skin may be effectively blocked by the superficial layers of the epidermis.

PRINCIPLES OF BIOPSY OF A SUSPICIOUS LESION IN THE HEAD AND NECK

The importance of the initial biopsy cannot be overstated. It is essential that every effort be made to perform an excisional biopsy, or at the very least, a large, representative, full-thickness sample of a large, suspicious lesion. Compromise of the biopsy is particularly common in the head and neck because of the many esthetic and functionally important structures in the area. In a study by Austin and colleagues, from M. D. Anderson Cancer Center, a retrospective analysis of 159 melanoma subjects who had a median follow-up

of 38 months was reviewed and matched for stage of disease, ulceration, location, thickness, and mode of biopsy. They found that 31% of subjects who had an incisional biopsy died of disease, whereas only 8.9% of the excisional group died of disease. This study suggests that the mode of biopsy of cutaneous melanomas of the head and neck may influence the clinical outcome.[11,12] However, these findings remain controversial; regardless of failure to perform an excisional biopsy, biopsy loses important prognostic information. With this fact in mind, the physician performing the initial biopsy should consider the following principles:

1. Excisional biopsy with 1 to 3 mm margins is preferred, taking care to avoid wide margins that might interfere with the subsequent lymphatic mapping.
2. Shave biopsy may compromise pathologic diagnosis and measurement of thickness, thereby forcing the treating surgeon to potentially submit patients to more surgical morbidity because of the uncertainty of the actual thickness of the primary.
3. If a punch biopsy is necessary because of location, it should be performed in the thickest portion of the lesion.
4. The specimen must be interpreted by someone who is experienced in interpreting pigmented lesion diagnosis.
5. The specimen must not be submitted for frozen section because this distorts cells, making definitive diagnosis difficult. The specimen should be submitted only for permanent section.

MANAGEMENT OF THE PRIMARY LESION

The mainstay of the initial treatment of melanoma has always been surgical, reserving radiation, chemotherapy, immunotherapy, or combinations of these adjunctive therapies for metastatic disease or prospective studies following a rigid protocol. As in other areas of the body, the treatment of the primary tumor is wide local excision with the margin dictated by its thickness. In the head and neck, there are many esthetically and functional sensitive structures.

There have been several prospective studies that provide the primary basis for the current recommendations for wide excision of melanomas up to 4 mm of thickness.[13] In situ disease should receive between 0.5 to 1 cm margins, with nodal observation, recent studies would suggest more generous margins controlled with staged excisions.[14] Thin lesions (<1 mm) should be widely excised with a 1 cm margin, whereas intermediate thickness

(1–4 mm) would require no more than a 2 cm margin. Lesions greater than 4 mm thick may occasionally need wider margins, although this is a point of controversy in the literature. Reconstruction of the defect from a primary excision is usually accomplished by applying basic principles of surgical reconstruction, using a local flap or a full thickness skin graft (FTSG).

Special locations, such as the ear, should have 1 or 2 cm margins, depending on the thickness of the primary. These margins can be closed primarily when on the helical rim of an otherwise normal-shaped ear. When located in the concha, the cartilage is the deep margin and a FTSG can be placed directly on the underlying dermis, producing a satisfactory esthetic result.

Mucosal melanomas, only 1% of all head and neck melanomas, develop more frequently in the nasal cavity and paranasal sinuses and less often in the oral cavity. Patients present with epistaxis, nasal obstruction, or polyposis with or without pigmentation. Melanoma of the paranasal sinuses are discovered at a more advanced stage. Nodal metastases are distinctly uncommon (<6%) in mucosal melanomas. Surgery is the keystone of therapy, but is frequently augmented with radiation.[8]

An unknown primary is defined as a melanoma that is first identified by its regional, nodal disease (70%) or a distant site (30%). Approximately 10% of head and neck melanomas present in this fashion. These melanomas are thought to have developed from a primary that has since regressed or overlooked. When diagnosed, an exhaustive systemic search should be made for the primary. If found, it is treated as noted earlier in this discussion, but if not uncovered, standard staging is performed and patients are treated as similar staged patients who have a known primary.[13]

Management of lentigo maligna can present a conundrum to the surgeon because of its unpredictable, subclinical extension of atypical disease well beyond the visible margins of the tumor. The work of Neuburg[14] and Jejurikar[15] has given us new insight into the treatment of this common variant of melanoma in the head and neck.

TREATMENT OF THE NECK

If there is metastatic disease to a regional lymph node, the prognosis worsens significantly. Elective lymphadenectomy in head and neck melanoma has been a source of controversy. In theory, removal of occult disease in a node could prevent the spread of disease to distant sites and lengthen survival. There are several large, nonrandomized studies that support this rationale.[13] Timing of the elective surgery, identification of which patients might benefit, and which nodal groups to remove all add to the difficulty of justifying an elective lymphadenectomy. Collectively, data from several trials of this topic would suggest that (1) not all patients benefit from elective lymphadenectomy, (2) patients who have thinner, intermediate thickness primary disease tend to have a survival advantage with the elective procedure, and (3) patients who have occult disease tend to do better with an early nodal dissection rather than waiting for the neck disease to evolve into a palpable node.[13] This problem has been obviated to a great extent with the advent of the sentinel lymph node biopsy (SLNB), which can dependably identify otherwise occult disease.

The role of the SLNB, useful in other anatomic areas, is more challenging in the head and neck area because of the varied drainage patterns and compact arborization of the nodal drainage basins. Some would argue that when a sentinel node is found to be located within the parotid gland, a superficial parotidectomy is the safest procedure to protect facial nerve function. There is also a much greater concentration of sentinel nodes in the head and neck, which further increases morbidity.[16] Regardless, studies have confirmed the accuracy (up to 95% in experienced hands) and safety of lymphoscintigraphy SLNB, when compared with other areas of the body.[16] SLNB remains a valuable diagnostic, but less useful as a therapeutic instrument. There are studies that suggest that, even in the head and neck, lymphatic territories coincide with the vascular territories and branchial origins and contradict the notion that lymphatic drainage in the head and neck is unpredictable or may involve multiple nodal basins.[17] SLNB work has produced the phenomena of the interval sentinel nodes, that is, nodes that are occasionally found outside the conventional nodal basin. In a report by Carling,[18] unequivocal interval sentinel nodes were identified in 8 of 374 subjects (2.1 percent). Three of these eight subjects had metastatic disease in the interval lymph node. In four of the eight subjects, the interval sentinel node was not located in the anticipated lymphatic pathway between the primary tumor and the expected lymph node basin. These findings would suggest that adequate preoperative lymphoscintigraphy and intraoperative recognition of these interval nodes are important in the definitive management of patients who have melanoma. The status of the sentinel node is significant for three reasons[1]: (1) It is the most valuable predictor of the burden of disease patients have and is therefore directly correlated with the prognosis[2]; (2) It can easily and efficiently, with great accuracy, identify patients at high risk who might be candidates for a complete lymphadenectomy or adjunctive treatment (eg, protocol directed)[3]; (3) It provides a measure of psychological benefit to patients when it does not show metastatic disease.[13] If the sentinel node is negative, a regional lymphadenectomy is not typically indicated, though some patients who are at stage III (those with a thick primary and no palpable nodes) might be offered an elective neck dissection.

The application of SLNB to thin (<1 mm) melanomas has been a point of controversy, but there is little question that with certain thin melanomas there is an increased risk for early regional disease and even late recurrence. Nahabedian and colleagues reported on a retrospective review of 24 subjects who had a thin (<1 mm) melanoma, Clark's level III or IV, tumor ulceration, or tumor regression who received regional lymphadenectomy. Two of 24 subjects, both of whom died of disease, had histologically positive metastases, with no recurrence in the other 22 subjects. This outcome led to the authors' recommendation that thin melanomas with ulceration, regression, or a deeper Clark level receive a SLNB.[19]

When regional disease is identified, a therapeutic lymphadenectomy is indicated, as it is curative for approximately 30% of patients. However, by the time regional nodes occur, 70% to 80% of patients have occult distant disease, which will eventually result in their death.[13] This fact should not be justification for not performing a potentially curative operation, but rather speaks to the worsened prognosis with nodal disease. A therapeutic neck dissection should include the node-bearing tissue immediately cephalic, lateral, and inferior to the sentinel node so that all associated lymphatic basins are cleared of potentially life-threatening disease. Palliative therapeutic neck dissection might be considered in selected patients who have distant disease because of the morbidity of uncontrolled loco-regional melanomas and its negative impact on dying patients.

ADJUNCTIVE THERAPY FOR MELANOMA OF THE HEAD AND NECK

Although completion of cervical lymphadenectomy is usually performed after SLNB for melanoma, there is some evidence that suggests that radiation therapy (XRT) might be effective for some patients in lieu of formal lymph-node dissection. Ballo and colleagues, from M. D. Anderson Cancer Center, reported on 36 subjects who had parotid or cervical nodal disease, treated with excision of only the nodal disease and postoperative XRT without formal nodal dissection. Radiation was delivered

to the primary site, the nodal site of excision, and the ipsilateral, undissected neck. With a median follow-up period of 5.3 years, disease recurred in the regional basin in only two subjects and at distant sites in 14 subjects. The 5-year regional control and distant metastases-free rates were 93% and 59%, respectively.[20]

On the other hand, to this point there has been no randomized trial that shows that chemotherapy increases the survival of patients who have melanoma and therefore it should not be considered as standard therapy outside of a clinical trial on protocol. The combination of chemotherapeutic agents and biologic therapies (interferon [IFN]-alpha or interleukin [IL]-2) has been performed in patients who have advanced melanoma, including those who have mucosal melanoma of the head and neck,[21] with some limited success.

In short, there is not conclusive evidence that any therapy adjunctive to standard surgical management is effective.

FOLLOW-UP AND SURVEILLANCE

As a result of developing melanoma of the head and neck, patients are at risk to develop a recurrence but are also at greater risk than the general population to develop a second primary; therefore, follow-up in conjunction with diligent surveillance is essential. This point must be stressed to patients and their families as part of the discussion of the management of the melanoma. Of course, the earlier the detection, the greater chance of definitive treatment of the new melanoma problem. Much of the head and neck is readily visible to patients, but some areas, such as the scalp and nape of the neck, are less so and a family member or spouse should be recruited to participate in the self examination.

For early, in situ (stage 0) disease, an annual skin examination associated with monthly self examinations is sufficient. With thin lesions (<1 mm) without ulceration and level II/III (Stage 1A), a history and physical (with emphasis on nodes and skin) every 3 to 12 months for 5 years and then annually, in association with self examination of the skin and node-bearing areas, is suggested. For all other disease, Stages 1B through IV, all of the above plus a chest X ray, lactic dehydrogenise (LDH), and an optional complete blood count (CBC) every 6 to 12 months for 3 to 4 years and then annually, is suggested. Routine imaging is not recommended unless there are specific indications or there is a high risk for metastases (eg, a thicker lesion with ulceration).[13]

Once there is a local, satellite, in-transit, or nodal recurrence, a more vigorous and diligent follow-up regimen is indicated.

REFERENCES

1. Garbe C, Buttner P, Bertz J, et al. Primary cutaneous melanoma: prognostic classification of anatomic location. Cancer 1995;75(10):2492–8.
2. Wanebo HJ, Cooper PH, Young DV, et al. Prognostic factors in head and neck melanoma: effect of lesion location. Cancer 1988;62:831–7.
3. Ringborg U, Afzelius LE, Lagerlof B, et al. Cutaneous malignant melanoma of the head and neck; analysis of treatment results and prognostic factors in 581 patients: a report from the Swedish Melanoma Study Group. Cancer 1993;71(3):751–8.
4. Myers E, Nemecheck D. Malignant melanoma. In: Myers E, Namecheck D, editors. Head and Neck Surgery – Otolaryngology. 4th edition. Baltimore: Lippincott, Williams and Wilkins; 2006. p. 383–401.
5. Kienstra MA, Paphya TA. Head and neck melanoma. Cancer Control 2005;12:242–6.
6. Schmalbach CE, Johnson TM, Bradford CR. The management of head and neck melanoma. Curr Probl Surg 2006;43:781–835.
7. Quinn MJ, Crotty KA, Thompson JF. Desmoplastic and desmoplastic neurotropic melanoma: experience with 280 patients. Cancer 1998;83(6):1128–35.
8. Meleti M, Leemans CR, deBree R, et al. Head and neck mucosal melanoma: experience with 42 patients, with emphasis on the role of postoperative radiotherapy. Head Neck 2008;30:1543–51.
9. Berwick M, Armstrong BK, Ben-Porat L, et al. Sun exposure and mortality from melanoma. J Natl Cancer Inst 2005;97(3):195–9.
10. Gandini S, Sera F, Cattaruzza MS, et al. Meta-analysis of risk factors for cutaneous melanoma: II. Sun exposure. Eur J Cancer 2005;41:45–60.
11. Austin JR, Byers RM, Brown WD, et al. Influence of biopsy on the prognosis of cutaneous melanoma of the head and neck. Head Neck 1996;18:107–17.
12. Balch CM, Buzaid AC, Soong S-J, et al. Final version of the American Joint Committee on cancer staging system for cutaneous melanoma. J Clin Oncol 2001; 19:3635–48.
13. Wagner JD, Gordon MS, Chuang TY, et al. Current therapy of cutaneous melanoma. Plast Reconstr Surg 2000;105:1774–99.
14. Bosbous MW, Dzwierzynski WD, Neuburg M. Staged excision of lentigo maligna melanoma: a 10-year experience. Plastic and Reconstructive Surgery [in press].
15. Jejurikar SS, Borschel GH, Johnson TM, et al. Immediate, optimal reconstruction of facial lentigo maligna and melanoma following total peripheral margin control. Plast Reconstr Surg 2007;120: 1249–55.
16. McMasters KM, Reintgen DS, Ross MI, et al. Sentinel lymph node biopsy for melanoma: controversy despite widespread agreement. J Clin Oncol 2001;19:2851–5.
17. Aydin AA, Okudan B, Aydin ZD. Lymphoscintigraphic drainage patterns of the auricle in healthy subjects. Head Neck 2005;27:893–900.
18. Carling T, Pan D, Ariyan S, et al. Diagnosis and treatment of interval sentinel lymph nodes in patients with cutaneous melanoma. Plast Reconstr Surg 2007; 119:907–13.
19. Nahabedian MY, Tufaro AP, Manson PN. Sentinel lymph node biopsy for the T1 (thin) melanoma: is it necessary? Ann Plast Surg 2003;50.601–6.
20. Ballo MT, Garden AS, Myers JN, et al. Melanoma metastatic to cervical lymph node: can radiotherapy replace formal dissection after local excision of nodal disease? Head Neck 2005;27:718–21.
21. Bartell HL, Bedkian AY, Papadopoulos NE. Biochemotherapy in patients with advanced head and neck mucosal melanoma. Head Neck 2008;30: 1592–8.

The Role of Lymphatic Mapping and Sentinel Lymph Node Biopsy in the Staging and Treatment of Melanoma

Wayne K. Stadelmann, MD, FACS

KEYWORDS
- Melanoma • Sentinel lymph node • Biopsy • Staging
- Lymphoscintigram

The incidence of malignant melanoma is increasing at an alarming rate, doubling in women and growing by more 300% in men during the past 25 years.[1] In the United States, the projected number of newly diagnosed cases of melanoma for 2008 is 62,000, with 8000 people expected to die from the disease.[2] Although the incidence of melanoma has increased over the last 25 years, mortality from the disease has not. This improvement is in part due to the great strides in greater public awareness, dermatologic screening examinations, and earlier diagnosis. The surgical treatment of melanoma has also undergone tremendous change with the establishment of recommended wide local excision margins determined by tumor thickness and based on prospective studies,[3–6] and the introduction of selective lymph node biopsy to allow the more accurate staging of clinically node-negative patients.[7] The importance of diagnosing nodal metastatic disease, with the ability to detect smaller and smaller volumes of tumor in the sentinel lymph nodes (SLNs) biopsied using immunohistochemical staining, has impacted the accurate staging and stratification of melanoma patients, allowing various treatment protocols to be rigorously compared and evaluated. Lastly, the development of effective chemotherapy in the form of FDA-approved interferon-α2b for high-risk primary melanomas and those with nodal disease has begun to show promise for extending survival in those with this highly lethal disease.[8]

The importance of nodal status featured prominently in the most recent American Joint Committee on Cancer (AJCC) staging system for melanoma, which was revised in 2002 and completely implemented in 2003 (**Table 1**).[9–11] The role that elective lymph node dissection now plays in staging the melanoma patient and determining subsequent treatment has been greatly diminished in favor of less morbid and less invasive techniques that have a higher degree of accuracy in detecting occult nodal disease.[12] This article explores what has driven the advent of selective or SLN biopsy, the rationale behind obtaining a preoperative lymphoscintigram, the technical details of the SLN procedure, and the refinement in the pathologic detection of ever smaller volumes of tumor in nymph node tissue removed. Finally, the role that these new modalities have played in changing the dynamic field of melanoma care is emphasized.

VARIABLES THAT INFLUENCE PROGNOSIS IN CUTANEOUS MELANOMA

There are many variables that have been found to predict clinical outcomes and therefore may influence the treatment of patients with melanoma.[13] Among the most prognostic variables in AJCC stage I and II (absence of nodal disease) that determine the risk for nodal involvement and 5-year survival are tumor thickness, the presence of tumor ulceration, anatomic location (extremity

Stadelmann Center for Plastic Surgery, 248 Pleasant Street, Suite 201, Concord, NH 03301, USA
E-mail address: nitro3706@aol.com

Clin Plastic Surg 37 (2010) 79–99
doi:10.1016/j.cps.2009.08.001
0094-1298/09/$ – see front matter © 2010 Elsevier Inc. All rights reserved.

Table 1
The most current AJCC staging system

Stage	Description
IA	Tumor ≤1.0 mm without ulceration and Clarks level II/III No lymph node involvement and no distant metastases
IB	Tumor ≤1.0 mm with ulceration and Clarks level IV/V Tumor 1.01–2.0 mm without ulceration No lymph node involvement and no distant metastases
IIA	Tumor 1.01 to 2.0 mm with ulceration Tumor 2.01 to 4.0 mm without ulceration No lymph node involvement and no distant metastases
IIB	Tumor 2.01–4.0 mm with ulceration Tumor >4.01 mm without ulceration No lymph node involvement and no distant metastases
IIC	Tumor >4.01 mm with ulceration No lymph node involvement and no distant metastases
IIIA	Tumor of any thickness without ulceration 1–3 positive micrometastatic lymph nodes
IIIB	Tumor of any thickness without ulceration with 1–3 positive macrometastatic lymph nodes Tumor of any thickness with ulceration with 1–3 positive micrometastatic lymph nodes Tumor of any thickness with 2–3 positive lymph nodes and in transit metastasis/satellite(s) metastasis
IIIC	Tumor of any thickness with ulceration with 1–3 positive macrometastatic lymph nodes Tumor of any thickness with 4 or more metastatic lymph nodes, or matted nodes, or in transit metastasis/satellite(s) metastasis
IV	Tumor of any thickness with any nodes and any distant metastases

Adapted from Balch CM, Buzaid AC, Soong S-J, et al. Final version of the American Joint Committee on Cancer staging system for cutaneous melanoma. J Clin Oncol 2001;19:3635–48; with permission.

versus trunk versus head and neck), surgical treatment of the primary tumor, and male gender.[14] If melanoma has been found to be metastatic to regional lymph nodes, the significance of the microscopic characteristics of the primary tumor as well as any clinical variables become significantly less important.[15] Once lymph node involvement is established, the 5-year survival rate drops precipitously by approximately 40% compared with those patients who demonstrate no nodal involvement.[16] Knowing the nodal status therefore has significant importance in discussing prognosis in melanoma patients and in orchestrating further treatments such as completion/therapeutic nodal basin dissection (TLND), meeting with a medical oncologist to discuss the possibility of starting chemotherapy, and also in qualifying for and subsequently enrolling in clinical trials.

THE SENTINEL LYMPH NODE CONCEPT

The relationship between the primary cancer location and the metastatic spread of that cancer to a specific regional lymph node was first described by Virchow[17] in 1863. In 1955 Seaman and

Powers,[18] using radiolabeled colloidal gold, described the metastatic spread of cancer cells to regional lymph nodes by way of lymphatic channels. The first use of the term "sentinel node" was in 1960 by Gould and colleagues[19] to describe the presence of a first lymph node or "sentinel node" in a nodal basin to which cancers would initially travel. Radiologic lymphatic mapping in the evaluation of cutaneous cancer metastases was first introduced clinically by Cabanas[20] in the treatment of penile carcinoma in 1977. Morton and colleagues[7] were the first to popularize the concept that lymphatic drainage was neither capricious nor random, and that melanoma nodal metastases occur in an orderly, stepwise fashion. These investigators also asserted that a sentinel node biopsy was representative of the nodal basin to which it belonged, and that a negative sentinel node correlated very closely to lack of metastatic involvement of the remaining lymph nodes in that basin. Further confirmatory studies published by Thompson and colleagues and Reintgen and colleagues[21–23] showed very similar results, indicating that the SLN biopsy provides equally reliable diagnostic data as that obtained by an elective lymph node basin dissection. If the SLN is found to be negative for metastatic disease then the negative predictive value for the remaining nodal basin is on the order of 95%.[24] The current use of the term sentinel node biopsy incorporates the preoperative localization of the nodal basin(s) at risk, the intraoperative harvesting of the sentinel node(s) usually using radioisotope as well blue dye localization, and the comprehensive pathologic evaluation of the nodal tissue once removed.

The concept of an SLN provides an elegant means to explain the pattern of metastatic disease in not only cutaneous cancers such as melanoma, squamous cell, basal cell, and Merkel cell carcinoma but also other organ-specific tumors such as breast, colon, and other visceral malignancies.[25–29] Melanoma typically metastasizes initially to regional lymph node basins and from there to distant sites such as the liver, bone, brain, and so forth. This fact was the primary driving force behind performing elective lymph node dissections (ELND) in the preselective lymph node biopsy era. The theory behind SLN mapping is that for any given area of skin, there is an afferent lymphatic channel that leads to a specific first-draining lymph node, the sentinel node. The sentinel node, therefore, is the first node to which melanoma would spread. Melanoma nodal metastases are believed to progress in an orderly and nonrandom fashion.[22,24] The SLN therefore accurately reflects the status of the lymph nodes contained in that nodal basin. The likelihood that the SLN is negative while another nonsentinel node in the same nodal basin is positive (a "skip" metastasis or false negative) is rare, occurring in less than 1% of SLNs removed.[7] Sentinel lymph node biopsies are particularly useful for melanomas in areas with ambiguous lymphatic drainage (eg, head and neck, the midline trunk) and where multiple SLNs are the rule rather than the exception. Failure to identify and subsequently remove all the SLNs represents an inadequate nodal staging procedure that may potentially place the patient at higher risk for nodal as well as visceral recurrences.[30]

THE DIMINISHING ROLE OF ELECTIVE LYMPH NODE BIOPSY IN FAVOR OF SELECTIVE LYMPH NODE BIOPSY

Controversy continues to surround the issue of how to address the possibility of occult regional nodal metastases in clinically node-negative melanoma patients (AJCC stages I and II). In the preselective node biopsy era, patients with thin melanomas (<1.00 mm) without clinical nodal involvement were believed to have a very good

chance for cure with local excision alone without a prophylactic or ELND (removal of a clinically negative nodal basin). In contrast, patients with thick melanomas (>4.00 mm) and no clinical nodal disease were not believed to benefit from ELND, as they exhibit a very high incidence of both regional and distant metastatic disease.[31] These individuals would be followed and if nodal disease developed, a therapeutic node dissection would be offered. Therefore, elective lymph node dissection had been advocated for the lymphatic basins draining the site of a primary melanoma of intermediate thickness (1.00–4.00 mm) in an attempt to remove occult nodal metastases before nodal spread became palpable. To date, of the 4 randomized prospective studies designed to evaluate the benefit of ELND in patients with 1.00- to 4.00-mm thick primary melanoma, none has demonstrated a clear survival advantage with this technique in this population of patients.[32–35] A major concern in performing an ELND is that only about 20% of patients will be found to have nodal metastases, and therefore 80% of patients undergoing an ELND will be subjected to the potentially significant morbidity of an operation that they did not require. Furthermore, in patients with melanoma primaries located in areas with ambiguous nodal drainage patterns such as over the head and neck and midline trunk, more than one nodal basin may need to be dissected. If these nodal basins are not discovered by preoperative lymphoscintigraphy, the ELND may be performed on nodal basins at low risk of harboring disease, decreasing the effectiveness of the operation even further. There are some data to suggest that elective lymph node dissection may improve survival in some patients mainly those with intermediate-thickness melanomas who have an ELND guided by preoperative lymphatic mapping.[36] A subgroup analysis of one such trial, the Intergroup Melanoma Surgical Trial, demonstrated improved survival rates in individuals with melanoma primaries between 1 and 2 mm thick located on the extremities in persons younger than 60 years.[37] If an SLN biopsy cannot be performed for whatever reason, these clinical guidelines should be considered in determining future surgical care (see later discussion).

Waiting until palpable disease develops in a nodal basin before performing a nodal basin dissection (a TLND) has been shown to correlate with a worse outcome (50%–60% for TLND vs 15%–35% for ELND).[36] Only patients who have a high likelihood of having nodal involvement ideally would be offered a full nodal basin dissection. This area is where sentinel node technology may have its greatest impact. With this relatively new technology, the indications for ELND are becoming increasingly limited, saving many melanoma patients the potential morbidity and costs associated with this type of a staging procedure. The prognostic value of a staging SLN biopsy is clearly demonstrated by the 5-year survival statistics from the AJCC melanoma database analyzing tumors greater than 1.0 mm.[38] With *clinical* node-negative staging the 5-year survival was 65%, for negative staging *based on ELND* it was 75%, while *based on negative SLN* data the survival rate was 90%.[39]

Regardless of the method used, local nodal basin evaluation is intended to provide regional lymph node staging based on pathologic tissue sampling, regional disease control, and provision of potential cure by removing nodal disease. These goals would ideally be met with the lowest morbidity possible, while still achieving a high diagnostic and prognostic yield.[40]

LYMPHATIC MAPPING

Blood vessels are porous to water and low molecular weight proteins, allowing the translocation of edema fluid into the interstitial space, thereby creating lymph. Lymphatic fluid is removed by lymphatic channels, which serve to return the third space fluid back to the venous and eventually to the arterial circulation. The lymphatic channels also channel the fluid to regional lymph nodes, where any foreign debris and bacteria are phagocytosed and removed by white blood cells. Most carcinomas use the lymphatic channels during their metastatic spread and become "trapped" in regional lymph nodes, where they may be subjected to the sterilizing action of immunocompetent cells. Taking into consideration the molecular weight of lymphatic fluid, liquids of similar composition can be injected intradermally around a cutaneous cancer site and can be traced to the regional nodal basin(s), identifying lymph nodes at risk for harboring metastatic cells. This process is called lymphatic mapping, and may be performed using either dyes or radioactive colloids. Both methods are used to perform an SLN biopsy when treating melanoma.

INCORPORATION OF PREOPERATIVE LYMPHOSCINTIGRAPHY

Sappey,[41] in 1864, described injecting mercury into human cadaver dermis and observing its migration to regional lymph nodes. The use of radioactive particles to map lymphatic spread was introduced in 1953 by Sherman and Ter-Pogossian[42] using radioactive gold. Radioactive gold was later replaced by ^{99m}Tc-sulfur colloid (termed radiocolloid) in the late 1960s and 1970s.[43,44] The agents used for lymphatic mapping should be compounds that have a small enough particle size to allow their translocation from the dermal location into the lymphatics. In addition, the agents should have a short radioactive half-life. Both of these requirements are met by ^{99m}Tc-labeled sulfur colloids, which travel to local lymph nodes relatively rapidly, emit γ-rays that image well, and have a half-life of only 6 hours and decay entirely after 2.5 days.[45]

Preoperative lymphatic mapping serves several important functions. First, it identifies all the nodal basins at risk for metastatic spread, allowing each nodal basin so identified to be evaluated with an SLN biopsy. Second, the number of sentinel nodes in a particular basin can also be estimated, allowing the surgeon to be more vigilant in the search for all nodes at risk for nodal disease. Third, preoperative mapping may identify in-transit nodes, such as the popliteal and epitrochlear sites, that would normally not be identified and removed, to detect nodal metastases.[46] Such interval nodes have the same incidence of harboring metastatic disease as an SLN retrieved from the neighboring nodal basin. The incidence of in-transit nodes ranges between 0.5% in the legs and up to 12% in the posterior trunk primaries.[47] Although extremity melanomas have been relatively easy to identify in lymphatic drainage basins, lymphatic mapping using radiocolloids has been especially valuable in identifying draining lymphatic basins, especially when the primary tumor is located in areas with ambiguous drainage pathways. This situation holds true particularly over the entire head and neck area, as well as over the shoulders and midline trunk regions (see later discussion).

On the day of the wide local excision and the SLN biopsy, preoperative lymphoscintigraphy typically is performed in the department of nuclear medicine, using 250 to 600 µCi of cold-filtered technetium-99m sulfur colloid injected intradermally in equal quadrants around the site of the primary tumor. On occasion the lymphoscintigram may be performed up to 24 hours before operative treatment to accommodate the nuclear medicine schedule or if an early start time is requested for the melanoma operation. The absolute counts are reduced by this maneuver; however, the SLNs are still able to be easily identified with the hand-held gamma probe and removed. Anterior-posterior and lateral radiographic views are then taken at 1 minute, 10 minutes, and 2 hours after injection using a large field-of-view gamma detection camera (**Fig. 1**). When lymphoscintigraphy was initially introduced in the treatment of melanoma, many cancer centers were performing the

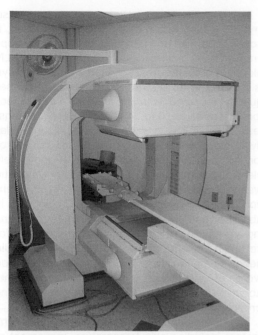

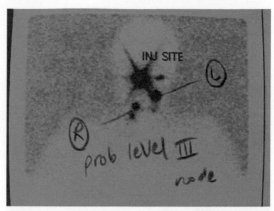

Fig. 2. The preoperative lymphoscintigrams can be hard to interpret for the novice sentinel node surgeon. In this head and neck lymphoscintigram, multiple nodes are seen and highlighted, and there is also bilateral drainage. Consulting with the radiologist to determine which nodes took up the radiocolloid first would be helpful in making an operative plan. In this situation, SLNs from each cervical area and the left parotid basin should be and were removed.

Fig. 1. The large-field-of-view gamma camera is essential for obtaining good-quality lymphoscintigraphic images.

preoperative lymphoscintigram several days before the SLN harvest. Radioactive sulfur colloid was again injected intradermally at the tumor site just before the wide local excision (WLE) to ensure high readings. This procedure is rarely performed today as the hand-held gamma probes are very sensitive at detecting even minute amounts of radioactive material, and the lymphoscintigrams are scheduled to occur on the day before or on the day of the operation and not days in advance. ^{99m}Tc-sulfur colloid has its greatest nodal concentration between 2 and 4 hours after injection, making localization of the SLN(s) on the day of the preoperative lymphoscintigram the most logical.[16] The images produced by the preoperative lymphoscintigram are somewhat "fuzzy" and may be hard to interpret for the novice SLN surgeon (**Fig. 2**). Discussing the findings with the nuclear radiologist may prove to be helpful in interpreting the images and planning the operative approach to harvesting the SLN(s). Current lymphoscintigraphic imaging provides a 2-dimensional imaging of the nodes to be removed but cannot localize their exact location in 3 dimensions. Newer scanners are being introduced that can provide images in "3D" by allowing the images to be manipulated and rotated 360°. Any markings made by the radiologist or the nuclear medicine technicians pertaining to the location of the SLNs should be confirmed by the surgeon

with the hand-held gamma probe before final patient positioning and prepping.

INCORPORATION OF VITAL BLUE DYE IN THE SENTINEL LYMPH NODE BIOPSY

Morton and colleagues[7,21] described using blue dye injected directly intradermally at the melanoma biopsy site to identify the afferent lymphatics and stain the SLN a brilliant blue color. Several dyes were initially investigated for their lymphatic transit times and staining patterns including fluorescein, patent blue-V, Cyalume, isosulfan blue, and methylene blue.[16] Isosulfan blue 1% aqueous solution proved to perform the best in terms of visualization with the unassisted eye in ambient operating room lighting; it has minimal collateral tissue diffusion, and has a rapid speed of migration to and retention within regional nodal basins (**Fig. 3**).

The use of intraoperative blue dye to identify an SLN is relatively safe; however, certain adverse effects are known to occur. Momeni and Ariyan,[48] in a series of 84 patients undergoing an SLN for melanoma, reported that 20% experienced a significant decline ($\geq$2%) in pulse oximetry oxygen saturations, reaching a nadir at about 23 minutes after the injection. Although the decline in oxygenation in erroneous, it could lead to unnecessary interventions and concern over the patients' well-being. The injection of isosulfan

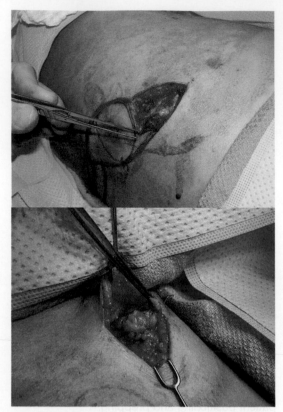

Fig. 3. Isosulfan blue dye is a good tracer as it stains the lymphatics a bright blue color, has little collateral tissue staining, and is retained by the lymph nodes during the duration of the operation. In these images, the lymphatics are seen leaving the primary site and then the dye is concentrated in an axillary SLN. This node also had high radiation counts and proved to be free of metastatic disease on immunohistochemical evaluation.

blue dye is associated with rare incidences of allergic reactions, ranging between 0.7% and 2.0%.[49–52] Montgomery and colleagues[52] described 3 grades of allergic reactions: grade 3 reactions are anaphylactoid with associated cardiovascular collapse and a systolic blood pressure of less than 70 mm Hg; grade 2 reactions are transient hypotension with blood pressure being maintained at greater than 70 mm Hg; and grade 1 reactions are defined as "blue hives" and as a generalized rash. Deaths associated with blue dye injections are very rare and probably reflect that the injections are done in a hospital/operating room setting with immediate availability of full resuscitative services. It is good practice to announce to the anesthesiologist exactly when the blue dye is being injected and to mention the rare risk of adverse effects on the blood pressure and pulse oximeter readings.

The intradermal injection of blue dye also imparts a blue tattoo at the injection site that, if not excised, can persist for many months postoperatively. This stain is mainly an issue when an SLN biopsy is done for breast cancer, and the blue dye is injected in an area of skin that is not subsequently resected with the mastectomy/lumpectomy procedure (**Fig. 4**). Over the distal legs, feet, and back where the lymphatic flow is relatively slow, the blue hue may persist for a prolonged time and may actually never completely clear. In the head and neck region, the lymphatic washout rates are typically high, making the retention on blue dye short-lived. The blue dye is absorbed and cleared by the renal system, imparting a greenish tint to the urine that may persist for several hours after the procedure (**Fig. 5**). To avoid needless phone calls and the need to provide words of reassurance, it is best to inform patients about the color change in their urine preoperatively.

The rate of lymph flow is dependent on several factors including skin temperature, movement of the body part, body location, and the presence of external pressure.[47] Under ideal conditions, the blue dye travels through the lymphatics relatively quickly at a rate ranging between 10 cm per minute in the lower extremity and foot to 1.5 cm per minute in the head and neck.[47] When the dye is injected before doing the surgical prep, enough time usually passes to allow the dye to reach a sufficient concentration in the nodal basin, making visual identification of the SLN simple; this is especially true in distal extremity primary sites. Massaging the injection site after the introduction of the dye also promotes dermal blood flow and associated lymph production, speeding the washout of the dye toward the nodal basin(s).[47]

INTRAOPERATIVE GAMMA PROBE SENTINEL LYMPH NODE LOCALIZATION

Without question, the introduction of the hand-held gamma probe has had a significant impact on the ease of use of SLN technology, and has made the technique more widely applicable to multiple tumor types. The gamma probe has also made the technique less technically demanding and thereby has opened up SLN mapping to a greater number of surgeons in academic as well as community practices. The first use of intraoperative lymphatic mapping to identify sentinel nodal tissue using a hand-held gamma detector was reported by Alex and colleagues and Krag and colleagues in 1993 and 1995, and by Van der Veen and colleagues in 1994.[53–55] Gamma probe localization was pursued because using

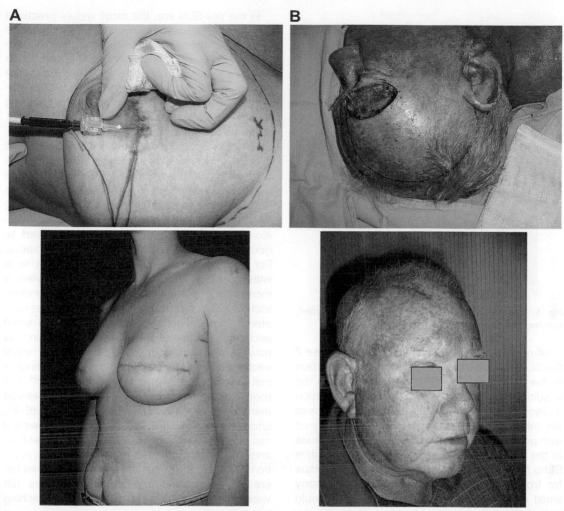

Fig. 4. (*A*) Isosulfan blue dye injected intradermally can result in a permanent blue-hue tattoo. In these images a women underwent an SLN biopsy at the time of her mastectomy for breast cancer. The injected skin was not excised and she was reconstructed immediately using saline breast implants. The lower image depicts the patient 1 year later. The blue hue can still be visualized. (*B*) In contrast to the previous image, SLN biopsies for melanoma typically remove all of the blue dye injected at the primary site. The patient is shown here 6 months after a resection of a right eyebrow melanoma and after a scalp rotation flap was used to reconstruct the defect with a full-thickness skin graft for the brow itself. There is no residual blue hue present.

blue dye alone as a sole modality to identify an SLN was often difficult, if not impossible, with only about 85% of SLN overall and considerably fewer in the head and neck region being retrieved.[40,56] Combining blue dye with intradermal [99mTc]-labled sulfur colloid has increased the overall retrieval rate from approximately 84% to 96% to 99% (**Table 2**).[36,57] Therefore, approximately 16% of melanoma patients who were treated with SLN biopsies using blue dye alone would have had an unsuccessful SLN biopsy, and would be at risk for having occult nodal disease undiagnosed and potentially undertreated. In this scenario, the option would be to adopt a "wait and watch" approach or proceed

to an ELND. With the combined modalities, the need to default to an ELND has been significantly reduced, as the successful retrieval rates are close to 100%.

STANDARDIZATION OF PATHOLOGIC EVALUATION

With the advent of SLN biopsy techniques, the amount of nodal tissue delivered to the pathologist has become increasingly small. The ability to accurately determine nodal involvement has also become increasingly more complex. Initially, SLNs were often examined using frozen section analysis while the surgeon waited to perform either

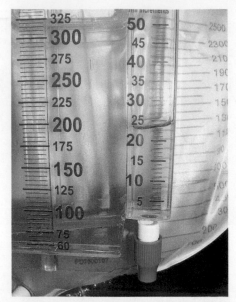

Fig. 5. The isosulfan blue dye is renally excreted, turning the urine an eerie green color.

a full nodal basin dissection for stage 3 disease if the SLN was positive, or to end the nodal portion of the operation if the SLN was negative.[7] In the ensuing years it was shown that frozen section analysis of the SLN has a low sensitivity, due to the inferior quality of frozen sections compared with permanent section analysis and also because of the low tumor burden present in most positive SLNs (typically <2 mm focus).[40,58] Preparing tissue for frozen section evaluation may also destroy small quantities of diagnostic tissue that would potentially be used to identify metastases by more sophisticated methods. At present, frozen section analysis should be performed only as a confirmatory maneuver for grossly positive lymph nodes that contain large quantities of metastatic disease (**Fig. 6**). Clinically benign nodes should be submitted to fixative for more intensive evaluation and not examined using frozen section techniques.

In the pre-SLN era, the most widely practiced permanent method of evaluating lymph nodes for metastatic disease was to submerge the specimen in fixative and then section the node once or twice in the central area, and stain the tissue with hematoxylin and eosin (H&E). In 1988 Cochran and colleagues[59] described simple bivalving of the nodes after fixation along with H&E staining. Although adequate for macroscopic nodal involvement, microscopic examination of nodes treated in such a manner examines less than 1% to 5% of the submitted specimen and is estimated to underdiagnose up to 5% to 15% of positive SLNs.[40] Incorporating serial sectioning (dividing the node multiple times at a prescribed thickness) along with routine H&E staining is believed to double number of nodes being read as positive. For micrometastatic disease, as with that seen with most SLN specimens, the diagnostic yield is increased further with the addition of immunohistochemical stains specific for melanoma-associated tumor antigens in combination with serial sectioning.[24] Immunohistochemical staining is now routinely performed in addition to serial sectioning and H&E staining to detect 1 melanoma cell in a background of 10^5 normal cells.[24] The most commonly used immunohistochemical markers used today are S-100 protein, HMB-45, and Melan-A/MART-1. The immunohistochemical markers MAGE3, the gp100 gene, tyrosinase, and reverse transcriptase-polymerase chain reaction (RT-PCR) are either of low diagnostic yield or are still considered experimental, and are not widely employed outside of academic teaching institutions.[40]

When performing pathologic examination on ELND specimens, the detailed use of these diagnostic tools is not common, due to the time required and expense involved in subjecting all the lymph nodes obtained to these techniques. With an SLN biopsy, the surgeon is delivering one or a few lymph nodes to the pathologist. These lymph nodes have been determined with

Table 2
Comparison between using blue dye alone and in combination with radiocolloid SLN localization

Improved localization of SLN using blue dye and radiolabeled colloid			
Basin	Dye Alone	Dye & Colloid	P Value
Cervical	56%	97%	0.002
Axillary	84%	98%	<0.00001
Inguinal	95%	100%	<0.03
Total	87%	99%	<0.00001

Data from Gershenwald JE, Tseng C-H, Thompson W, et al. Improved sentinel lymph node localization in patients with primary melanoma with the use of radiolabeled colloid. Surgery 1998;124:203–10.

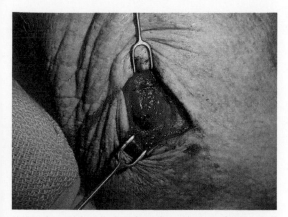

Fig. 6. A grossly positive lymph node was found that was blue stained and radioactive. The patient had no clinical adenopathy preoperatively. In this situation, a confirmatory frozen section analysis would be warranted if a cervical node dissection was going to be done immediately. In this case, this was not done and the patient indeed was found to have nodal disease. He later returned to the operating room for a formal functional neck dissection.

preoperative lymphoscintigraphy and intraoperative lymphatic mapping to be representative of the entire nodal basin. The pathologist accordingly is able to subject these nodes to more intensive scrutiny to determine the presence of metastatic disease. SLN biopsies are therefore believed to render more precise diagnostic information than performing an ELND.

WHEN TO OFFER A SENTINEL LYMPH NODE BIOPSY

The rationale for offering an SLN biopsy include: it potentially reduces the risk of regional recurrence; it is minimally invasive and is associated with low morbidity; if positive, the patient would be eligible for further treatment such as completion nodal dissection, interferon-α2b treatment, or enrollment in investigational trials; and the SLN status is

a strong prognostic indicator of survival. Reasons to not offer an SLN biopsy include: no survival advantage has been documented to date; there are additional costs and possible morbidity; and not all patients are candidates for completion nodal basin dissection, interferon therapy, or are eligible to enroll in clinical trails.

Although to date SLN biopsies have not definitively been shown to impact ultimate survival, accurate staging is very useful in guiding care in terms of further completion lymph node basin dissection as well as instituting adjuvant therapy. Of note, SLN status is highly predictive of future survival. In one study incorporating 1487 melanoma patients with a mean tumor thickness of 1.5 mm, those with a positive SLN had a 5-year survival of 73% whereas a negative SLN had an associated 5-year survival of 97%.[36] This result also holds true for thick melanomas greater than 4 mm.[60] Other investigators remain uncertain as to the true benefit that SLN plays in predicting overall survival, even though there is proven predictive value in evaluating disease-free survival at 5 years.[61] When the SLN is found to harbor micrometastatic disease with a nonulcerated primary, the 5-year survival is 69%. Compare this to palpable nodal disease with 3 or more positive nodes and an ulcerated primary tumor, for which the 5-year survival is only 13%.[38] Given these numbers, it is generally believed that any individual with a melanoma thicker than 1.00 mm and having no evidence of clinical nodal or visceral organ involvement should be offered an SLN biopsy, as the incidence of positive nodes is directly related to the thickness of the primary tumor (**Table 3**).[24,56]

The question arises often as to when to offer melanoma patients an SLN diagnostic procedure when the diagnostic yield becomes ever less fruitful as the melanoma primary becomes thinner. Very thin melanomas (<0.76 mm) may, however, have a positive SLN. Bleicher and colleagues[62] reported an incidence of 1.7% positive SLN biopsy specimens in 1661 patients with very thin primary

Table 3
Incidence of positive SLN biopsies in relation to primary tumor thickness

TumorThickness in Millimeters	Percentage of Positive SLN Biopsied
≤1.00	3.2
1.01–2.00	10.3
2.01–3.00	19.8
3.01–4.00	37.7
≥4.01	44.3

Data from Gershenwald JE, Tseng C-H, Thompson W, et al. Improved sentinel lymph node localization in patients with primary melanoma with the use of radiolabeled colloid. Surgery 1998;124:203–10.

tumors. For melanomas between 0.75 mm to 1.00 mm, SLN biopsies were positive 8% of the time,[63] whereas other studies have shown that the incidence of a positive SLN in thin melanomas (<1.00 mm) is between 5% and 6%.[64,65] Even in thin melanomas less than 1 mm thick, SLN status remains highly prognostic, yet offering this diagnostic test to every melanoma patient with thin tumors is neither practical nor a good use of resources.[66] The decision to do an SLN biopsy in thin melanoma patients may therefore be based on the presence of poor prognostic indicators of the primary tumor such as ulceration, a positive primary deep margin, severe tumor regression, Clark level of III or higher, male gender, young age, microsatellitosis, higher mitotic rate, vertical growth phase, axial anatomic location and a primary tumor over the head, scalp, and neck, and if diagnostic screening tests (chest radiography, lactate dehydrogenase, liver function tests) are not suggestive of metastatic disease.[64] Sondak and colleagues[64] reported a strong correlation between tumor thickness, tumor mitotic rate, and age less than 35 years and positivity in the SLN biopsied. Therefore, they suggested that young patients younger than 35, with a high tumor mitotic rate and a tumor thickness 1.0 mm or less, should be considered for SLN. An absolute thickness below which an SLN biopsy should not be performed cannot as of yet be derived from their data. Chao and colleagues[67] noted an inverse relationship between age and positive SLN biopsies, even though older age clearly carries a worse prognosis. There remain conflicting data that obscure the clear indications to perform an SLN biopsy. In a review of 146 patients with thin melanomas 1.00 mm or less, Stitzenberg and colleagues[68] found 4% had a positive SLN with a primary tumor thickness between 0.4 and 0.9 mm who had *no* evidence of primary tumor ulceration and *no* evidence of regression. In the author's own practice, the presence of ulceration, axial or head and neck primary location, and male gender are the strongest clinical variables that sway the decision toward offering an SLN biopsy.

Another factor that needs to be taken into consideration, yet is almost impossible to quantify, is the patient's desire to know his or her nodal status even though the risk of nodal involvement is low. These requests are not infrequent, and are driven in part by the growing awareness in the population at large as to the poor prognostic implications once nodal disease is discovered. If a patient has an overwhelming desire to know his or her nodal status for quality of life or financial planning purposes, or simply to have peace of mind, in the absence of firm scientific guidelines the topic of SLN biopsy should at least be discussed.

The risks associated with the biopsy as well as the costs associated with the procedure need to be strongly considered when weighing with the patient the decision to perform an SLN biopsy. At present, the incidence of experiencing a complication with SLN biopsy is reported at 6% and therefore a diagnostic yield below this rate should be considered as an indication to not offer the procedure.[69] Compared with performing an ELND, SLN biopsy has a reduced risk of lymphedema, pain, hematoma, loss of range of motion, and sensory loss.[70] Nevertheless, these complications can and do occur, and should be kept in mind and discussed with the patient for what is still regarded as a diagnostic procedure.

SENTINEL LYMPH NODE BIOPSY AS A DIAGNOSTIC AND NOT YET A THERAPEUTIC PROCEDURE

Although SLN biopsy is becoming the standard of care at most large cancer centers in North America, Australia, and Europe, it has not been fully endorsed by all members of the larger medical community.[71–74] Much of the skepticism is centered around the fact that there are no prospective randomized studies to date that have definitively shown a survival advantage for patients receiving an SLN biopsy. This fact has not escaped the recognition of those surgeons who perform these procedures for the patients they treat. It has long been hoped that SLN biopsies would prove to impart some therapeutic benefit, and this may actually prove to be the case. Until large prospective randomized scientific trials prove this, however, SLN biopsies should be viewed as having no therapeutic benefit. The SLN procedure should be seen as a diagnostic tool designed to assess the status of the regional lymph nodes and determine the appropriateness of further treatment. McMasters[75] argues appropriately that no other diagnostic test (such a positron emission tomography scan or computed tomography scan) is held to the high standard of improving outcome. The diagnostic benefit of SLN biopsy has been proven in melanoma, colon cancer, breast cancer, and any solid cancer that is known to spread to lymphatic basins.[76] McMasters writes that there are 4 main reasons to perform an SLN biopsy in melanoma patents, primarily to more accurately provide staging information for the disease. First, the SLN biopsy provides critical prognostic information for the treating physician and more importantly, the patient, that allow him or her to make major treatment and life-planning decisions. Second, the results of the SLN biopsy can direct treatment toward a TLND, which may have survival implications as well as quality of life value in limiting the incidence of uncontrolled nodal basin disease that can be debilitating, painful, and socially handicapping. Third, a positive SLN biopsy identifies those patients who would potentially benefit most from adjuvant chemotherapy using interferon-α2b.[8] Last, McMasters contends that the results of the SLN biopsy can be used as a selection criteria for patients to enter into important and valuable clinical trials that may potentially prolong survival and shed greater insight on the disease process.

HOW MANY SENTINEL NODES SHOULD BE REMOVED?

The number of SLNs identified depends on the anatomic location of the primary tumor and the number of draining nodal basins identified on preoperative lymphoscintigraphy. Published reports indicate that the average number of SLNs removed overall is on the order of 2.3.[77] It should be emphasized that each basin identified to harbor an SLN must be evaluated separately, and any SLN identified in a basin should be sampled independently of the radiation counts or blueness of nodes biopsied from unrelated nodal basins elsewhere. Although predictive of further nodal involvement in the same basin, an SLN biopsy from one basin has no predictive power for a neighboring basin that reveals radiotracer uptake. When doing an SLN biopsy procedure, frequently there are multiple nodes that have high radioactive tracer activity or are blue staining. The question arises as to how many nodes to remove. This question is especially pertinent in the head and neck area, where multiple draining basins are frequently encountered. Morton and colleagues[7] originally emphasized that the nodes that were blue staining had the greatest predictive value. As the use of radioactive colloid showed tremendous localization advantages, the radiation counts of the nodes biopsied began to assume more significance. McMasters and colleagues[78] have advocated removing all radioactive nodes until the background counts of the undissected nodes decrease to below 10% of those of the hottest node. Other investigators have suggested that removing the 3 hottest nodes and all blue-staining nodes is able to detect 100% of positive SLNs. In addition, removing lymph nodes with less than 30% of the radioactivity of that of the hottest node was found to be of no value.[79] A node or its afferent lymphatics occasionally are obstructed

by tumor cells, preventing the radiocolloid and the blue dye from entering and subsequently identifying that node as an SLN. The radioactive tracer and blue dye flow may be diverted from that node to secondary echelon nodes, resulting in lower counts and less intense blue staining within the true sentinel node.[77] It has been shown that node was the most radioactive tissue biopsied only 80% of the time when a biopsied node was positive.[80] Therefore, simply removing the hottest or the most blue-staining lymph node may potentially miss the true sentinel nodal tissue in roughly 20% of patients, resulting in potentially adverse consequences.

ABERRANT AND UNUSUAL LYMPHATIC DRAINAGE PATTERNS

Cutaneous lymphatic drainage patterns had been thought to be somewhat predictable except over an area 5 cm wide along the midline, and along a circumferential band between the umbilicus and L2 termed Sappey's line.[16] Early lymphatic drainage studies, however, were performed in cadavers using gold injections, and they did not reliably predict lymphatic flow characteristics in live patients. More recent investigations using lymphoscintigraphy have determined that the entire head and neck area and a wide band of 10 cm from the midline and 10 cm from Sappey's line should be considered watershed regions where lymphatic drainage is not very predictable.[81] In a series of 1086 patients with melanoma primaries over the posterior trunk, lymphatic drainage was found to travel to the axilla in 91% of patients and to the groin in 11%; contralateral drainage was noted in 35%, and 20% of patients with shoulder melanomas drained to the neck.[47] The head and neck area is notorious for seemingly random nodal drainage patterns.[47,81,82] SLN mapping in the head and neck area is particularly challenging for several reasons. First, the rich lymphatic network and ambiguous drainage patterns makes multiple SLN in more than one basin the rule rather than the exception.[81–83] On average, 2.83 SLNs are removed per head in melanoma patients, which is more than for any other primary site.[83] Second, the close proximity of the melanoma primary to the nodal basin often makes using the intraoperative gamma probe very difficult due to scatter from the radioisotope deposited as a bolus during the preoperative lymphoscintigram (**Fig. 7**). Third, the lymph nodes in the head and neck are very small, often being only a few millimeters in diameter (**Fig. 8**),[47] which is particularly true with intraparotid lymph nodes. Also, the rate of discordance between the clinically

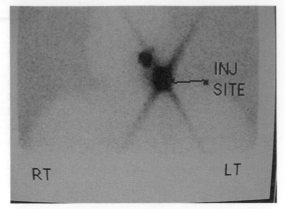

Fig. 7. In the head and neck area a tremendous amount of "scatter" is obtained from the primary site. Because the nodal basins are so closely juxtaposed in this region, any SLN located in the vicinity of the primary may be overshadowed. Finding all the SLN in these scenarios can be very difficult, time consuming, and frustrating.

predicted lymphatic basin and the actual drainage as demonstrated by the use of preoperative lymphoscintigraphy is great, reflecting complex drainage pathways and overlapping drainage patterns.[83] Uren[47] noted that with head and neck melanomas, 33% of patients mapped preoperatively drained to nodal basins not predicted clinically and 10% drained across the midline. Wells and colleagues[82] noted an 84% discordance rate over the head and neck, whereas Berman and colleagues[84] noted a 64% discordance rate in the head, 73% over the neck, 21% for the shoulder, and 35% for primaries over the trunk. Failure to predict the nodal drainage patterns clinically leads to a change in the operative plan (additional nodal basins dissected or contralateral

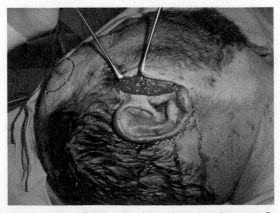

Fig. 8. A parotid SLN is found in the posterior superficial portion of the gland. These nodes are typically small, but are very radioactive and often deeply blue staining.

dissections performed) in as many as 62% of patients.[57]

Lymphoscintigrams for head and neck cutaneous malignancies occasionally fail to identify any SLNs at all. The exact incidence of SLN nonlocalization is not well documented in the literature, but is believed to be in the range of 5% to 10%.[85–87] In one series of 74 consecutive head and neck melanoma and Merkel cell carcinoma patients treated with preoperative lymphoscintigraphy, 6.8% failed to demonstrate any concentration of the tracer in any nodal basin.[85] The failure to localize a sentinel node preoperatively makes intraoperative localization of an SLN particularly difficult. Unlike other locations where the ability to identify an SLN using blue dye alone is in the neighborhood of 90% to 95%, single-modality methods to localize an SLN in the head and neck are not as successful, ranging anywhere between 50% and 92%.[7,12,13,17] In addition, the preoperative lymphoscintigram identifies the nodal basin(s) at risk for potential metastatic disease. Therefore, if the nodal basin at risk is known but an SLN cannot be found intraoperatively, the decision can be made to perform an ELND. At present, accepted general guidelines for pursuing an ELND are a tumor thickness between 1 and 2 mm, age younger than 60 years, and no evidence of tumor ulceration.[32] If the nodal basin is not known, this plan of action cannot be pursued and a "wait and watch" posture is assumed. In these situations, it is generally suggested that the wide local excision and immediate reconstruction only be performed. For those patients at particularly high risk of metastatic disease (tumor thickness greater than 4.0 mm, ulceration, Clark level IV or V), thought should be given to adjuvant immunochemotherapy and referral to a medical oncologist should be offered. Radiation therapy may also be considered, but again the lack of knowledge as to which basin is at greatest risk makes this form of treatment questionable in the face of clinically node-negative disease.[88]

Primary melanomas that demonstrate lymphatic drainage to the region of the parotid gland deserve special attention. Although it is richly invested with lymphatic tissue, the parotid gland is not a lymphatic organ and there is no oncologic or physiologic reason to remove the entire gland during what must be regarded as a staging procedure. Routine superficial parotidectomy is a potentially morbid procedure, with complication rates being reported as high as 69%.[89] The technique of performing an SLN biopsy accordingly is ideally suited for this complex anatomic area. Ninety percent of the lymph nodes in the parotid are in the superficial lobe and are therefore superficial to the facial nerve and parotid duct, minimizing the risk of damaging these structures during the SLN biopsy procedure.[90] Most of the nodes are located in the posterior portion of the gland in the superficial lobe, making extensive dissection unnecessary and making it usually unnecessary to expose the parotid-massenteric fascia and the facial nerve branches. Wells and colleagues[91] demonstrated that SLN biopsies can be easily and reliably obtained from the parotid gland with minimal morbidity and associated facial nerve damage. In general, a standard face-lift incision coursing over the pretragal region is used to gain access to the parotid gland (**Fig. 9**). All the usual precautions used to safeguard the facial nerve during any parotid operation are used, including avoiding using lidocaine in the locally delivered epinephrine solution, having the anesthesiologist avoid the use of a muscle relaxant during the parotid gland dissection, having the hemiface fully exposed to

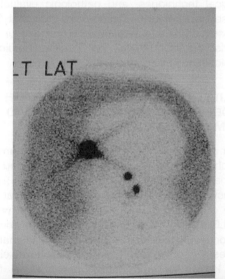

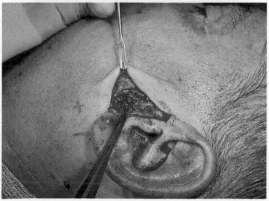

Fig. 9. A standard facelift incision is used to gain access to most SLNs located in the parotid region.

allow any muscle twitching to be observed, and using a nerve stimulator as needed.[92]

THE STATUS OF THE SENTINEL LYMPH NODE

The presence of nodal involvement is the single most powerful prognostic indicator in determining 10-year survival.[9] In the latest AJCC staging system, the number of nodes involved, and not node diameter, was factored into the TNM classification: one positive node is now N1, 2 to 3 positive nodes are N2, and 4 or more positive nodes are classified as N3. After the number of positive nodes involved, the next most significant prognostic indicator is the presence of palpable clinically apparent or macroscopic versus microscopic or clinically occult nodal disease.[11] In 2001, Balch and colleagues[38] documented the huge variation between these 2 groups of patients who both had stage III disease. In patients with nonulcerated primaries and a single microscopic focus of tumor in an SLN, the 5-year survival was 69%. In contrast, if the primary tumor was ulcerated and there were 3 or more clinically apparent nodes, the 5-year survival was a mere 13%. Tumor burden within a positive lymph node will certainly become more important as SLN biopsy becomes more widespread and patients are more accurately stratified according to their respective risk subgroups.[36]

Tumor thickness, ulceration, male gender, younger age, and mitotic index have been shown to be associated with a positive lymph node biopsy.[64,93] Of all these predictors, tumor thickness has been shown to correlate most accurately with SLN status. For thin melanomas 0.5 mm to 1.0 mm thick the probability of a positive SLN is roughly 6%, for intermediate thickness melanomas 1.01–2.0 mm thick the risk is 16%, for intermediate thickness tumors between 2.01 and 4.0 mm thick the risk is 34%, and for thick melanomas ≥ 4 mm the risk is about 55%.[94]

What should be done if the SLN biopsy is positive? Several studies have shown that the overall incidence of positive nonsentinel lymph nodes at the time of TLND is about 10% to 20%.[30,95] Therefore a completion nodal dissection is strongly considered whenever an SLN biopsy is positive; this is also important because the local nodal basin recurrence rates are very low in a previously dissected regional basin.[96] A strong argument may then be made that an SLN biopsy and subsequent TLND can be done to control regional disease and spare patients with nodal disease from the pain, hygiene problems, threat of imminent loss of limb viability or hemorrhage from vessel erosion, as well as social isolation associated with ulcerating nodal disease.

It has been proposed that SLN with a micrometastasis less than 0.2-mm focus of tumor should be regarded as node negative [N0(i+)] and any positive lymph node with a greater than 0.2-mm focus of tumor be classified as stage III disease.[97,98] Other investigators have questioned the need for performing a therapeutic node dissection because of the low probability of further positive nodes being obtained.[99] In a review of 1318 melanoma patients who underwent an SLN biopsy, Scheri and colleagues[100] demonstrated that 214 had positive nodes and 57 harbored foci of tumor <0.2 mm, and 52 went on to a TLND. At TLND, 12% of the 52 patients were shown to have tumor involvement of nonsentinel nodes. As a group, the 57-month recurrence rate was higher in the microscopically positive group than in the tumor-negative SLN group. These data reveal that even micrometastatic disease should warrant a discussion of the merit of performing a TLND and instituting adjuvant chemotherapy.

PATTERNS OF FAILURE AFTER SELECTIVE LYMPHADENECTOMY

As important as it is to identify patients with a positive SLN, it is equally important to identify individuals with negative nodal involvement. If the SLN is negative, the lymphatic basin is observed for the development of clinical nodal involvement and no further surgical treatment is indicated to address regional nodal disease. If patients with negative SLN are compared with patients with positive SLN involvement with tumor, the 3-year disease-free survival rates are 88.5% and 55.8%, respectively.[101] The negative predictive value of any staging test is vital to the power of the study and the ability to make treatment decisions. SLN evaluation has an overall false-negative rate of approximately 3%.[102] Many investigators have noted that the false-negative rate, that is, having a recurrence in a previously node-negative basin by SLN, is very close to, if not at, 0%.[82,87,102] Low false-negative results allow patients at risk for nodal metastases to be followed with a high degree of certainty that their disease will not recur locally. By performing a completion nodal dissection only for those patients who are found to harbor nodal metastases, unnecessary ELNDs are avoided in as many as 83% of patients.[87]

Recurrences in negative SLN basins do occur in a small number of patients. These false-negative results were initially attributed to skip metastases. Later work by Thompson and colleagues[23] showed that 77% of node-negative SLN patients

who went on to have recurrent nodal disease had undiagnosed micrometastases when the SLNs were reexamined. Refining the pathologic evaluation of the SLN using serial sectioning and immunohistochemical staining has come about partially as a result of these findings. In a 5-year retrospective review of 773 patients with negative SLN biopsies using serial sectioning and immunohistochemical staining, 8.9% developed a recurrence but only 1.7% had a recurrence in the SLN basin.[102] Similar findings were also reported by Gershenwald and colleagues,[103] looking at the nodal recurrence rates in previously node-negative SLN biopsied basins. With appropriate pathologic evaluation, the nodal recurrence rate was 3%, once again proving the validity of the SLN evaluation of basins at risk for nodal metastases. Thompson and colleagues[21] note that major cancer centers are now reporting false-negative rates as high as 15%, and whereas this does not mean that the SLN concept is flawed, there may be ongoing shortcomings in nuclear medicine, surgical techniques, and pathologic evaluation. These drawbacks underscore the fact that SLN biopsies constitute a multispecialty endeavor that needs the coordination of nuclear medicine, surgical specialties, and pathology.

UTILITY OF PERFORMING A SENTINEL LYMPH NODE BIOPSY AT A POINT IN TIME REMOVED FROM THE WIDE LOCAL EXCISION

After a WLE has been performed, the surrounding lymphatic pathways may be damaged and the drainage patterns may be altered.[104] An SLN biopsy ideally should therefore be done at the time of the WLE. There are scenarios in which a WLE is performed when the extent of the primary tumor level of invasion, presence of ulceration, regression, or lymphovascular invasion was either not known or was underappreciated. A SLN biopsy was therefore not incorporated into the initial operative plan. The question arises as to whether an SLN biopsy is still possible and if so, how predictive are the results compared with a standard SLN biopsy performed at the time of the WLE.

Leong and colleagues[104] found that performing an SLN biopsy in patients who had a previous WLE on the extremities still provides useful diagnostic data, and these findings supported similar findings reported by Kelemen and colleagues[105] Neither of these groups noted an increased rate of regional recurrences, suggesting that the true SLNs were removed when the SLN biopsies were done at a time remote from the WLE. Similar findings have been reported for melanomas located over the head and neck area. Wells and colleagues[106] showed that there was no difference in the prognostic significance of SLN biopsied at the time of the WLE or remotely at a later date. On average, more nodes were harvested and the difficulty of the procedure was greater.

RISKS ASSOCIATED WITH USING TECHNETIUM-99M RADIOCOLLOID IN THE OPERATING ROOM

^{99m}Tc-sulfur radiocolloid is a short-lived radio-pharmaceutical having a half-life of about 6 hours. However, measurable radiation levels are detectable in removed WLE specimens for almost 3 days after they are harvested and for 16 to 48 hours in any SLN procured.[107] Because of the low levels of radiation emitted, special precautions such as radiation exposure tags and lead shielding are not required. The United States Nuclear Regulatory Commission (NRC) has defined the maximal acceptable extremity skin radiation exposure as 50 rem per year, with radiation monitoring being required if the anticipated radiation exposure will exceed 10% of this amount annually. Miner and colleagues[107] estimated that the average surgeon would have to perform 5000 SLN procedures annually to reach the NRC limit, and only after 500 procedures were done would radiation monitoring be needed. In addition, no significant radiation levels were found in the operating room trash after a WLE and SLN biopsy, obviating the need for special disposal protocols. Because almost all injections of ^{99m}Tc-sulfur colloid are done in nuclear medicine departments, special handling and disposal protocols do not to be implemented in the operating suites. It is recommended, however, that the WLE specimens be labeled as radioactive and kept isolated for 72 hours before further handling. For SLN, the same protocol should be followed for 36 hours for permanent section analysis.[107] The delay in obtaining final pathologic readings should be explained to the patient before hand.

TECHNICAL DETAILS OF SENTINEL LYMPH NODE BIOPSY

On the day of the planned WLE and SLN biopsy, the patient is injected with ^{99m}Tc-sulfur radiocolloid by the radiologist. If the surgeon wishes to do the injections, licensing issues and hospital protocols will have to be established beforehand. Later that day, the patient is seen in the preoperative holding area and the findings of lymphoscintigram are discussed with the patient. This discussion should include the basins to be explored and the incisions used to remove the nodes. Also, the author usually

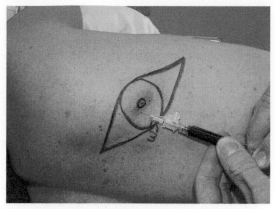

Fig. 10. When injecting the blue dye, it is helpful to use a small-gauge needle to facilitate intradermal injections and avoid the subcutaneous space. The small-gauge needle, however, generates a tremendous amount of back pressure, making the needle prone to "pop" off the syringe, creating a mess. A Luer-Lok syringe will prevent this from happening.

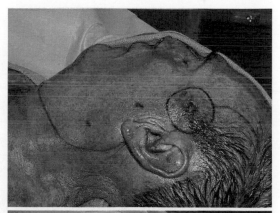

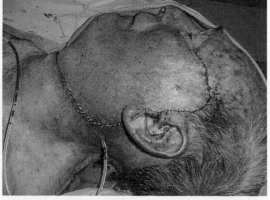

Fig. 11. A primary melanoma located over the left temple with an SLN identified in the parotid gland and level 3 cervical nodes. The wide local excision, the SLN biopsies, and the cervicofacial flap reconstruction were all able to be performed using a standard facelift incision. Postoperatively the cosmetic result was good, with almost inconspicuous scars.

takes this opportunity to again inform the patient of the potential risks associated with operating on the nodal basins in question. For example, a melanoma over the temple may show radiocolloid localization to the parotid region, the entire cervical chain, or the postauricular and the occipital nodes. Once the lymphoscintigram is done, if the tracer is confined to the parotid region, the risks involved to the facial nerve and the parotid duct are again explained, as well as that a face-lift type incision will be used to harvest the node(s). Once in the operating room, all nodal basins at risk for possible lymphatic drainage from the primary tumor are checked with the gamma probe as well as any potential in-transit nodes before the initiation of the procedure. Ensuring that there are no in-transit nodes is important when the primary tumor is near the nodal basin and the scatter from the lymphoscintigram overshadows the region between the primary and the nodal basin. Before prepping, the blue dye is injected intradermally in 4 quadrants, typically using 2 to 3 mL of dye (**Fig. 10**). A 3-mL syringe with

a Luer-Lok hub and a 27-gauge needle are preferred to avoid spillage of the dye or inadvertent injection into the subcutaneous space. Gentle massage is then used to promote lymphatic drainage, and the patient is prepped and draped. When the primary tumor is located in close proximity to the nodal basin to be explored, the radioactive signal emitted from the primary may be so intense that locating the sentinel node becomes very difficult. In this situation the WLE in performed first but even when this is done, a significant amount of the radiocolloid may have migrated into the surrounding deep tissues, making the background scatter a factor to contend with. This scenario frequently occurs with melanoma situated over the parotid gland. When this is the case, the radiologist in the nuclear medicine department is usually instructed to use less ^{99m}Tc-sulfur colloid to minimize the scatter yet still allow the SLN to be identified.

The length of the incisions used to harvest the SLN(s) depends on the anatomic location as

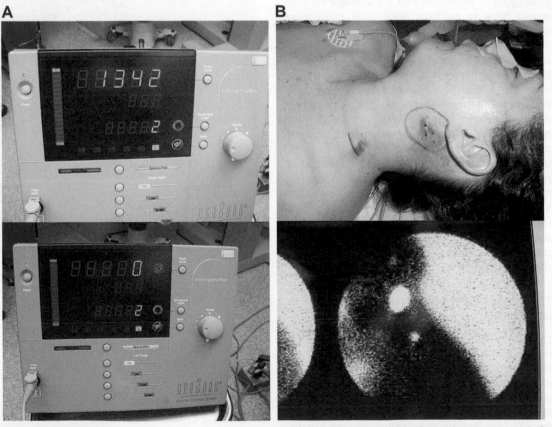

Fig. 12. (*A*) The gamma probe, here shown localizing a radioactive node (*top*). After the node was removed, the counts went to zero, indicating that all the radioactive nodal tissue had been removed (*bottom*). (*B*) The corresponding clinical (*top*) and lymphoscintigraphic (*bottom*) status, showing a solitary bright lymph node which, once removed, rendered the basin free of any residual radioactive tracer activity.

well as the planned flap closure being used. For example, a cheek melanoma WLE defect may be closed with a cervicofacial rotation advancement flap elevated along the pre-auricular and cervical skin over the sternocleidomastoid muscle. In this situation the SLN biopsies can be performed in the parotid and cervical area after the flap has been elevated (**Fig. 11**). The author finds that fine jeweler's bipolar forceps work extremely well for performing a precise and hemostatic dissection of the SLN. Any blue staining lymphatic is controlled with hemoclips or suture ligatures to minimize the risk of postoperative lymphoceles. It is important to remove the entire SLN, as only a small segment of the node may harbor metastatic disease. Removing the whole node is sometimes tricky in the head and neck because the nodes are very closely juxtaposed and often difficult to separate cleanly. The hand-held gamma probe is then used to measure the radioactivity of the SLN and also to check the nodal basin for significant residual radiation (**Fig. 12**). If the background counts are higher than 10% of the hottest node removed, further exploration and SLN harvesting is pursued. The author usually makes mention of the radiation counts and the blue staining pattern of the SLNs as they are removed, and includes these details in the operative notes. The nodes are submitted to pathology in formalin for permanent section analysis. Frozen sections are almost never requested. The incision(s) are then closed in layers with or without a drain. In men, in the head and neck location, the author is more inclined to use a drain because of the increased risk of postoperative hemorrhage, especially if the patient has a history of hypertension.

SUMMARY

The treatment of melanoma has changed significantly over the past 25 years. With the introduction of better public awareness campaigns, earlier diagnosis is more common. The establishment of ever narrower recommended margins of excision has made the surgical treatment of the primary cancer much less morbid and disfiguring. The introduction of sentinel node technology has rendered ELND procedures unnecessary in the vast majority of patients, thereby limiting the morbidity and disfigurement associated with what must still be considered a staging procedure. The improved pathologic evaluation of nodal tissue removed using immunohistochemical stains and serial sectioning has gone hand in hand with the emergence of less invasive techniques used to perform staging analysis. Lastly, the emergence

of potentially more effective chemotherapy for high-risk patients and those with metastatic disease has given hope to those who have this potentially lethal disease. Ongoing research trials and emerging new treatment options will continue to shed light on the disease process, and provide better and more focused patient-specific therapeutic alternatives. Melanoma care is truly a multidisciplinary team effort, with each link being vital to the overall strength of the treatment rendered.

REFERENCES

1. Lens MB, Dawes M. Global perspectives of contemporary epidemiological trends of cutaneous malignant melanoma. Br J Dermatol 2004;150: 179–85.
2. National Cancer Institute. Cancer stat fact sheets. Available at: www.seer.cancer.gov/statfacts. 2008.
3. Veronesi U, Cascinelli N. Narrow excision (1 cm margins). A safe procedure for thin cutaneous melanoma. Arch Surg 1991;126:438–41.
4. Balch CM, Urist MM, Karakousis CP, et al. Efficacy of 2 cm surgical margins for intermediate-thickness melanomas (1 to 4 mm). Ann Surg 1993;218:262–9.
5. Heaton KM, Sussman JJ, Gershenwald JE, et al. Surgical margins and prognostic factors in patients with thick (>4.0 mm) primary melanoma. Ann Surg Oncol 1998;5:322–8.
6. Kenady DE, Brown BW, McBride CM. Excision of underlying fascia with a primary malignant melanoma: effect on recurrence and survival rates. Surgery 1992;92:615–8.
7. Morton DL, Wen D-R, Wong JH, et al. Technical details of intraoperative lymphatic mapping for early stage melanoma. Arch Surg 1992;127:392–9.
8. Kirkwood JM, Strawderman MH, Ernstoff MS, et al. Interferon-alfa-2b adjuvant therapy of high-risk resected cutaneous melanoma: the Eastern Cooperative Oncology Group Trial EST 1684. J Clin Oncol 1996;14:7–17.
9. Balch CM, Buzaid AC, Soong S-J, et al. Final version of the American Joint Committee on Cancer staging system for cutaneous melanoma. J Clin Oncol 2001;19:3635–48.
10. Balch CM. Cutaneous melanoma. In: Greene FL, Page DL, Fleming ID, et al, editors. AJCC cancer staging manual. 6th edition. New York: Springer Verlag; 2002. p. 209–17.
11. Balch CM, Soong S-J, Atkins MB, et al. An evidence-based staging system for cutaneous melanoma. CA Cancer J Clin 2004;54:131–49.
12. Doubrovsky A, de Wilt JHW, Scolyer RS, et al. Sentinel node biopsy provides more accurate staging than elective lymph node dissection in

patients with cutaneous melanoma. Ann Surg Oncol 2004;11:829–36.

13. Stadelmann WK, Rapaport DP, Soong SJ, et al. Prognostic. Clinical and pathologic features. In: Balch CM, editor. Cutaneous melanoma. 3rd edition. St Louis (MO): Quality Medical Publishing; 1998. p. 11–35.

14. Soong SJ. A computerized mathematical model and scoring system for predicting outcome in patients with localized melanoma. In: Balch CM, Houghton AN, Milton GW, et al, editors. Cutaneous melanoma. 2nd edition. Philadelphia: JB Lippincott; 1992. p. 200.

15. Stadelmann WK, Reintgen DS. Prognosis in malignant melanoma. Hematol Oncol Clin North Am 1998;12:767–96.

16. Reintgen DS, Rapaport DP, Tanabe KK, et al. Lymphatic mapping and sentinel lymphadenectomy. In: Balch CM, editor. Cutaneous melanoma. 3rd edition. St Louis (MO): Quality Medical Publishing; 1998. p. 227–44.

17. Starz H, Siedlecki K, Balda B-R. Sentinel lymphadenectomy and S-classification: a successful strategy for better prediction and improvement of outcome of melanoma. Ann Surg Oncol 2004;11: 162S–8S.

18. Seaman W, Powers W. Studies on the distribution of radioactive colloidal gold in regional lymph nodes containing cancer. Cancer 1955;8:1044–6.

19. Gould EA, Winship T, Pholbin PH, et al. Observations on a "sentinel node" in cancer of the parotid. Cancer 1960;13:77–8.

20. Cabanas RM. An approach for the treatment of penile carcinoma. Cancer 1977;39:456–66.

21. Thompson JF, Stretch JR, Uren RF, et al. Sentinel node biopsy for melanoma: where have we been and where are we going. Ann Surg Oncol 2004; 11:147S–51S.

22. Reintgen DS, Cruse CW, Wells KE, et al. The orderly progression of melanoma nodal metastases. Ann Surg 1994;220(6):759–67.

23. Thompson JF, McCarthy WH, Bosch CM, et al. Sentinel lymph node status as an indicator of the presence of metastatic melanoma in regional lymph nodes. Melanoma Res 1995;5:255–60.

24. Reintgen DS, Albertini J, Miliotes G, et al. The accurate staging and modern day treatment of malignant melanoma. Cancer Res Ther Control 1995;4: 183–97.

25. Stadelmann WK, Javaheri S, Cruse CW, et al. The use of sentinel lymph-adenectomy in squamous cell carcinoma of the wrist. A case report. J Hand Surg Am 1997;22:726–31.

26. Javaheri S, Cruse CW, Stadelmann WK, et al. Sentinel node excision for the diagnosis of metastatic neuroendocrine carcinoma of the skin: a case report. Ann Plast Surg 1997;39:299–302.

27. Leong SPL. Paradigm of metastasis for melanoma and breast cancer based on the sentinel lymph node experience. Ann Surg Oncol 2004;11: 192S–7S.

28. Saha S, Dan AG, Berman B, et al. Lymphazurin 1% versus 99mTc sulfur colloid for lymphatic mapping in colorectal tumors: a comparative analysis. Ann Surg Oncol 2004;11:21–6.

29. Kitajima M, Kitagawa Y. Universal applications of sentinel node technology. Ann Surg Oncol 2004; 11:144S–6S.

30. Scolyer RA, Thompson JF, Li L-XL, et al. Failure to remove true sentinel nodes can cause failure of the sentinel node biopsy technique: evidence from antimony concentrations in false-negative sentinel nodes from melanoma patients. Ann Surg Oncol 2004;11:174S–8S.

31. Crowley NJ, Seigler HF. The role of elective lymph node dissection in the management of patients with thick cutaneous melanoma. Cancer 1990;66: 2522–7.

32. Balch CM, Soong SJ, Bartolucci AA, et al. Efficacy of an elective regional lymph node dissection of 1 to 4 mm thick melanomas for patients 60 years of age and younger. Ann Surg 1996;224:255.

33. Sim FH, Taylor WF, Ivins JC, et al. A prospective randomized study of the efficacy of routine elective lymphadenectomy in management of malignant melanoma: preliminary results. Cancer 1978;41: 948.

34. Veronesi U, Adamus J, Bandiera DC, et al. Delayed regional lymph node dissection in stage I melanoma of the skin of the lower extremities. Cancer 1982;49:2420–30.

35. Cascinelli N, Morabito A, Santinami M, et al. Immediate or delayed dissection of regional nodes in patients with melanoma of the trunk: a randomized trial—WHO Melanoma Programme. Lancet 1998; 351:793–6.

36. Pawlik TM, Gershenwald JE. Sentinel node biopsy for melanoma. Contemp Surg 2005;61(4):175–82.

37. Balch CM, Soong S, Ross MI, et al. Long-term results of a multi-institutional randomized trial comparing prognostic factors and surgical results for intermediate thickness melanomas (1.0 to 4.0 mm). Intergroup Melanoma Surgical Trial. Ann Surg Oncol 2000;7:87–97.

38. Balch CM, Soong SJ, Gershenwald J, et al. Prognostic factors analysis of 17,600 melanoma patients: validation of the new American Joint Committee on Cancer melanoma staging system. J Clin Oncol 2001;19:3622–34.

39. Dessureault S, Soong SJ, Ross MI, et al. Improved staging of node-negative patients with intermediate to thick melanomas (>1.0 mm) with the use of lymphatic mapping and sentinel lymph node biopsy. Ann Surg Oncol 2001;8:749–51.

40. Pawlik TM, Ross MI, Gershenwald JE. Lymphatic mapping in the molecular era. Ann Surg Oncol 2004;11:362–74.

41. Sappey MPC. Anatomie, physiologie, pathologie, des vaisseaux lymphatiques considérés chez l'homme et les vertègres. Paris (France): A. Delahaye & E. Lecrosnier; 1864.

42. Sherman AI, Ter-Pogossian M. Lymph node concentration of radioactive colloidal gold following interstitial injection. Cancer 1953;6:1238–40.

43. Hauser W, Atkins HL, Richards P. Lymph node scanning with ^{99m}Tc-sulfur colloid. Radiology 1969;92:1369.

44. Meyer CW, Lecklitner ML, Logic JR, et al. Technetium-99m sulfur-colloid cutaneous lymphoscintigraphy in the management of truncal melanoma. Radiology 1979;131:205–9.

45. Ali-Salaam P, Ariyan S. Lymphatic mapping and sentinel lymph node biopsies. Clin Plast Surg 2000;27:421–9.

46. McMasters KM, Chao C, Wong SL, et al. Interval sentinel lymph nodes in melanoma. Arch Surg 2002;137:543–7 [discussion: 7–9].

47. Uren RF. Lymphatic drainage of the skin. Ann Surg Oncol 2004;11:179S–85S.

48. Momeni R, Ariyan S. Pulse oximetry declines do to intradermal isosulfan blue dye: a controlled prospective study. Ann Surg Oncol 2004;11(4):434–7.

49. Cimmino VM, Brown AC, Szocik JF, et al. Allergic reactions to isosulfan blue during sentinel node biopsy—a common event. Surgery 2001;130:439–42.

50. Komenaka IK, Bauer VP, Schnabel FR, et al. Allergic reactions to isosulfan blue dye in sentinel lymph node mapping. Breast J 2005;11:70–2.

51. Raut CP, Hunt KK, Akins JS, et al. Incidence of anaphylactoid reactions to isosulfan blue dye during breast carcinoma lymphatic mapping in patients treated with preoperative prophylaxis. Cancer 2005;104:692–9, published online.

52. Montgomery LL, Thorne AC, Van Zee KJ, et al. Isosulfan blue dye reactions during sentinel lymph node mapping for breast cancer. Anesth Analg 2002;95:385–8.

53. Alex JC, Weaver DL, Fairbank JT, et al. Gamma-probe-guided lymph node localization in malignant melanoma. Surg Oncol 1993;2:303–8.

54. Krag DN, Meijer SJ, Weaver DL, et al. Minimal-access surgery for staging of melanoma. Arch Surg 1995;130:654.

55. Van der Veen H, Hoekstra OS, Paul MA, et al. Gamma probe-guided sentinel node biopsy to select patients with melanoma for lymphadenectomy. Br J Surg 1994;81:1769–70.

56. Gershenwald JE, Tseng C-H, Thompson W, et al. Improved sentinel lymph node localization in patients with primary melanoma with the use of radiolabeled colloid. Surgery 1998;124:203–10.

57. Albertini JJ, Cruse CW, Rapaport D, et al. Intraoperative radiolymphoscintigraphy improves sentinel lymph node identification for patients with melanoma. Ann Surg 1996;223:217–24.

58. Koopal SA, Tiebosch AT, Albertus PD, et al. Frozen section analysis of sentinel lymph nodes in melanoma patients. Cancer 2000;89:1720–5.

59. Cochran AJ, Wen DR, Morton DL. Occult tumor cells in the lymph nodes of patients with pathologic stage I malignant melanoma: an immunohistochemical study. Am J Surg Pathol 1988;12:612–8. Bedrosian.

60. Ferrone CR, Panagaes KS, Busam K, et al. Multivariate prognostic model for patients with thick cutaneous melanoma: importance of sentinel lymph node status. Ann Surg Oncol 2002;9:637–45.

61. Essner R, Chung MH, Bleicher R, et al. Prognostic implications of thick (≥4-mm) melanoma in the era of intraoperative lymphatic mapping and sentinel lymphadenectomy. Ann Surg Oncol 2001;9:754–61.

62. Bleicher RJ, Essner R, Foshag LJ, et al. Role of sentinel lymphadenectomy in thin invasive cutaneous melanoma. J Clin Oncol 2003;21:1326–31.

63. Wong SL, Brady MS, Busam KJ, et al. Results of sentinel lymph node biopsy in patients with thin melanoma. Ann Surg Oncol 2006;13:302–9.

64. Sondak V, Taylor JMG, Sabel MS, et al. Mitotic rate and younger age are predictors of sentinel lymph node positivity: lessons learned from the generation of a probabilistic model. Ann Surg Oncol 2004;11:247–58.

65. Bedrosian I, Faries MB, Guerry D IV, et al. Incidence of sentinel node metastasis in patients with thin primary melanoma (≤1 mm) with vertical growth phase. Ann Surg Oncol 2000;7:262–7.

66. Ranieri JM, Wagner JD, Wenck S, et al. The prognostic importance of sentinel lymph node biopsy in thin melanoma. Ann Surg Oncol 2006;3:927–32.

67. Chao C, Martin RCG, Ross MI, et al. Correlation between prognostic factors and increasing age in melanoma. Ann Surg Oncol 2004;11:259–64.

68. Stitzenberg KB, Groben PA, Stern S, et al. Indications for lymphatic mapping and sentinel lymphadenectomy in patients with thin melanoma Breslow thickness ≤1.0 mm. Ann Surg Oncol 2004;11:900–6.

69. Wrightson WR, Reintgen DS, Edwards MJ, et al. Morbidity of sentinel lymph node biopsy for melanoma. Annual Meeting of the Society of Surgical Oncology, Washington, DC, March 15-18, 2001 [abstr 28].

70. Wrightson WR, Wong SL, Edwards MJ, et al. Sunbelt Melanoma Trial Study Group. Complications

associated with sentinel lymph node biopsy for melanoma. Ann Surg Oncol 2003;10:676–80.

71. McMasters KM, Reintgen DS, Ross MI, et al. Sentinel node biopsy for melanoma controversy despite widespread agreement. J Clin Oncol 2001;11:2851–5.

72. World Health Organization declares lymphatic mapping to be the standard of care for melanoma. Oncology 1999;13:288.

73. Medalie NS, Ackerman B. Sentinel lymph node biopsy has no benefit for patients with primary cutaneous melanoma metastatic to a lymph node: an assertion based on comprehensive, critical analysis. Part I. Am J Dermatopathol 2003;25: 399–417.

74. Medalie NS, Ackerman B. Sentinel lymph node biopsy has no benefit for patients with primary cutaneous melanoma metastatic to a lymph node: an assertion based on comprehensive, critical analysis. Part II. Am J Dermatopathol 2003;25:473–84.

75. McMasters KM. Editorial. What good is sentinel lymph node biopsy for melanoma if it does not improve survival? Ann Surg Oncol 2004;11(9): 810–2.

76. Morton DL. Sentinel node mapping and an international sentinel node society: current issues and future directions. Ann Surg Oncol 2004;11: 137S–43S.

77. Nieweg OE, Estourgie SE. What is a sentinel node and what is a false-negative sentinel node? Ann Surg Oncol 2004;3:169S–73S.

78. McMasters KM, Reintgen DS, Ross MI, et al. Sentinel lymph node biopsy for melanoma: how many radioactive nodes should be removed? Ann Surg Oncol 2001;8:192–7.

79. Abou-Nukta F, Ariyan S. Sentinel lymph node biopsies in melanoma: how many nodes do we really need? Ann Plast Surg 2008;60:416–9.

80. Martin RC, Fey J, Yeung H, et al. Highest isotope count does not predict sentinel node positivity in all breast cancer patients. Ann Surg Oncol 2001; 8:592–7.

81. Norman J, Cruse CW, Espinosa C, et al. Redefinition of cutaneous lymphatic drainage with the use of lymphoscintigraphy for malignant melanoma. Am J Surg 1991;162:432–7.

82. Wells KE, Cruse CW, Daniels S, et al. The use of lymphoscintigraphy in melanoma of the head and neck. Plast Reconstr Surg 1994;93:757–61.

83. Chao C, Wong SL, Edwards MJ, et al. Sentinel lymph node biopsy for head and neck melanomas. Ann Surg Oncol 2003;10(1):21–6.

84. Berman CG, Norman J, Cruse CW, et al. Lymphscintigraphy in malignant melanoma. Ann Plast Surg 1992;28:29–32.

85. Stadelmann WK, Cobbins L, Lentsch EJ. Incidence of nonlocalization of sentinel lymph nodes using preoperative lymphoscintigraphy in 74 consecutive head and neck melanoma and Merkel cell carcinoma patients. Ann Plast Surg 2004;52:546–50.

86. Medina-Franco H, Beenken SW, Heslin MJ, et al. Sentinel node biopsy for cutaneous melanoma in the head and neck. Ann Surg Oncol 2001;8:716–9.

87. MacNeill KN, Ghazarian D, McCready D, et al. Sentinel lymph node biopsy for cutaneous melanoma of the head and neck. Ann Surg Oncol 2005;12:726–32.

88. Trotti A, Peters LJ. The role of radiotherapy in the primary management of cutaneous melanoma. Ann Plast Surg 1992;28:39–44.

89. O'Brien CJ, Petersen-Schaefer K, Papadopoulos T, et al. Evaluation of 107 therapeutic and elective parotidectomies for cutaneous melanoma. Am J Surg 1994;168:400–3.

90. McKean ME, Lee K, McGregor IA. The distribution of lymph nodes in and around the parotid gland: an anatomical study. Br J Surg 1985;38:1–5.

91. Wells KE, Stadelmann WK, Rapaport DP, et al. Parotid selective lymphadenectomy in malignant melanoma. Ann Plast Surg 1999;43:1–6.

92. Stadelmann WK, McMasters KM, Digenis AG, et al. Cutaneous melanoma of the head and neck: new advances in evaluation and treatment. Plast Reconstr Surg 2000;105(6):2105–26.

93. Rousseau DL Jr, Ross MI, Johnson MM, et al. Revised Joint Committee on Cancer staging criteria accurately predict sentinel lymph node positivity in clinically node-negative melanoma patients. Ann Surg Oncol 2003;10:569–74.

94. Vuylsteke RJCLM, van Leeuwen PAM, Muller MGS, et al. Clinical outcome of stage I/II melanoma patients after selective lymph node dissection: long-term follow-up results. J Clin Oncol 2003;21: 1057–65.

95. Elias N, Tanabe KK, Sober AJ, et al. Is completion lymphadenectomy after a positive sentinel lymph node biopsy for cutaneous melanoma always necessary? Arch Surg 2004;139:400–4.

96. Chao C, Wong SL, Ross MI. Patterns of early recurrence after sentinel lymph node biopsy for melanoma. Am J Surg 2002;184:520–4.

97. Sigletary SE, Greene FL, Sobin LH. Classification of isolated tumor cells: clarification of the 6th edition of the American Joint Committee on Cancer Staging Manual. Cancer 2003;90:2740–1.

98. Schuchter LM. Review of the 2001 AJCC staging system for cutaneous malignant melanoma. Curr Oncol Rep 2001;3:332–7.

99. van Akkooi AC, de Wilt JH, Verhoef C, et al. Clinical relevance of melanoma micro metastases (<0.1 mm) in sentinel nodes: are these nodes to be considered negative? Ann Oncol 2006;17:1578–85.

100. Scheri RP, Essner R, Turner RR, et al. Isolated tumor cells in the sentinel node affect long-term

prognosis of patients with melanoma. Ann Surg Oncol 2007;14:2861–6.

101. Gershenwald JE, Thompson W, Mansfield PF, et al. Multi-institutional melanoma lymphatic mapping experience: the prognostic value of sentinel lymph node status in 612 stage I or II melanoma patients. J Clin Oncol 1999;17: 976–83.

102. Zogakis TG, Essner R, Wang H-J, et al. Natural history of melanoma in 773 patients with tumor-negative sentinel lymph nodes. Ann Surg Oncol 2007;14:1604–11.

103. Gershenwald JE, Colome MI, Lee FE, et al. Patterns of recurrence following a negative sentinel lymph node biopsy in 243 patients with stage I or II melanoma. J Clin Oncol 1998;16:2253–60.

104. Leong SP, Thelmo MC, Kim RP, et al. Delayed harvesting of sentinel lymph nodes after previous wide local excision of extremity melanoma. Ann Surg Oncol 2003;10(2):196–200.

105. Kelemen PR, Essner R, Foshag LJ, et al. Lymphatic mapping and sentinel lymphadenectomy after wide local excision of primary melanoma. J Am Coll Surg 1999;189:247–52.

106. Wells KE, Joseph E, Ross M, et al. Lymphatic mapping for melanoma before and after wide local excision: 4th World Conference on Melanoma. Sydney, Australia: Melanoma Research, 1997:S105.

107. Miner TJ, Shriver CD, Flicek PR, et al. Guidelines for the safe use of radioactive materials during localization and resection of the sentinel lymph node. Ann Surg Oncol 1999;6:75–82.

Evaluation of Sentinel Lymph Nodes for Melanoma Metastases by Pathologists

Vinod B. Shidham, MD, FIAC, FRCPath[a,b]

KEYWORDS

- Melanoma • Sentinel lymph node • Immunocytochemistry
- MCW melanoma cocktail • Tyrosinase
- Intraoperative cytology • Micrometastasis
- Benign capsular nevi

Many studies emphasize the role of sentinel lymph node (SLN) biopsy in the management of cutaneous melanoma.[1–12] The pathologic evaluation of SLNs for melanoma metastases, however, is not without significant challenges. It is affected by significant variation in approaches, which may compromise the final interpretation, leading to nonrepresentative spurious results. Because of this, conclusions derived from most of the clinical trials and studies, based on older evaluation methods with older immunomarkers, may not be realistic. Some of the causes for concern include inadequate grossing/cutting of the SLNs, proportion of SLNs evaluated, selection of immunomarkers to detect the rare event of melanoma micrometastases, and application of some practices inadvertently compromising the final evaluation, such as frozen section analysis (FS).

The conventionally used melanoma immunomarkers, such as S-100 protein and HMB-45, have significant drawbacks when applied to evaluation of SLN for melanoma micrometastasis. MCW melanoma cocktail (MMC), a mixture of monoclonal antibodies to MART-1 {1:500}, Melan-A {1:100}, and tyrosinase {1:50}, has demonstrated an excellent discriminatory immunostaining pattern with significant advantages.[9,13–16]

Melanoma metastases are located predominantly along the capsule of SLN and in the hilar area. Because of this, it is critical to evaluate a maximum portion of the subcapsular area. Transecting the lymph node perpendicular to the long axis and bread-loafing it into 2-mm thick sections achieves maximum exploration of this location.

Although the most precise approach would be to examine the entire SLN tissue, that is prohibitively expensive and unrealistic. Many studies have explored different approaches to address this issue with variable rates of detectability of melanoma metastases.[10,17] Although evaluation of more levels increases the number of positive SLNs, the most practical approach is to evaluate three step levels at intervals of 200 μm.[9] The section adjacent to the hematoxylin-eosin (H & E)–stained section at each level should be evaluated by immunostaining with optimum melanoma immunomarkers, such as MMC. All three levels

Different areas of research referred to in this article were supported in part by a multidisciplinary grant from the Cancer Research Center of the Medical College of Wisconsin, Milwaukee, Wisconsin, and in part by the Armour family grant through the Chicago Marathon and Ann's Hope Foundation through the Cancer Research Center of the Medical College of Wisconsin, for single-step MCW melanoma cocktail for easy and rapid intraoperative evaluation of sentinel lymph nodes for melanoma micrometastases to prevent second surgery, currently under development.

[a] Department of Pathology, Medical College of Wisconsin, 9200 West Wisconsin Avenue, Milwaukee, WI 53226, USA
[b] CytoJournal, USA
E-mail address: vshidham@mcw.edu

may be immunostained simultaneously and evaluated. Alternatively, only the middle level is immunostained and evaluated initially, followed by immunostaining and evaluation of the other two levels if the middle level is negative. Or, all the three sections are evaluated together if they are small enough to be mounted on a single slide. An additional approach is to include SLN gamma counts in the algorithm with processing of SLNs proportionate to their level of gamma counts (examining more sections of hotter SLNs as compared with fewer sections for colder SLNs).[10]

Because of its clean discriminatory immunostaining pattern in lymph nodes, MMC can also be applied for rapid intraoperative evaluation of SLNs for detection of melanoma micrometastases in imprint smears.[18] In positive cases, this provides the opportunity to complete regional lymphadenectomy during the same surgical event and avoid additional surgical intervention at a later date. This article discusses these approaches along with recommended dos and don'ts for optimum evaluation of SLNs for melanoma metastases.

PERSPECTIVE
General

Although the clinical relevance of SLN metastases is still evolving and not entirely understood, the status of SLNs is considered one of the most important prognostic factors in the management of cutaneous melanoma.[1–12] Patients undergoing an immediate complete lymph node dissection after a positive sentinel node evaluation demonstrated a longer 5-year survival rate (72.3%), as compared with a statistically significant lower survival rate (52.4%) for those in whom the lymphadenectomy was delayed until the lymph nodes were clinically detectable.[19]

Patients with morphologically positive SLNs may not progress to clinically widespread disease, so it is suggested that SLN biopsy may contribute to considerable biologic false positivity.[20] Because individual tumor cells vary biologically, melanoma cells in a particular SLN may not have acquired the genotype to support their survival in distant sites. This concern is applicable, however, to many morphology-based scenarios in oncopathology.

Grossing of Sentinel Lymph Notes

It is usually recommended that a SLN is bisected along its long axis and submitted for formalin-fixed paraffin-embedded (FFPE) tissue sectioning. Larger nodes are cut parallel to the meridian at 1-mm intervals.[19] Melanoma metastases are located predominantly along the capsule and in the hilar area. Because of this, it is crucial to evaluate most of the subcapsular area of the SLNs.

As demonstrated by calculations and sketches in **Fig. 1**, the total surface area evaluated by any cutting approach is not significantly affected, but the proportion of the circumference available for microscopic evaluation is markedly variable with different cutting methods. Bread-loafing the lymph nodes perpendicular to the long axis (see **Fig. 1**A) explores maximum circumference, as compared with bisecting along the long axis (see **Fig. 1**C) or bread-loafing along the long axis (see **Fig. 1**B).[21]

Identifying and Confirming Sentinel Lymph Node Status

Currently only a physician mapping the SLN and performing its biopsy can validate the sentinel status of the biopsied node. Pathologists may suggest the sentinel nature of the lymph node, if the node under evaluation is blue during grossing, but cannot confirm it objectively. Sentinel nodes may not be positive for metastases and other non-sentinel nodes may be positive for tumor cells. Because of this, presence or absence of metastasis cannot decide the sentinel node status.[22]

To confirm the sentinel status of biopsied lymph node objectively, carbon particles have been included in the dye used for lymph node mapping. Identification of carbon particles in the lymph node during histomorphologic evaluation would allow confirmation of sentinel status of the biopsied lymph node.[22] This approach, however, cannot be applied to cases where a carbon-based black tattoo is located in the same anatomic area as the primary melanoma, because it may share overlapping or identical lymphatic drainage.[19] To avoid this challenge in the future, other colored nanoparticles may be used to replace carbon particles in the injected dye used for sentinel lymph node mapping.

How to and How Many Levels to Evaluate

Cases without grossly identifiable metastasis require the application of a more sensitive approach.[9,19,23,24] If intraoperative evaluation is planned, FS should not be performed, to avoid introduction of freezing artifacts and significant loss of SLN tissue during FS procedure. These negatively affect the final morphologic and immunohistochemical evaluation. Multiple serial sections at different levels are evaluated with H&E stain and immunocytochemistry. The number of sections to be evaluated with H&E and immunohistochemistry is a nagging dilemma with variable approaches.[10,17]

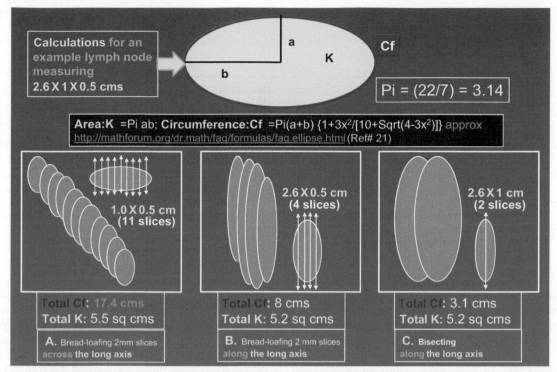

Fig. 1. Method of grossing SLNs—bread-loafing *across* the long axis. (A) Bread-loafing 2 mm slices *across* the long axis, (B) bread-loafing 2 mm slices *along* the long axis, (C) bisecting *along* the long axis. (*From* Shidham VB. Recent advances in pathologic evaluation of melanoma sentinel lymph nodes. Available at: http://www.slideshare.net/vshidham/recent-advances-in-pathologic-evaluation-of-melanoma-sentinel-lymph-nodes-sl-ns-v-shidham-presentation; with permission. Accessed January 7, 2009.)

IMMUNOHISTOCHEMICAL EVALUATION

Currently, morphologic examination with immuno-histochemistry is the most reliable means of SLN evaluation, especially for the detection of melanoma micrometastases and for distinguishing them from benign nevus inclusions.[6,21,23,25]

Conventionally applied immunomarkers for sentinel lymph node evaluation

Although S-100 protein and HMB-45 are excellent conventional melanoma immunomarkers, they can be ineffective in evaluation of SLNs for melanoma micrometastases.[13–15]

S-100 protein (immunostain dendritic cells in the lymph nodes)[15] and HMB-45 (immunostain mast cells)[9] have a high noise-to-signal ratio in SLNs, with a less reliable interpretation than some of the recent melanoma immunomarkers, especially regarding melanoma micrometastases.[9,13,15,18] Due to the previous biopsy procedure for the primary melanoma in the draining lymphatic field, reactive cells, including dendritic cells and mast

cells, are relatively prominent in SLNs, further enhancing this noise factor.

Recent immunomarkers for evaluation of melanoma sentinal lymph nodes

Recently, MART-1, Melan-A, and tyrosinase were reported as melanoma immunomarkers without confounding immunostaining of different components in the reactive lymph nodes.[9,13,14,26] A standardized cocktail can evaluate multiple epitopes and antigens in a single histologic section. This avoids challenges associated with evaluation of coordinate immunoreactivity for individual components in the cocktail in different sections. A mixture of these immunomarkers in the proportions standardized previously as MMC (**Table 1**) showed an excellent discriminatory immunostaining pattern in lymph nodes, with improved detection and interpretation of melanoma cells (**Fig. 2**).[9,13,15]

Evaluation of other melanoma immunomarkers, such as HMB-45[13] and microphthalmia transcription factor,[27] suggested that they would introduce nonspecificity if included in the cocktail.[13] Although a cocktail of HMB-45 along with Melan-A

Table 1
MCW melanoma cocktail

Melanoma Immuniomarker	Clone	Source	Concentration in the Final Cocktail[a]
MART-1	M2-7C10	Signet Laboratories (Dedham, Massachusetts)	1:500
Melan-A	A103	Dako Corporation (Carpinteria, California)	1:100
Tyrosinase	T311	Novocastra Laboratories (Newcastle upon Tyne, UK)	1:50

[a] To 9.68 mL of DAKO antibody diluent (Dako Corporation, Carpinteria, California) add 20 μL MART-1, 100 μL Melan-A, and 200 μL tyrosinase.

Modified from Shidham VB, Qi D, Rao RN, et al. Improved immunohistochemical evaluation of micrometastases in sentinel lymph nodes of cutaneous melanoma with 'MCW melanoma cocktail'—a mixture of monoclonal antibodies to MART-1, melan-A, and tyrosinase. BMC Cancer 2003;3:15:1–9.

and tyrosinase has been used in some studies,[28] such cocktails have the potential for nonspecific immunostaining of certain cells in reactive lymph nodes (such as mast cells by HMB-45 component),[15,26,29,30] and affect the final interpretation (especially in cases with scant tumor cells).

Although MMC is an excellent immunomarker for evaluation of melanoma micrometastases and covers a wider spectrum of melanoma epitopes and antigens than any single immunomarker (three epitopes in two antigens, Melan-A and MART-1, are two epitopes of the same antigen), it has a few relative limitations. Special variants of melanoma, such as desmoplastic melanoma and clear cell melanoma, are known to demonstrate variable immunoreactivity for different melanoma immunomarkers, including S-100 protein. This should not be a limiting concern because the diagnosis of melanoma is known at the time of SLN biopsy, and the purpose of evaluation of SLN is primarily to detect the metastases of a known melanoma. If the primary melanoma is a rare variant, the surgical pathology of the primary lesion should be evaluated

for comparative review along with its immunoreactivity for MMC. If the primary melanoma is nonimmunoreactive for MMC, other melanoma immunomarkers (to which the primary tumor is immunoreactive) should be used with the caveat of accepting the limitations associated with that particular immunomarker. Usually, S-100 protein covers most melanomas and may be the immunomarker of choice in these rare situations, with a caution that the possibility of false positivity exists in interpreting scant micrometastases because of immunoreactivity of other nonmelanoma constituents, such as dendritic cells.

Immunohistochemical Evaluation of Sentinel Lymph Nodes for Melanoma Micrometastases in Paraffin-Embedded Tissue Sections

The details of the protocol for immunostaining 3-μm–thick, paraffin-embedded, tissue sections with MMC were reported previously.[13] Applicable to most of the melanoma markers, MMC also

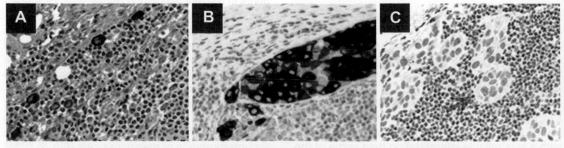

Fig. 2. Melanoma micrometastases in FFPE tissue sections of SLN immunostained with the MMC: (*A*) as single cells; (*B*) as groups of cohesive cells; (*C*) negative control-SLN with metastases of mammary carcinoma (*arrow*). Note the nonimmunoreactivity of mammary carcinoma and adjacent lymphoid tissue for the cocktail. Immunostaining with hematoxylin counterstain. (*Reproduced from* Shidham VB, Qi D, Rao RN, et al. Improved immunohistochemical evaluation of micrometastases in sentinel lymph nodes of cutaneous melanoma with 'MCW melanoma cocktail'—a mixture of monoclonal antibodies to MART-1, melan-A, and tyrosinase. BMC Cancer 2003;3:15:1–9.)

immunostains benign capsular nevi (BCN) in 4% to 10% of SLNs (in addition to melanoma cells).[13,14,31]

Distinguishing BCN from melanoma metastases is one of the most significant diagnostic challenges during evaluation of melanoma SLNs.[9,13,15,23] Currently, morphologic evaluation, with some assistance from immunochemistry, is the only approach to distinguish them. BCNs are generally nonimmunoreactive or weakly immunoreactive for HMB-45, and it has been suggested as an immunomarker to differentiate capsular nevi from melanoma micrometastases.[23] Several melanomas are also nonimmunoreactive for HMB-45. A strong immunoreactivity for HMB-45 favors melanoma metastases and may rule out capsular nevus. Nonimmunoreactivity for HMB-45, however, does not equate with BCN.

Thus, morphology is the most reliable distinguishing feature. BCN are usually seen as cohesive groups of spindle shaped benign melanocytes, mostly along the capsule, and have been reported in variable numbers, ranging from 4% to 22 % of lymph nodes.[9,13,14,31,32]

This challenge is enhanced further by the observation that singly scattered MART-1 or Melan-A immunoreactive parenchymal cells may be observed even in lymph nodes from nonmelanoma cases. One study reported such cells in 11 lymph nodes (two lymph nodes also had associated BCN, four lymph nodes from same case with squamous cell carcinoma) out of 217 lymph nodes from nonmelanoma cases.[32] Because of this reason, non–in situ molecular methodologies, such as reverse transcriptase–polymerase chain reaction,[33–38] without morphologic input are not adequate for separating out BCN from melanoma metastases. Nonmorphology-based molecular tests alone have higher false-positive results, introducing significant nonspecificity, so are not reliable.[21,39]

Although the immunohistochemical features (discussed previously) may be considered, morphology is an important primary tool for correct interpretation of capsular melanocytic nevi in the current situation.[9,13,15,23,32] Cytologic atypia along with location in the subcapsular sinus favors micrometastases.[31] Scant isolated cells with MART-1 or Melan-A immunoreactivity in melanoma SLNs without associated cytologic atypia, comparable to that of the primary melanoma lesion in H&E stained sections, should be interpreted with caution. This highlights the crucial role of morphology in SLN work-up with caution regarding nonmorphology based molecular tests.

INTRAOPERATIVE EVALUATION OF SENTINEL LYMPH NODES

Regional lymphadenectomy after a positive sentinel node result is the recommended practice.[40] Evaluation of SLN for melanoma micrometastases intraoperatively permits completion of regional lymphadenectomy if the results are positive for metastasis. Depending on the flexibility of operative scheduling at individual institutions, intraoperative evaluation of the SLN for metastatic melanoma is strongly recommended to extend the opportunity to complete the concurrent regional lymphadenectomy. This prevents additional surgery for regional lymphadenectomy at a later stage in significant proportion of cases. Because some initially negative cases may show positive results on permanent sections, the chance of returning to the operating room for completion of lymphadenectomy remains. This is related to the phenomenon of sampling artifact with nonretrieval of a rare event in the examined material on the slides during initial rapid intraoperative evaluation. Patients should be educated about this possibility during preoperative consultation.

Intraoperative evaluation has to be rapid, without compromising the final evaluation or definitive results in cases with negative intraoperative results. A few alternatives to rapid intraoperative evaluation of SLN for melanoma micrometastases are discussed briefly. Most of these are unreliable and may compromise the final precise evaluation.[18,25,28,41–44]

Frozen section analysis is not sensitive, with loss of a significant proportion of SLN tissue during this technique. Because of this and other drawbacks, FS evaluation of SLN is strongly discouraged.[45] Similarly, although evaluation of SLN for melanoma metastases with immunostaining of frozen sections has been reported,[28] it is also discouraged because of the same reason and because of the relative difficulty of achieving good quality of immunostaining of frozen sections.[18] These approaches are less sensitive and exhibit higher false-negative rates with the additional potential of introducing freezing artifacts and loss of significant sample material, both of which negatively compromise the quality of tissue for final evaluation with permanent sections.[25,28,41–44]

Imprint cytology with morphologic evaluation is another alternative for rapid intraoperative evaluation.[40] Evaluation of imprint smears does not have the drawbacks associated with FS and is less expensive with rapid turnaround times. The cytomorphologic evaluation of imprint smears, however, is subjective and training dependent, with a low sensitivity, especially for detecting melanoma micrometastases. The melanoma cells have a significantly deceptive resemblance with a variety of reactive cells, such as reactive histiocytes, lymphocytes, fibroblasts, and endothelial cells, which are usually abundant in SLNs.

Recommended Approach (Rapid Immunocytochemical Evaluation of Imprint Smears of Sentinel Lymph Nodes for Melanoma Micrometastases)

Currently, rapid intraoperative immunocytochemical evaluation of imprint smears of SLN sections, without compromising the final evaluation in negative cases, is the most optimal alternative. Conventional melanoma immunomarkers, such as S-100 protein and HMB-45, however, demonstrate significant nonspecificity due to the presence of many nonmelanoma cells immunoreactive for these immunomarkers in most of the lymph nodes.[9]

MMC showed a significantly clean discriminatory immunostaining pattern in lymph nodes.[9,13] Because of this, MMC could be used for rapid

intraoperative immunostaining of imprint smears of SLNs for evaluation of melanoma metastases.[18] If the results are positive (**Fig. 3**), the patient may undergo regional lymphadenectomy synchronously during the same procedure, thus preventing additional surgery at a later time under separate anesthesia.

A rapid protocol for immunostaining of air-dried imprint smears of SLNs with MMC was standardized, with input from the author's and colleagues' previous experiences (**Box 1**)[46,47] (reported by the author and colleagues in detail elsewhere).[18] The cohesive cells of the melanocytic nevi in the capsule and fibrous septa of lymph nodes seem to lack exfoliation onto glass slides during preparation of imprint smears, thus preventing false positivity in all studied cases. This information about lack of exfoliation is a distinct benefit during final morphologic interpretation of benign melanocytic nevi.

Depending on experience, cytomorphologic evaluation can be adapted by any surgical pathologist or cytopathologist after a brief initial learning curve related to preparation, processing, and interpretation of smears.

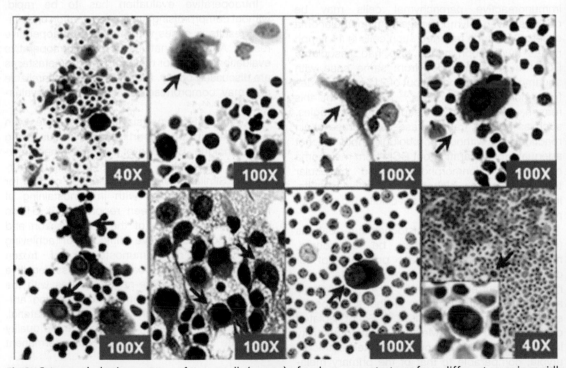

Fig. 3. Cytomorphologic spectrum of tumor cells (*arrows*) of melanoma metastases from different cases in rapidly immunostained air-dried imprint smears with the MMC, after saline rehydration and postfixation in alcohol-formalin. The tumor cells were large and showed high nuclear to cytoplasmic ratios, with nongranular cytoplasmic staining, usually exhibiting clear nuclear details. The chromatin did not resemble the chromatin of adjacent lymphocytes in the background. The cell margins were well defined. (*Reproduced from* Shidham VB, Komorowski R, Macias V, et al. Optimization of immunostaining protocol for rapid intraoperative evaluation of melanoma sentinel lymph nodes imprint smears with the 'MCW melanoma cocktail.' CytoJournal 2004;1:2.)

Box 1
Recommended rapid intraoperative immunostaining protocols

1. Rehydrate air-dried imprint smear with 0.9% saline—15 seconds (approximately 10 slow dips)
2. Postfix the rehydrated smear in alcoholic formalin[a]—5 slow dips and then for 1 minute
3. Rinse the postfixed smear with 95% ethanol (may store in this for a short time up to 30 minutes)
4. 3% H_2O_2 in water—slow dips for 1 minute
5. Deionized water—10 dips
6. Tris buffer (PH 7.6)—10 dips
7. Immunostaining steps

   a. MMC—5 minutes
   b. Rinse in 0.2% Tween 20 (Polysorbate 20) in distilled water (DW.)
   c. HRP-linker antibody[b]—5 minutes
   d. Rinse in tap water
   e. Chromogen diaminobenzidine (DAB)[c]—3 minutes
   f. Rinse in tap water

8. Azure B (blue solution of Diff-Quik), to change brown melanin or other brown pigments into blue gray—1 minute[d]
9. Rinse in tap water
10. Counter-stain with Harris hematoxylin—30 seconds
11. Rinse in tap water—10 dips
12. Dehydrate in ascending concentration of ethanol
13. Clear in xylene
14. Coverslip the smear with the mounting medium.

[a] 50 mL of formalin (38%–40% formaldehyde) to 350 mL of 95% ethanol and 100 mL of distilled water.[46]
[b] May be replaced by Envision + Monoclonal HRP detection kit (DAKO Cat.# K4007). along with Nova Red chromogen (Vector, Cat.# SK-4800).
[c] May be replaced by Nova Red chromogen (Vector, Cat.# SK-4800) with Envision + Monoclonal HRP detection kit (DAKO Cat.# K4007).
[d] May be omitted if the problem of interference due to melanophages is not expected, such as when Nova Red is used as chromogen-indicator system (brick red color).
Modified from Shidham VB, Komorowski R, Macias V, et al. Optimization of immunostaining protocol for rapid intraoperative evaluation of melanoma sentinel lymph nodes imprint smears with the 'MCW melanoma cocktail.' CytoJournal 2004;1:2.

A few structures may interfere with morphologic evaluation of immunostained imprint smears in some cases. They include melanophages, with passively carried melanin and rare mast cells

(**Fig. 4**). Because of the rapid nature of the immunostaining protocol, endogenous peroxidase activity may not be inactivated completely by the short endogenous peroxidase blocking step, and some nonmelanoma cells, such as mast cells (with high endogenous peroxidase), may show coarsely granular cytoplasmic brown staining (or a different color depending on the chromogen) (see **Fig. 4**). The selection of a nonbrown chromogen indicator system may overcome the interference due to the brown-black melanophages. This may also be achieved simply by counterstaining the immunostained smear with azure B, which stains the melanin blue to gray.[9]

SUMMARY OF METHODOLOGY
Grossing the Sentinel Lymph Nodes

Thus, at grossing it is important to transect the lymph node perpendicular to the long axis to get at least 2-mm thick sections (see **Fig. 1**A) to achieve thorough evaluation of most of the subcapsular area (**Fig. 5**).

Intraoperative Evaluation—Dos and Don'ts

Methods used for intraoperative rapid evaluation should not compromise the final definitive evaluation to be continued if the initial results are negative. The quality of FS sections is generally suboptimal with loss of significant proportion of the tissue during FS procedure. In addition, the freezing artifacts compromise the final evaluation of melanoma micrometastases in permanent sections. Because of this, rapid evaluation of melanoma micrometastasis by FS (for H & E–stained sections or immunoperoxidase stained sections of SLNs) is strongly discouraged.[9,41,45]

Selection of Immunomarker (Yesterday, Today, and Tomorrow)

Yesterday
S-100 protein and HMB-45 have been the traditional immunomarkers used for evaluation of melanoma SLNs, but, as discussed previously, they are not optimal due to several drawbacks.

Today
Many new melanoma markers, such as Melan-A, MART-1, and tyrosinase, display cytoplasmic immunoreactivity. They have demonstrated excellent discriminatory immunostaining patterns in lymph nodes, restricted almost entirely to the melanoma cells.[9,13,15] MMC as the prototypical cocktail of these immunomarkers, saves cost and overcomes the interpretative challenges related to the evaluation of coordinate immunoreactivity in multiple serial sections.

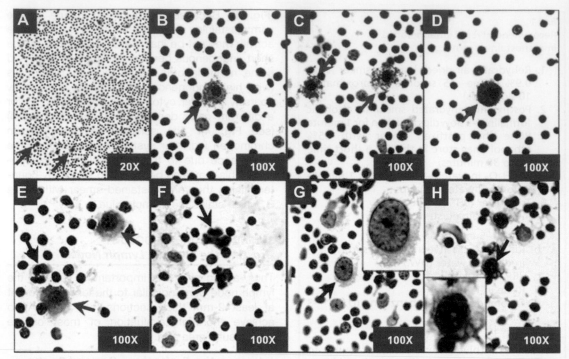

Fig. 4. Morphologic spectrum of nontumor structures in rapidly immunostained, air-dried imprint smears with MMC, after saline rehydration and postfixation in alcohol formalin. (A–E) Mast cells (*brown arrows*) show a low nuclear/cytoplasmic ratio, with granular staining of cytoplasm and fuzzy cell borders. The chromatin is clumped and simulates the chromatin of lymphocytes in the background. (F) Non-nucleated, ill-defined structures (*black arrows*). (G, H) Cells with immunoreactive nuclei (*blue arrow*); zoomed cells with unequivocally negative cytoplasm but with brown staining of the nuclei (*insets*). (*Reproduced from* Shidham VB, Komorowski R, Macias V, et al. Optimization of immunostaining protocol for rapid intraoperative evaluation of melanoma sentinel lymph nodes imprint smears with the 'MCW melanoma cocktail.' CytoJournal 2004;1:2.)

Although currently micrometastases can be highlighted and detected, the biologic categorization of these cells cannot be performed for further prognostic or therapeutic purposes. Such cells may be a component of benign melanocytic nevus inclusions.[9,32,48] Objective molecular or immunohistochemical alternatives other than morphologic evaluation are lacking.

Tomorrow
Future markers for biologic categorization of melanocytic cells in melanoma SLN are indicated. Some techniques, such as laser capture microdissection of cells and their analysis with special studies, may be performed for such evaluation. Simultaneous in situ application of multiple markers facilitating detection and categorization of the melanoma cells in SLN would be of additional biologic and therapeutic significance.

Rapid Intraoperative Evaluation (Yesterday, Today, and Tomorrow)

Yesterday
Due to the many limitations (described previously), rapid intraoperative evaluation of SLNs for melanoma micrometastases not possible in the past without compromising the integrity of SLN biopsy material for final interpretation.

Today
Immunocytochemical evaluation performed on imprint smears for intraoperative evaluation can be performed with an indirect immunocytochemistry method (see **Box 1**).[18] For the best outcome, this requires a relatively complex infrastructure, preferably with an automated immunostainer. Such a set-up may not be available in FS laboratories at many institutions.

Blocking of endogenous enzymes, such as endogenous peroxidase (with reference to HRP indicator system), in a rapid protocol is another significant challenge. Although this problem is

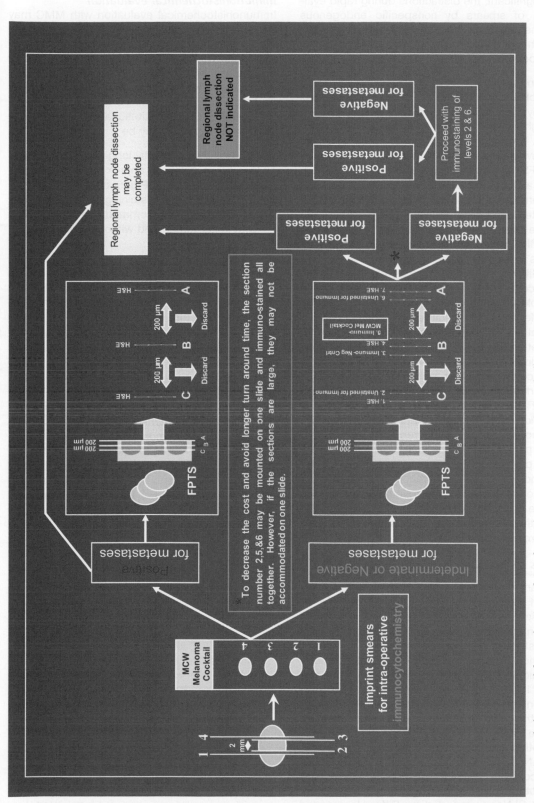

Fig. 5. Recommended protocol for evaluation of SLN for melanoma metastases. (*From* Shidham VB. Recent advances in pathologic evaluation of melanoma sentinel lymph nodes. Available at: http://www.slideshare.net/vshidham/recent-advances-in-pathologic-evaluation-of-melanoma-sentinel-lymph-nodes-sl-ns-v-shidham-presentation; with permission. Accessed January 7, 2009.)

less significant, the distractions during rapid evaluation of smears by nonspecific endogenous enzyme activity may slow down and interfere with the rapid microscopic interpretation during intraoperative evaluation.

Tomorrow

A cocktail consisting of individual antibodies directly conjugated to an indicator enzyme system through polymer for optimum sensitivity is indicated. It may be used for direct immunostaining in a few simple steps, which could be performed in a FS laboratory with basic staining set-up. Such a direct immunostaining protocol not only shortens the immunostaining time by decreasing the steps but also allows its application with routine intraoperative resources in a FS laboratory. This MMC with directly conjugated individual antibodies is currently being engineered.

Additional technology, such as microwaving and liquid cover slipping, may be incorporated in single portable equipment for onsite use in FS laboratoires for rapid intraoperative immunocytochemical evaluation. The same equipment may be used for evaluation of SLNs related to other cancers, including breast, Merkel cell tumor, and so forth, in concert with suitable antibodies and protocols.

Interference by the endogenous peroxidase in the HRP indicator system may be overcome by specific inhibitors/blocking agents. Such an inhibitor should nullify the interference by the endogenous peroxidase in the mast cells during the rapid protocol without interfering with the cytomorphology and immunoreactivity properties of melanoma cells. This improvement would also reduce indeterminate interpretations by simplifying the learning curve for distinguishing mast cells from melanoma tumor cells.

Levels to Examine

Permanent sections, at least three levels at intervals of 200 μm, should be evaluated (see **Fig. 5**). The section adjacent to each H & E–stained section at each level is selected for immunoperoxidase staining. All three levels may be evaluated by immunostaining concurrently or by evaluating only the middle level initially, followed by other two levels if the middle level is negative. If all three sections are small enough to be mounted on single slide, they may be immunostained simultaneously on one slide.

Another approach is to consider gamma counts of SLN specimens and implement a suitable protocol, with evaluation of more levels-sections for hotter SLNs and fewer levels-sections for colder SLNs, as reported by Riber-Hansen and colleagues.[10]

Immunohistochemical evaluation

Immunohistochemical evaluation with MMC may be performed intraoperatively on imprints of the cut surfaces of a transected SLN. If the results are negative, the lymph nodes are evaluated for melanoma micrometastasis by immunohistochemical evaluation with MMC on permanent sections.

Depending on the institutional choices, the recommended protocol may be

1. Sequential with slightly longer turnaround time (additional delay of approximately 24 hours) with lower cost (see **Fig. 5**) or
2. Concurrent immunostaining if all the three sections can be accommodated on one slide (with faster turnaround without additional cost) or
3. Concurrent immunostaining of all the three levels on different slides simultaneously if all sections cannot be accommodated on fewer glass slides (with faster turnaround but at higher cost) (see **Fig. 5**).

ACKNOWLEDGMENTS

I thank Dr Dzwierzynski (plastic surgery) and Dr Neuburg (dermatology) for their multidisciplinary clinical support as coinvestigators for the evaluation of the MMC. I thank Dr Saul Suster, Dr Jose Plaza, Dr Richard Komorowski, Dr George Varsegi, and Dr Krista D'Amore for their input in improving the manuscript. I also thank Anushree Shidham for copy editing support. The technical support of John R. Kuhnmuench, BS; Dr Farrukh Ghazala, MD; and Glen Dawson, BS, HT, IHC(ASCP), from my research group is highly appreciated.

REFERENCES

1. Salti GI, Das Gupta TK. Predicting residual lymph node basin disease in melanoma patients with sentinel lymph node metastases. Am J Surg 2003; 186:98–101.
2. Nowecki ZI, Rutkowski P, Nasierowska-Guttmejer A, et al. Sentinel lymph node biopsy in melanoma patients with clinically negative regional lymph nodes—one institution's experience. Melanoma Res 2003;13:35–43.
3. Manca G, Facchetti F, Pizzocaro C, et al. Nodal staging in localized melanoma. The experience of the Brescia Melanoma Unit. Br J Plast Surg 2003; 56:534–9.
4. Rutkowski P, Nowecki ZI, Nasierowska-Guttmejer A, et al. Lymph node status and survival in cutaneous malignant melanoma—sentinel lymph node biopsy impact. Eur J Surg Oncol 2003;29:611–8.

5. Wagner JD, Ranieri J, Evdokimow DZ, et al. Patterns of initial recurrence and prognosis after sentinel lymph node biopsy and selective lymphadenectomy for melanoma. Plast Reconstr Surg 2003;112:486–97.

6. Zapas JL, Coley HC, Beam SL, et al. The risk of regional lymph node metastases in patients with melanoma less than 1.0 mm thick: recommendations for sentinel lymph node biopsy. J Am Coll Surg 2003; 197:403–7.

7. Pu LL, Wells KE, Cruse CW, et al. Prevalence of additional positive lymph nodes in complete lymphadenectomy specimens after positive sentinel lymphadenectomy findings for early-stage melanoma of the head and neck. Plast Reconstr Surg 2003; 112:43–9.

8. Reintgen DS, Cruse CW, Glass F, et al. In support of sentinel node biopsy as a standard of care for patients with malignant melanoma. Dermatol Surg 2000;26:1070–2.

9. Shidham VB, Chang CC, Komorowski R. 'MCW melanoma cocktail' for evaluation of metastases in sentinel lymph nodes of cutaneous melanoma (invited review article). Expert Rev Mol Diagn 2005; 5(3):281–90.

10. Riber-Hansen R, Sjoegren P, Hamilton-Dutoit SJ, et al. Extensive pathological analysis of selected melanoma sentinel lymph nodes: high metastasis detection rates at reduced workload. Ann Surg Oncol 15(5):1492–1501.

11. Morton DL, Thompson JF, Cochran AJ, et al. Sentinel-node biopsy or nodal observation in melanoma. N Engl J Med 2006;355:1307–17.

12. Gershenwald JE, Thompson W, Mansfield PF, et al. Multiinstitutional melanoma lymphatic mapping experience: the prognostic value of sentinel lymph node status in 612 stage I or II melanoma patients. J Clin Oncol 1999;17:976–83.

13. Shidham VB, Qi D, Rao R, et al. Improved immunohistochemical evaluation of micrometastases in sentinel lymph nodes of cutaneous melanoma with MCW melanoma cocktail—a mixture of monoclonal antibodies to MART-1, Melan-A, and Tyrosinase. BMC Cancer 2003;3(1):15, 1–9. Available at: http://www.biomedcentral.com/qc/1471-2407/3/15.

14. Qi D, Acker S, Kampalath B, et al. Detection of melanoma micrometastases in sentinel lymph nodes: evaluation of MART-1 and Melan-A in comparison to traditionally used immunomarkers [abstract no. 8]. Am J Clin Pathol 2000;114:629–59.

15. Shidham VB, Qi D, Acker S, et al. Evaluation of micrometastases in sentinel lymph nodes of cutaneous melanoma: higher diagnostic accuracy with Melan-A and MART-1 compared to S-100 protein and HMB-45. Am J Surg Pathol 2001;25:1039–46.

16. Shidham V, Macias V, Neuberg M, et al. Rapid intraoperative immunocytochemical evaluation of cutaneous melanoma sentinel lymph nodes for melanoma metastases with 'MCW Melanoma Cocktail' [abstract no. 191]. Acta Cytol 2003;47:938.

17. Gietema HA, Vuylsteke RJ, de Jonge IA, et al. Sentinel lymph node investigation in melanoma: detailed analysis of the yield from step sectioning and immunohistochemistry. J Clin Pathol 2004; 57(6):618–20.

18. Shidham VB, Komorowski R, Macias V, et al. Optimization of immunostaining protocol for rapid intraoperative evaluation of imprint smears of melanoma sentinel lymph nodes with 'MCW melanoma cocktail'. CytoJournal 2004;1:2. DOI:10.1186/1742-6413-1-2 Free full text is Available at: http://www.cytojournal.com/content/1/1/2.

19. Cochran AJ, Ohsie SJ, Binder SW. Pathobiology of the sentinel node. Curr Opin Oncol 2008;20:190–5.

20. Thomas JM. Prognostic false-positivity of the sentinel node in melanoma. Nat Clin Pract Oncol 2008;5:18–23.

21. Ellipse & parabola formulas, ask Dr Math: FAQ, the math forum @ Drexel. Available at: http://mathforum.org/dr.math/faq/formulas/faq.ellipse.html. Accessed: January 1, 2009. Archived by WebCite at: http://www.webcitation.org/5dVtGAVxS.

22. Haigh PI, Lucci A, Turner RR, et al. Carbon dye histologically confirms the identity of sentinel lymph nodes in cutaneous melanoma. Cancer 2001;92:535–41.

23. Cochran AJ. Surgical pathology remains pivotal in the evaluation of 'sentinel' lymph nodes. Am J Surg Pathol 1999;23:1169–72.

24. Cochran AJ, Wen DR, Herschman HR, et al. Detection of S-100 protein as an aid to the identification of melanocytic tumors. Int J Cancer 1982; 30:295–7.

25. Gibbs JF, Huang PP, Zhang PJ, et al. Accuracy of pathologic techniques for the diagnosis of metastatic melanoma in sentinel lymph nodes. Ann Surg Oncol 1999;6:699–704.

26. Jungbluth AA, Iverson K, Coplan K, et al. T311—an anti-tyrosinase monoclonal antibody for the detection of melanocytic lesions in paraffin embedded tissues. Pathol Res Pract 2000;196(4): 235–42.

27. Miettinen M, Fernandez M, Franssila K, et al. Microphthalmia transcription factor in the immunohistochemical diagnosis of metastatic melanoma: comparison with four other melanoma markers. Am J Surg Pathol 2001;25:205–11.

28. Eudy GE, Carlson GW, Murray DR, et al. Rapid immunohistochemistry of sentinel lymph nodes for metastatic melanoma. Hum Pathol 2003;34: 797–802.

29. Shidham VB, Susnik B, Rao RN, et al. HMB45 immunoreactive single cells in sentinel lymph nodes negative for melanoma micrometastases are mast cells [abstract no. 1528]. Mod Pathol 2004;17(Suppl 1):1a–388a.

30. Mahmood MN, Lee MW, Linden MD, et al. Diagnostic value of HMB-45 and anti-Melan A staining of sentinel lymph nodes with isolated positive cells. Mod Pathol 2002;15(12):1288–93.

31. Yu LL, Flotte TJ, Tanabe KK, et al. Detection of microscopic melanoma metastases in sentinel lymph nodes. Cancer 1999;86:617–27.

32. Yan S, Brennick JB. False-positive rate of the immunoperoxidase stains for MART1/MelanA in lymph nodes. Am J Surg Pathol 2004;28:596–600.

33. Blaheta HJ, Ellwanger U, Schittek B, et al. Examination of regional lymph nodes by sentinel node biopsy and molecular analysis provides new staging facilities in primary cutaneous melanoma. J Invest Dermatol 2000;114:637–42.

34. Blaheta HJ, Paul T, Sotlar K, et al. Detection of melanoma cells in sentinel lymph nodes, bone marrow and peripheral blood by a reverse transcription-polymerase chain reaction assay in patients with primary cutaneous melanoma: association with Breslow's tumour thickness. Br J Dermatol 2001;145:195–202.

35. Ghossein R, Rosai J. Polymerase chain reaction in the detection of micrometastases and circulating tumor cells. Cancer 1996;78:10–6.

36. Ribe A, McNutt NS. S100A6 protein expression is different in Spitz nevi and melanomas. Mod Pathol 2003;16(5):505–11.

37. Shivers SC, Wang X, Li W, et al. Molecular staging of malignant melanoma: correlation with clinical outcome. JAMA 1998;280:1410–5.

38. Sung J, Li W, Shivers S, et al. Molecular analysis in evaluating the sentinel node in malignant melanoma. Ann Surg Oncol 2001;8(Suppl 9):29S–30S.

39. Rimoldi D, Lemoine R, Kurt AM, et al. Groupe Mélanome Lémanique. Detection of micrometastases in sentinel lymph nodes from melanoma patients: direct comparison of multimarker molecular and immunopathological methods. Melanoma Res 2003;13:511–20.

40. Soo V, Shen P, Pichardo R, et al. Intraoperative evaluation of sentinel lymph nodes for metastatic melanoma by imprint cytology. Ann Surg Oncol 2007; 14:1612–7.

41. Clary BM, Lewis JJ, Brady MS, et al. Should frozen section analysis of the sentinel node be performed in patients with melanoma? Eur J Nucl Med 1999; 26:S68.

42. Tanis PJ, Boom RP, Koops HS, et al. Frozen section investigation of the sentinel node in malignant melanoma and breast cancer. Ann Surg Oncol 2001;8: 222–6.

43. Creager AJ, Shiver SA, Shen P, et al. Intraoperative evaluation of sentinel lymph nodes for metastatic melanoma by imprint cytology. Cancer 2002;94: 3016–22.

44. Hocevat M, Bracko M, Pogacnik A, et al. Role of imprint cytology in the intraoperative evaluation of sentinel lymph nodes for malignant melanoma. Eur J Cancer 2003;39:2173–8.

45. Stojadinovic A, Allen PJ, Clary BM, et al. Value of frozen-section analysis of sentinel lymph nodes for primary cutaneous malignant melanoma. Ann Surg 2002;235:92–8.

46. Shidham VB, Chang CC, Rao RN, et al. Immunostaining of cytology smears: a comparative study to identify the most suitable method of smear preparation and fixation with reference to commonly used immunomarkers. Diagn Cytopathol 2003;29:217–21.

47. Shidham V, Kampalath B, England J. Routine air drying of all the smears prepared during fine needle aspiration and intraoperative cytology studies. An opportunity to practice a unified protocol, offering the flexibility of choosing variety of staining methods. Acta Cytol 2001;45:60–8.

48. Abrahamsen HN, Hamilton-Dutoit SJ, Larsen J, et al. Sentinel lymph nodes in malignant melanoma: extended histopathologic evaluation improves diagnostic precision. Cancer 2004;100(8):1683–91.

Complete Lymph Node Dissection for Regional Nodal Metastasis

William W. Dzwierzynski, MD, FACS

KEYWORDS

- Axillary dissection • Groin dissection
- Ilioinguinal dissection • Complete lymph node dissection
- Therapeutic lymph node dissection • Lymphedema

Melanoma is now the sixth most common cancer, and more than 8000 patients die from the disease each year. Stage I and II melanoma remains a highly curable disease, but stage III melanoma is a significant threat to life.[1] The basics of surgical treatment for advanced disease have not changed significantly in the last century. In 1892 Snow proposed lymph node dissection as a method to control regional nodal metastasis for early stage melanoma.[2] Surgical resection remains the only proven treatment for local and advanced melanoma.

Sentinel node biopsy (SNB) has been the most significant advance in the treatment of melanoma. This procedure can help identify patients with early stage III disease who may benefit from complete node dissection. Before the advent of sentinel lymph node biopsy, elective lymph node dissection (ELND) was advocated for many patients with intermediate-depth melanoma of the extremity, yet the benefit of ELND remained unproven. Several non-randomized studies suggested a survival benefit to ELND, yet all randomized studies of ELND showed no proven survival benefit.[3,4] ELND also carries a significant risk of morbidity. This is problematic, most notably in patients who were node negative. Since occult disease was identified in only 20% to 33% of ELNDs, many patients were subjected to this morbidity unnecessarily.[4,5] The era of ELND ended with the advent of SNB. In 1999 the World Health Organization declared SNB as the standard of care in melanoma in patients with no clinical evidence of metastasis.[6]

The Multicenter Selective Lymphadenectomy Trial (MSLT) was initiated in 1993 to determine whether intraoperative lymphatic mapping followed by selective lymphadenectomy would effectively prolong overall survival.[7] Subset analysis of the data suggested that for patients with tumors of intermediate thickness and occult metastasis, disease-free survival is better among those patients who undergo immediate lymphadenectomy compared with those who delay lymphadenectomy until after the clinical appearance of nodal metastasis.[8]

The terminology used for node dissections is confusing, with references to complete lymph node dissections (CLNDs), ELNDs, therapeutic lymph node dissections (TLNDs), and radical lymph node dissection (RLNDs). The term TLND is used if clinically positive lymphadenopathy is identified on physical examination. ELND is referred to only if the nodal status is unknown and the dissection is performed prophylactically. Since the advent of SNB, this procedure has virtually been abandoned. CLND and RLND are often used interchangeably. The terms complete and radical are used to differentiate these dissections from node-sampling procedures performed for other diseases, such as breast cancer. Unlike nodal sampling for breast cancer, which is a staging procedure, CLND for melanoma is performed as a curative resection with a goal of removing all of the lymph nodes and metastatic disease in a lymphatic basin. Young surgeons, with training in heavy breast oncology, often fail to realize the difference between these surgical procedures and to understand the much more extensive dissection required for the CLND.

Department of Plastic Surgery, Medical College of Wisconsin, 8700 Watertown Plank Road, Milwaukee, WI 53226, USA
E-mail address: billd@mcw.edu

Clin Plastic Surg 37 (2010) 113–125
doi:10.1016/j.cps.2009.07.002
0094-1298/09/$ – see front matter © 2010 Elsevier Inc. All rights reserved.

NATIONAL COMPREHENSIVE CANCER NETWORK RECOMMENDATIONS

The National Comprehensive Cancer Network (NCCN) guidelines recommend CLND for patients with clinical stage III disease or with nodal metastasis found after SNB.[9,10] The guidelines recommend that all nodal tissue be sent for permanent evaluation since frozen sections are not reliable. CLND should be performed in all patients with a positive sentinel lymph node biopsy unless they are participating in a clinical trial or have severe comorbidities. This procedure offers a chance of a surgical cure for patients with disease localized to the regional nodes, but also offers decreased morbidity for patients with extensive nodal involvement or patients with distal metastatic disease. CLND removes extensive tumor deposits, which can cause ulceration, pain, and significant disability. CLND virtually eliminates regional lymph node recurrences and the associated morbidity.

Bilimoria and colleagues[1] reviewed the national cancer database of patients with stage I, II, and III melanomas, to determine compliance with the NCCN guidelines. More than 44,000 patients with melanoma were identified between 2004 and 2005. Nodal metastasis was identified in 17% of these patients (2942 of 7524) after sentinel lymph node biopsy. Only 50% of these patients underwent CLND. Patients with lower extremity melanomas and those older than 75 years had a significantly lower chance of undergoing CLND. Of patients without nodal metastases, 17% did have a CLND. It is unclear why a patient with a negative sentinel lymph node would be subjected to a CLND. This may be because surgeons do not understand the rationale of SNB compared with ELND, or possibly surgeons early in their SNB career may not yet feel comfortable with their biopsy technique. Using the National Cancer Institute (NCI) Surveillance, Epidemiology and End Results database, Cormier found that the rate of patients undergoing CLND decreased from 76% to 66% from 1998 to 2001, and the rate from 2003 to 2004 was only 50%.[11] This suggests that physicians are unaware of the current guidelines or are rejecting them. Further information is required to answer these questions.

DO WE NEED A COMPLETE NODE DISSECTION IN ALL PATIENTS WITH A POSITIVE SENTINEL NODE?

SNB followed by CLND has reduced the need for unnecessary node dissections in 80% of patients who may have been eligible for an ELND. When CLND is performed after SNB, metastases to nonsentinel lymph nodes (non-SLNs) are found in 7% to 28% of patients.[11,12] The necessity of CLND has been questioned by many practitioners, especially in patients with micrometastases.[13] The Multicenter Selective Lymphadenectomy Trial 2 (MSLT-2) is designed to answer the question "Is sentinel node biopsy alone enough?" The results of the MSLT-2 trial will not be available for many years; it is hoped that when this study is fully analyzed, the benefit of CLND in sentinel lymph node positive patients will be better known.[9] Until that time many researchers have tried to determine if there is a group of patients who have a positive sentinel node yet may not need a CLND.

Independent risk factors for involvement of non-SLNs have been analyzed by several groups. Clinical pathologic risk factors have included primary tumors in the head and neck or lower extremity, Breslow depth (>2 or >4 mm depending on the study), number of positive SLNs, and tumor satellitosis.[14–17] Risk factors specific to the SLN pathology include angiolymphatic invasion, extranodal extension, tumor seen on hematoxylin and eosin (H&E) stain, and tumor burden.[15,16,18–21] The most promising predictor of non-SLN metastasis is sentinel lymph node tumor burden. Frankel found tumor burden of greater than 1% of surface area of the lymph nodes statistically correlated with finding tumor-spread to non-SLNs.[20] Satzger identified tumor burden greater than 10% of the total lymph node tissue along with metastasis identified by H&E stain alone, and perinodal intralymphatic tumor invasion had a high correlation with positive non-SLN involvement.[22] However, in 5 of 28 (18%) patients with non-SLN involvement, all three of these parameters were negative. Even when only isolated tumor cells are seen in the sentinel node, further positive non-SLNs can be found on CLND.[21] Non-SLN positivity before CLND cannot be predicted.[16] Analysis of previous studies shows there is no absolute factor that correlates with non-SLN positivity or negativity, and therefore at least until the results of the MSLT-II trial are known, the decision not to perform a CLND should be made cautiously and probably only as part of a clinical trial.

TECHNIQUES OF SNB
Axillary Dissection

The goal of axillary CLND is to remove all lymph node–bearing tissue. This includes all lymphatic-bearing tissue anterior, posterior, superior, and inferior to the axillary vessels. The limits of the dissection extend superiorly from the subclavius muscle inferiorly to the level of the thoracodorsal nerve insertion into the latissimus dorsi muscle, approximately at the level of the areola. The medial limit of the dissection is the first rib (medial to the edge of the pectoralis minor muscle), extending laterally to the edge of the latissimus dorsi muscle. Included in the dissection is the nodal tissue above the pectoralis major muscle, between the pectoralis major and minor muscles (Rotter node), and between the pectoralis major and latissimus dorsi muscles. Dissection of levels 1, 2, and 3 lymph nodes is recommended. Removal of the fascia of the pectoralis muscles, the subaxillary fat pad, the interpectoral space, and lateral chest wall is also recommended. The intercostal brachial nerves should be resected, but the long thoracic and thoracodorsal nerves must be preserved unless overly involved in tumor.[6]

The operation is performed under general anesthesia. After intubation no further muscle relaxation is used to allow identification of the motor nerves. A preoperative dose of cefazolin is used along with appropriate deep vein thrombosis prophylaxis. The patient is placed in the supine position with a rolled towel under the ipsilateral scapula to facilitate access to the axillary cavity. There is no consensus on the optimal surgical approach for axillary lymph node dissection. There are three incision choices: a transverse incision, extending from the edge of the pectoralis major to the border of the latissimus dorsi muscle; a U-shaped incision; or an extended S-shaped incision following the contour of the pectoralis major into the axillary apex and down the border of the latissimus dorsi muscle.[23] The author uses an S-shaped incision starting just behind the pectoralis major muscle, posterior under the level of the axillary hairline and then inferiorly over the anterior edge of the latissimus dorsi muscle (**Fig. 1**). This incision gives excellent access to the axillary contents and is well hidden under the pectoral fold. Although the straight transverse

incision may appear to give better cosmesis, if it extends beyond the pectoral fold it is obvious. The biopsy site from the SNB should be incorporated in the incision. Skin flaps should be 4 to 5 mm thick initially and progressively thicker as the dissection approaches its base. Initial dissection is performed with the monopolar cautery, but as the muscle and axillary vessels are approached, bipolar cautery allows a safer dissection. Flaps are developed anteriorly above the level of the pectoralis major muscle and inferiorly to the edge of the latissimus dorsi muscle.

The adipose tissue above the pectoralis major muscle is dissected along with the fascia of the pectoralis major muscle; dissection proceeds laterally to the edge of the pectoralis major muscle and in the space between the major and minor muscles (**Fig. 2**). If there are palpable nodes in the axilla, the pectoralis minor is divided; if no palpable nodes are present, the pectoralis minor is preserved. The limit of the dissection is the medial edge of the pectoralis muscle where the medial pectoral nerve and artery pierce the pectoralis on the minor and major muscles. The nerve must be spared to preserve the function of the pectoralis muscles. The interpectoral fat and Rotter node are mobilized toward the specimen. To reach level 3, the assistant adducts the extremity over the patient's head to relax the pectoralis major muscle (**Fig. 3**). The fascia is divided with tenotomy scissors and the bipolar electrocautery and the axillary contents are exposed. The axillary vein is exposed and skeletonized. The adipose tissue and lymph nodes over the plexus are mobilized; a stick sponge or a right-angle clamp is helpful during this portion of the dissection. The assistant strongly retracts the pectoralis minor muscle with a Richardson retractor to allow access to the most medial portion of the dissection. Tributaries to the vein and lymphatics are

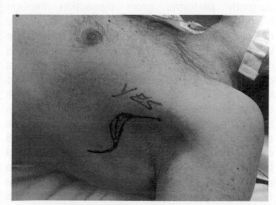

Fig. 1. Marking for axillary node dissection, the incision from the SNB is incorporated in the "S" incision.

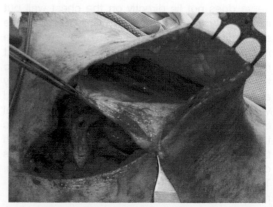

Fig. 2. The pectoralis fascia and lymphatic tissue is elevated en-bloc with the axillary contents.

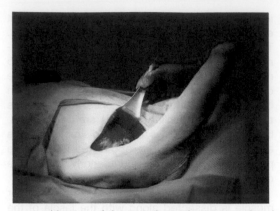

Fig. 3. Adduction of the arm above the patient's head facilitated access to level 3 lymph nodes.

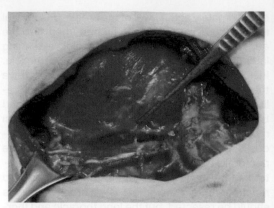

Fig. 4. Completion of the axillary CLND. The axillary vessels are seen. The forceps points out the long thoracic nerve overlying the serratus anterior muscle. The thoracodorsal nerve and vessels are seen at the lower aspect of the incision. The lymphatic tissue has been removed between the two nerves.

clipped with hemaclips and the axillary contents are mobilized laterally; the inferior flap is developed to the surface of the serratus anterior muscle.[24] The skeletonization of the axillary vein continues to the first rib, and the adipose tissue and lymph nodes are dissected from the vein. At this point before approaching the long thoracic nerve, the assistant stops adducting the arm, and the inferior and posterior portions of the dissection are performed. Dissection proceeds down to the level of T6, or roughly the level of the nipple. The posterior dissection identifies the edge of the latissimus dorsi muscle, dissecting medially over the muscle to the thoracodorsal vessels. The assistant once again adducts the arm to continue the dissection of the axillary contents. The intercostal brachial nerves and vessels are identified coursing laterally from the chest wall; these are clipped and divided close to the chest wall. This results in persistent numbness in the axilla, which is usually well tolerated by the patient. Two important nerves are encountered. The first is the long thoracic nerve. The nerve does not lie directly on the chest wall but in the fatty tissue slightly above it; direct gentle stimulation with a forceps can help identify the nerve. Lateral to the long thoracic nerve, the next nerve encountered is the thoracodorsal nerve to the latissimus dorsi muscle. This nerve is closely accompanied by the thoracodorsal artery and vein (**Fig. 4**); the nerve lies just inside the lateral edge of the latissimus dorsi muscle. The lymphatic tissue between these two nerves is dissected with the specimen. The lateral edge of the latissimus dorsi marks the posterior extent of the dissection. The en-bloc dissection is then removed from inferior to superior.

After completion of the dissection, meticulous hemostasis is obtained. One or two closed-suction

drains are placed in the axilla through separate stab incisions. Fibrin glue has been used, but has not been shown to decrease seroma formation or complications. Patients are usually admitted overnight for recovery and discharged home the next morning. The drains are left in place until they produce less than 30 mL of fluid a day. Drainage can continue for up to 4 to 6 weeks. Postoperative antibiotics are not used. Patients are encouraged to begin range of motion of the arm immediately, but aggressive therapy is withheld until the drains are removed. Although lymphedema in the upper extremity is uncommon after CLND, the patients are referred to a lymphedema-certified therapist for exercises and prophylactic care.

Inguinal Dissection

The options for skin incisions include transverse, vertical, oblique, or sigmoidal.[24–26] The author currently performs groin dissection through a limited transverse incision. Although technically more demanding, this approach has fewer wound-healing complications. The incision is made 1 to 2 fingerbreadths above the inguinal crease (**Fig. 5**). The incision may be varied to incorporate the scar from the SNB. Scars in the crease are more likely to develop complications from skin maceration. The superior limit of the dissection for a superficial node dissection is 5 cm above the inguinal ligament. The medial border of the adductor longus muscle, and the pubic tubercle are the medial extent of the dissection. The lateral border of the dissection is the sartorius muscle and the anterior superior iliac spine. The inferior limit of the dissection is the

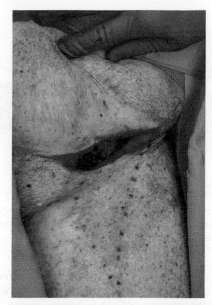

Fig. 5. Transverse approach to the inguinal CLND. The incision is placed above the groin crease. The surface markings are the adductor longus muscle (*right*) and the sartorius muscle (*left*).

confluence of the sartorius and adductor longus muscle, this is where the greater saphenous vein is encountered.[25] Three-millimeter flaps are developed. At the origin of the sartorius muscle over the anterior superior iliac spine, the lateral femoral cutaneous nerve lies in front of the sartorius muscle, and this should be preserved. The motor branches of the femoral nerve and the saphenous nerve, which courses next to the femoral artery, should be preserved. The sheath of the femoral artery is entered and dissection continues within the sheath of the artery, mobilizing the anterior half of the sheath toward the specimen. Small branches of the artery are ligated. Inferiorly the dissection is continued to the confluence of the sartorius and adductorlongus muscles. Here the saphaneous vein is encountered and must be ligated. A small incision directly over the vein at this point may aid the ligation. The dissection is performed to the inguinal ligament and Cloquet node is dissected. If the groin dissection is done for a positive sentinel node, it is stopped at this point.

One melanoma center uses the results of lymphoscintigrams, obtained during sentinel lymph node biopsy, to determine the extent of their groin dissection.[27] A combined superficial and deep dissection is performed when the lymphoscintigram shows second-echelon nodes in the deep lymph node area. Otherwise, only a superficial dissection is performed. If nodal metastasis proceeds in a stepwise fashion, and a second-echelon node is a deep

node, patients with positive sentinel nodes are more likely to develop deep lymphatic nodal spread. The value of the Cloquet node alone in predicting pelvic nodal status is debatable. A tumor-positive Cloquet node had a sensitivity of only 65% to predict involvement of deep nodes and a negative predictive value of 78%.[13,27–30]

If there is tumor metastasis in the Cloquet node or palpable involvement of the inguinal nodes, the dissection is continued with the deep inguinal dissection in continuity with the superficial dissection. The inguinal ligament is divided 2 cm superior and medial to the anterior superior iliac spine. The external oblique and inguinal ligaments are divided and internal oblique, transverse abdominis, and transversalis fasciae are divided. The retroperitoneal space is entered and the peritoneum is mobilized. The inferior epigastric artery and vein are ligated and divided. The peritoneum is retracted medially and the obturator lymph nodes and lymph nodes along the internal and common iliac vessels are exposed. Dissection is performed inferiorly down to the external iliac lymph nodes. Medially, the iliac nodes are separated from the bladder. The obturator nerve and vessels are exposed. The transversalis, abdominis, and internal oblique are closed with permanent suture, and the inguinal ligament is reconstructed. Regardless of whether a superficial or deep dissection is performed, the sartorius muscle is mobilized to cover the femoral vessels (**Fig. 6**). The risk of vessel exposure is small but a sartorius flap has minimum morbidity and is quick to perform. The fascia over the sartorius muscle is excised superiorly and the muscle is divided from its insertion on the anterior superior iliac spine. The 1 or 2 most superior perforating vessels from the femoral artery and vein are divided and the muscle is mobilized medially and inset onto the inguinal ligament. A drain is placed and is brought out through a separate stab wound or the inferior incision if one was made for the saphenous vein ligation.

Modified inguinal node dissections have been described with 2 transverse incisions and preservation of the saphenous vein and femoral sheath.[31] Parallel skin incisions 4 to 5 cm above and below the inguinal ligament are used in an attempt to then decrease wound necrosis. Combined endoscopic and open ilioinguinal node dissections have also been used.[32] The deep pelvic portion of dissection is performed using an endoscopic peritoneal approach, and the superficial inguinal dissection is performed using a conventional approach. This technique is similar to an endoscopic extraperitoneal hernia repair.[27]

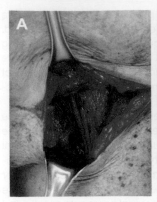
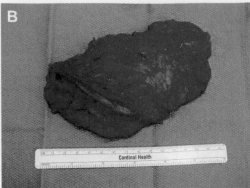
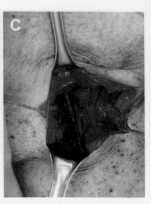

Fig. 6. (*A*) Completion of the superficial inguinal dissection. Structures from medial to lateral, the pectineus muscle, femoral vein, femoral artery, femoral nerve, and sartorius muscle. (*B*) Surgical specimen from the inguinal lympadenectomy. (*C*) The sartorius muscle (in forceps) is mobilized to cover the femoral vessels.

Unusual Sites of Metastasis

Interval sentinel nodes have been reported in 1% to 15% of sentinel node biopsies.[33–35] The most common locations of these nodes are in the popliteal fossa, epitrochlear fossa, and supraclavicular neck. Melanoma metastasis to these areas can occur. There is controversy about the proper treatment for these areas of metastasis and for the distal site of lymphatic drainage. The implications of a positive interval SLN are the same as those of positive SLN in other sites. Patients with positive SLN are at higher risk for recurrence and death due to melanoma and may benefit from lymph node dissection. Drainage to interval nodes is an infrequent but important event that has significant implications for patient treatment. Generally, a node dissection should be performed in the interval area. Whether a complete node dissection should be performed in the more distal nodal basin is debatable.[36] The question arises whether an axillary dissection should be performed for a positive SLN in the epitrochlear area if there is a negative finding in the SLN in the axilla. Careful consideration of each individual case is needed.

Adequacy of Dissection

The NCCN guidelines recommend that 15 or more nodes should be resected in an axillary dissection and 10 or more nodes should be resected in the inguinal dissection.[9] The parameters for inclusion in MSLT-1[8] require more than 15 lymph nodes for an axillary dissection, more than 8 nodes for inguinal dissection, and more than 6 nodes for a pelvic node dissection.

Spillane and colleagues from the Sydney Melanoma Unit reviewed 2363 RLNDs. Surgery performed by experienced melanoma unit surgeons had an average of 21.9 lymph nodes removed

from the axilla. Surgery by non-melanoma unit surgeons averaged 17.8 nodes. In groin dissections, an average of 14.5 lymph nodes were removed by melanoma unit surgeons and 12.0 nodes by non-melanoma unit surgeons.[37] Spillane and colleagues found a significant prognostic value to the number of positive lymph nodes resected. They postulate that a CLND should increase the chance of removing all regional disease and accurately assessing the number of nodes that contain melanoma metastases. Chan and Morton reviewed the database of 8700 melanoma patients from 1971 to 1999 who had TLND at the John Wayne Cancer Institute.[38] Of these, 548 patients underwent regional lymph node dissection. The extent of lymph nodes dissected ranged from 1 to 98 lymph nodes. Chan and Morton divided the lymph node dissections into quartiles for each nodal basin. The 5-year survival rate in patients who had the greatest number of lymph nodes removed was improved compared with the less complete dissections. They conclude that the extent of the lymph node dissection is important, especially in patients with higher tumor burdens. Yet the NCI database review from 2004 to 2005 found only 69% of the 1470 CLNDs had more than 10 lymph nodes resected.[1] Cases with low lymph node counts should be assessed critically, and acceptable standards should be reproducible among surgeons.

Complications

The aim of CLND is to achieve radical control of microscopic and macroscopic disease, and to prevent the unnecessary morbidity of an ELND. CLND is not an innocuous procedure; the risk of surgical complications is high.[39] Complication rates range from 30% to more than 80%. Wound-related complications include skin necrosis, infections, hematomas, seromas, and prolonged lymph fluid drainage. Long-term complications include nerve injuries, stiffness, and chronic lymphedema.

Wound Morbidity

Wound complications are reported frequently after CLND. After axillary dissections, rates are reported from 19% to more than 50% (**Table 1**).[3,40,42–44] Complications from inguinal dissections have been reported in up to 90% of patients (**Table 2**).[3,40,42–46] The reasons for these complications are varied, but most commonly are related to the disruption of the lymphatics or the thinness of the skin flaps. Several studies have implicated radiation as a significant cause of increased morbidity,[24,48,49] but this does not adequately explain the high rate of complications, because radiation is used infrequently as an adjuvant procedure in melanoma. Other risk factors that have been implicated are previous SLNB, obesity, patient age, and type of incision. Wound infections have been reported to be more common in CLND after SNB compared with TLND without SNB,[47] presumably as a result of the combination of two surgical manipulations. However, others note fewer complications in CLND after SNB compared with TLND.[30,39] Obesity has also been implicated as a cause of increased morbidity.[3,30,43] Poos and colleagues reviewed short-term complications in 139 groin TLNDs in an 18-year period. At least one wound-related complication was reported in 49.7%[19] of patients. These included hematomas (2.1%), wound infections (20.7%), wound necrosis (17.5%), and seromas (21.8%). The complication rate was higher than that previously reported by these investigators for TLND performed between 1970 and 1984. They believed this was because of higher body mass index (BMI, calculated as weight in kilograms divided by the square of height in meters) in the later group of patients. Being older than 70 years has also been implicated as an increased cause of healing problems.[40] None of these factors are controllable, at least in the time available to perform the CLND safely. The only controllable surgical factor may be the type of surgical incision. For inguinal node dissections, sigmoidal incisions are associated with a greater risk of wound necrosis and infection.[24,31,44] A linear incision directed transversely or vertically can theoretically reduce these complications (**Fig. 7**). Another factor controllable by surgeons is the thickness of the skin flaps. Relatively thin flaps are required to remove all the lymph-bearing tissue adequately, and the flaps should be of uniform thickness with gradual

Table 1
Complication rates of axillary dissections

Author	Year	Number of Procedures	Wound Necrosis (%)	Wound Infection (%)	Seroma (%)	Hematoma (%)	Lymphedema (%)	Overall Complications (%)
Serpell et al[39]	2002	37	6	6	32	1	6	47
Van Akkooi et al[3]	2007	50	6[a]	[a]	12	2	2	—
Kretschmer et al[40]	2008	70	15	21	19	0	19	53
Neuss et al[41]	2008	58	0	5	10	2	12	—
Guggenheim et al[42]	2008	47	0	46	44	—	—	47

[a] Wound infection/necrosis grouped together.

Table 2
Complication rates of groin dissections

Author	Year	Number of Procedures	Wound Necrosis (%)	Wound Infection (%)	Seroma (%)	Hematoma (%)	Lymphedema (%)	Overall Complications (%)
Beitsh & Balch[45]	1992	177	26	29	14	3	44	—
Karakousis & Driscoll[46]	1994	205	8	16	5	—	40	—
Serpell et al[39]	2002	28	25	25	46	0	29	71
Tonouchi et. al[44]	2003	25	52	24	32	4	40	—
deVries et al[47]	2006	14	7	29	7	7	64	50
Van Akkooi et al[3]	2007	129	29[a]	[a]	20	2	30	—
Sabel et al[30]	2007	212	19[a]	[a]	—	—	30	—
Poos et al[43]	2008	139	18	21	22	2	—	50
Kretschmer et al[40]	2008	45	49	30	57	0	62	84
Guggenheim et al[42]	2008	43	7	33	42	—	—	48

[a] Wound infection/necrosis grouped together.

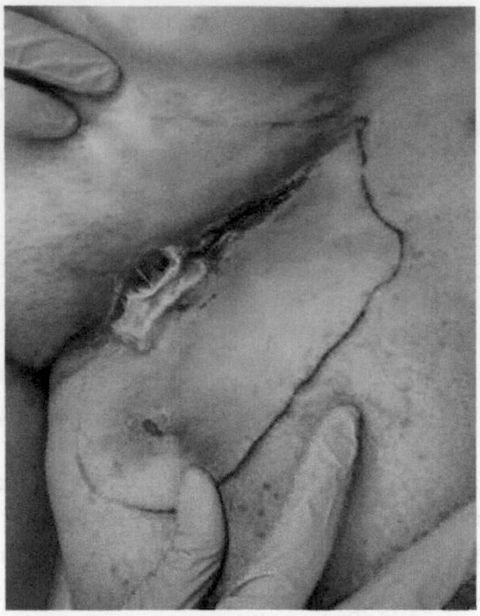

Fig. 7. Wound necrosis and infection. This incision was placed in the inguinal crease. The use of a transverse incision reduces the risk of femoral vessel exposure.

thickening toward the base. Uneven flaps or buttonholing can lead to increased wound complications.[24]

Drains are advocated after all CLNDs; early routine removal of drains has been associated with increased seroma formation and drainage. Drains should be retained until their drainage is minimal, less than 30 mL in a 24-hour period.[24] The use of fibrin glue has been advocated as a method to decrease seroma and complications related to lymph leaks. In the author's own experience and several studies reported in the literature there is no decrease in seromas or reduction in complications with the use of these agents.[40–42] For groin dissections many surgeons routinely mobilize the sartorius muscle to cover the femoral vessels. Muscle-flap mobilization has been advocated as a method to decrease lymph flow, but sartorius-flap transposition has not been shown to decrease lymph flow or complications.[50] Regardless of this, the flap has not been shown to increase morbidity and may prevent vessel exposure in the event of skin necrosis and should routinely be performed.

Lymphedema

The most feared long-term complication is the development of chronic lymphedema. Lymphedema is significantly more common in inguinal dissections than in axillary dissections. Lymphedema is rare after axillary CLND for melanoma, occurring in 3% to 10% of patients. This is in contrast with axillary lymph node dissections after mastectomy, in which rates of more than

25% are reported.[40] The triad often associated with lymphedema is surgery, radiation, and infection.[24] With one of these factors alone, lymphedema is not common; the combination of any two factors significantly increases the risk of lymphedema. Several series appear to confirm that radiation leads to a significantly higher rate of long-term lymphedema.[48,49] In the absence of radiation therapy, Karakousis found only a 2% risk of lymphedema. Lymphedema was not seen with ancillary procedures such as skeletonizing the axillary vein, exposing level 3 nodes, removing the fat pads above the level of the axilla, or removing node the fascia of the serratus latissimus or subscapularis muscles.[24] When radiation is used, lymphedema can be found in more than 50% of patients.[49]

Even in the absence of radiation in the lower extremities, lymphedema is found in 30% of patients after inguinal node dissections.[43] The incidence of lymphedema increases with thin flaps and wide resection of the primary melanoma below the knee. No increased risk of lymphedema is reported with ilioinguinal dissections compared with superficial groin dissections.[26] Careful dissection, avoiding excessive lateral dissection, and a good postoperative therapy regimen are advocated to minimize lymphedema.[24]

Outcome

The utility of CLND can best be evaluated by two criteria: overall survival and reduction of regional recurrence. Surgeons desire to cure patients and strive for improvements in survival rates. Even for patients who cannot be cured by CLND, prolonged survival and better quality of life are hoped for.

Regional Control

CLND reduces the risk of regional recurrence. This seems intuitive since CLND eliminates the nodal basin. Regional recurrence after CLND ranges from 4% to 34% (**Tables 3** and **4**).[56] A broad mix of patients is included in these studies: some with large bulky metastases and some with micronodal metastases. Early series were performed exclusively for TLNDs, although later series had a mix of TLNDs and CLND after SNB. One series from Germany reported a significantly high rate of regional recurrence.[54] That series considered in its analysis regional recurrence occurring before nodal dissection and after systemic metastases. All patients in the series had TLNDs for palpable disease. Even with these differences there are few data suggesting a difference in regional control between patients undergoing CLND for clinically evident disease or not. There is debate concerning the extent of surgery for node dissection. Current recommendations are complete level I, II, and III dissections for the axilla. Some authors advocate level III dissections only if there are suspicious nodes on intraoperative inspection (**Fig. 8**).[39,42] These series, although relatively small, have rates of regional control comparable to other studies with more extensive dissections; however, their complication rate does not differ significantly from series that advocate a more complete dissection.

For groin dissections only a superficial dissection is recommended by most studies, unless visible disease is identified. Ilioinguinal dissections may reduce local recurrence and have been suggested as the standard of care. Santinami and colleagues[29] conclude that radical dissection including groin, obturator, and external iliac obturator nodes should be considered the standard treatment of care until further data are obtained.

Analysis of factors associated with regional recurrences suggests that tumor load is the greatest risk factor associated with recurrence.[12,36] Extracapsular extension of the lymphatic metastasis is predictive for tumor recurrence.[17]

Table 3
Nodal recurrence after axillary dissections

Author	Year	Number of Patients	Nodal Recurrence (%)
Calabro et al[51]	1989	438	15
Karakousis et al[52]	1990	66	17
Gadd et al[53]	1992	225	13
Kretschmer et al[54]	2001	63	9.5
Serpell et al[39]	2002	34	5.9
Lawton et al[55]	2002	119	3
Nathansohn et al[56]	2005	86	8.1
Guggenheim et al[42]	2008	46	4.3

Table 4
Nodal recurrence after groin dissections

Author	Year	Number of Patients	Nodal Recurrence (%)
Calabro et al[51]	1989	276	17
Singletary et al[57]	1992	264	15
Gadd et al[53]	1992	224	9
Karakousis & Driscoll[58]	1995	48	4
Hughes et al[59]	2000	132	5
Kretschmer et al[54]	2001	104	34
Serpell et al[39]	2002	28	10.7
Lawton et al[55]	2002	93	2
Nathansohn et al[56]	2005	62	8.1
Sabel et al[30]	2007	212	9.4
Guggenheim et al[42]	2008	43	11.9

Survival

Analysis of patients with stage III melanoma shows a disparate survival rate ranging from 13% to 69%.[23,42,56,60,61] The current classification system for stage III melanomas is stratified by the number of metastatic lymph nodes and the clinical appearance of metastasis (substage a or b). Although surgery is the only recognized treatment for stage III melanoma, there is no prospective evidence that surgery is effective at curing melanoma. Several nonrandomized studies show only a questionable benefit to CLND.[30,42] The previous prospective studies have looked at the survival benefit of only ELND, and these were before the acceptance of SLNB and improved pathologic identification of the nodal metastasis. CLND is performed under the premise that there is a survival advantage in the subset of patients who have their regional disease eradicated when it is at a microscopic level. Nowecki and colleagues[17] assessed the survival benefit of CLND after SLNB and TLND in a retrospective analysis of 544 consecutive patients between 1994 and 2005. In patients with tumor thickness between 1 mm and 4 mm, they found a significantly improved 5-year overall survival for patients undergoing CLND after SNB (57.2%) compared with those with TLND (37.9%). In patients with tumors less than 1 mm or those greater than 4 mm there was no difference in survival. Survival rates for patients with stage N1a and N2a (micrometastasis) were better than for patients with macrometastasis (N1b to N2b).

Factors that have been associated with worse prognosis in CLND are male gender, being older than 50 years, primary tumor site in the trunk, deeper Breslow thickness, ulceration, extracapsular invasion, and the number of involved lymph nodes.[3,25,61] Patients with regional melanoma metastasis from an unknown primary site have a more favorable prognosis. TLND can cure up to one-third of patients with metastatic melanoma in the regional lymph nodes.[61]

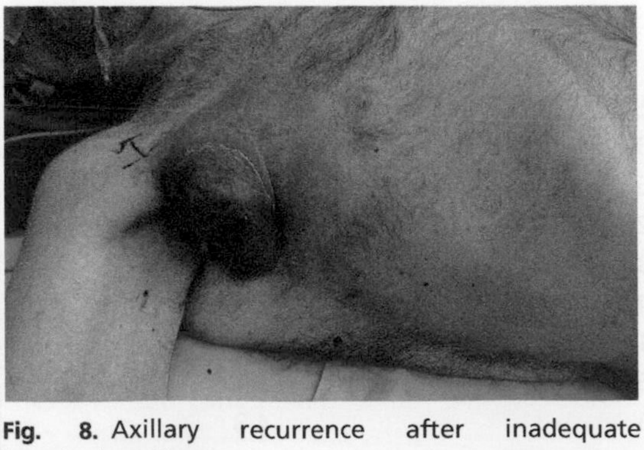

SUMMARY

Clinical controversy still exists as to whether CLND improves survival or if it is necessary for all patients with stage III disease. Current recommendations call for CLND for all patients with stage III disease, whether it is clinically apparent or found after SNB. A subset of patients may exist that has an improved overall survival benefit from CLND, yet conclusive evidence of this is not available. At minimum, CLND yields important information on prognosis and may be useful in selecting patients for adjuvant clinical trials.

Fig. 8. Axillary recurrence after inadequate lymphadenectomy.

ACKNOWLEDGMENTS

The author thanks Deborah Bruening and Beth Kaczmarek for copy-editing support.

REFERENCES

1. Bilimoria KY, Balch CM, Bentrem DJ, et al. Complete lymph node dissection for sentinel node-positive melanoma: assessment of practice patterns in the United States. Ann Surg Oncol 2008;15(6):1566–76.

2. Neuhaus SJ, Clark MA, Thomas JM, et al. Dr Herbert Lumley Snow, MD, MRCS (1847–1930): the original champion of elective lymph node dissection in melanoma. Ann Surg Oncol 2004;11(9):875–8.

3. van Akkooi ACJ, Bouwhuis MG, van Geel AN, et al. Morbidity and prognosis after therapeutic lymph node dissections for malignant melanoma. Eur J Surg Oncol 2007;33:102–8.

4. Sim FH, Taylor WF, Ivins JC, et al. A prospective randomized study of the efficacy of routine elective lymphadenectomy in the management of malignant melanoma: preliminary results. Cancer 1978;41:948–56.

5. Veronesi U, Adamus J, Bandiera DC, et al. Inefficacy of immediate node dissection in stage 1 melanoma of the limbs. N Engl J Med 1977;297:627–30.

6. Karakousis CP. Therapeutic lymph node dissection and malignant melanoma. Semin Surg Oncol 1998; 14:291–301.

7. Morton DL. John Wayne Cancer Institute. A clinical study of wide excision alone versus wide excision with intraoperative lymphatic mapping and selective lymph node dissection in the treatment of patients with cutaneous invasive melanoma. 2009. Available at: http://clinicaltrials.gov/ct2/show/NCT00275496?intr=%22Complete+Lymph+Node+Dissection%22&rank=1. Accessed April 30, 2009.

8. Morton DL, Thompson JF, Cochran AJ, et al. Selective lymphadenectomy trial group. Interim results of the Multicenter Selective Lymphadenectomy Trial (MSLT-I) in clinical stage I melanoma. J Clin Oncol 2005;23:7500–710.

9. In: Practice guidelines in oncology, vol. 2. National Comprehensive Cancer Network-Melanoma; 2009. Available at: http://www.nccn.org/professionals/physician_gls/PDF/melanoma.pdf. Accessed January 21, 2009.

10. Cormier JN, Xing Y, Ding M, et al. Population-based assessment of surgical treatment trends for patients with melanoma in the era of sentinel lymph node biopsy. J Clin Oncol 2005;23(25):6054–62.

11. Haddad FF, Stall A, Messina J, et al. The progression of melanoma nodal metastasis is dependent on tumor thickness of the primary lesion. Ann Surg Oncol 1999;6(2):144–9.

12. Wagner JD, Corbett L, Park HM, et al. Sentinel lymph node biopsy for melanoma: experience with 234 consecutive procedures. Plast Reconstr Surg 2000;105(6):1956–66.

13. Pu LLQ, Cruse CW, Wells KE, et al. Superficial femoral lymph node dissection after positive sentinel lymphadenectomy for early-stage melanoma of the lower extremity. Ann Plast Surg 2003; 51(1):69–76.

14. Page AJ, Carlson GW, Delman KA, et al. Prediction of nonsentinel lymph node involvement in patients with a positive sentinel lymph node in malignant melanoma. Am Surg 2007;73(7):674–8 [discussion: 678–9].

15. Satzger I, Völker B, Meier A, et al. Criteria in sentinel lymph nodes of melanoma patients that predict involvement of nonsentinel lymph nodes. Ann Surg Oncol 2008;15(6):1723–32.

16. Guggenheim M, Dummer R, Jung FJ, et al. The influence of sentinel lymph node tumour burden on additional lymph node involvement and disease-free survival in cutaneous melanoma – a retrospective analysis of 392 cases. Br J Cancer 2008;98:1922–8.

17. Nowecki ZI, Rutkowski P, Michej W, et al. The survival benefit to patients with positive sentinel node melanoma after completion lymph node dissection may be limited to the subgroup with a primary lesion Breslow thickness greater than 1.0 and less than or equal to 4 mm. Ann Surg Oncol 2008;15(8):2223–34.

18. Wagner JD, Gordon MS, Chuang TY, et al. Predicting sentinel and residual lymph node basin disease after sentinel lymph node biopsy for melanoma. Cancer 2005;89(2):453–62.

19. Wagner JD, Davidson D, Coleman JJ 3rd, et al. Lymph node tumor volumes in patients undergoing sentinel lymph node biopsy for cutaneous melanoma. Ann Surg Oncol 1999;6(4):398–404.

20. Gershenwald JE, Andtbacka RHI, Prieto VG, et al. Microscopic tumor burden in sentinel lymph nodes predicts synchronous nonsentinel lymph node involvement in patients with melanoma. J Clin Oncol 2008;26(26):4296–303.

21. Carlson GW, Murray DR, Lyles RH, et al. The amount of metastatic melanoma in a sentinel lymph node: does it have prognostic significance? Ann Surg Oncol 2003;10(5):575–81.

22. Frankel TL, Griffith KA, Lowe L, et al. Do micromorphometric features of metastatic deposits within sentinel nodes predict nonsentinel lymph node involvement in melanoma? Ann Surg Oncol 2008; 15(9):2403–11.

23. Mack LA, McKinnon JG. Controversies in the management of metastatic melanoma to regional lymphatic basins. J Surg Oncol 2004;86:189–99.

24. Karakousis CP. Surgical procedures and lymphedema of the upper and lower extremity. J Surg Oncol 2006;93:87–91.

25. Karakousis CP. Therapeutic node dissection in malignant melanoma. Ann Surg Oncol 1998;5(6): 473–82.

26. Allan CP, Hayes AJ, Thomas JM, et al. Ilioinguinal lymph node dissection for palpable metastatic melanoma to the groin. ANZ J Surg 2008;78:982–6.

27. van der Ploeg IM, Valdes olmos RA, Kroon BB, et al. Tumor-positive sentinel node biopsy of the groin in clinically node-negative melanoma patients: superficial or superficial and deep lymph node dissection? Ann Surg Oncol 2008;15(5):1485–91.

28. Karakousis CP, Driscoll DL. Positive deep nodes in the groin and survival in malignant melanoma. Am J Surg 1996;171:421–2.

29. Santinami M, Carbone A, Crippa F, et al. Radical dissection after positive groin sentinel biopsy in melanoma patients: rate of further positive nodes. Melanoma Res 2009;19(2):112–8.

30. Sabel MS, Griffith KA, Arora A, et al. Inguinal node dissection for melanoma in the era of sentinel lymph node biopsy. Surgery 2007;141(6):728–35.

31. Pearlman NW, Robinson WA, Dreeiling LK, et al. Modified ilioinguinal node dissection for metastatic melanoma. Am J Surg 1995;170:647–50.

32. Schmeider C, Brodersen JP, Scheuerlein H, et al. Combined endoscopic and open inguinal dissection for malignant melanoma. Arch Surg 2003;388:42–7.

33. McMasters KM, Chao C, Wong SL, et al. Interval sentinel lymph nodes in melanoma. Arch Surg 2002;137:543–9.

34. Karakousis CP. The technique of popliteal node dissection. Surg Gynecol Obstet 1980;151:420–3.

35. Sholar A, Martin RC, McMasters KM. Popliteal lymph node dissection. Ann Surg Oncol 2005;12:189–93.

36. Matter M, Lalonde MN, Allaoua M, et al. The role of interval nodes in sentinel lymph node mapping and dissection for melanoma patients. J Nucl Med 2007;48(10):1607–13.

37. Spillane AJ, Cheung BL, Stretch JR, et al. Proposed quality standards for regional lymph node dissections in patients with melanoma. Ann Surg 2009; 249(3):473–80.

38. Chan AD, Essner R, Wanek LA, et al. Judging the therapeutic value of lymph node dissections for melanoma. J Am Coll Surg 2000;191(1):16–22.

39. Serpell JW, Carne PWG, Bailey M, et al. Radical lymph node dissection for melanoma. ANZ J Surg 2003;73:294–9.

40. Kretschmer L, Thomas KM, Peeters S, et al. Postoperative morbidity of lymph node excision for cutaneous melanoma – sentinel lymphonodectomy versus complete regional lymph node dissection. Melanoma Res 2008;18(1):16–21.

41. Neuss H, Raue W, Koplin G, et al. Intraoperative application of fibrin sealant does not reduce the duration of closed suction drainage following radical axillary lymph node dissection in melanoma

patients: a prospective randomized trial in 58 patients. World J Surg 2008;32:1450–5.

42. Guggenheim MM, Hug U, Jung FJ, et al. Morbidity and recurrence after completion lymph node dissection following sentinel lymph node biopsy in cutaneous malignant melanoma. Ann Surg 2008;247(4):687–93.

43. Poos HP, Kruijff S, Bastiaannet E, et al. Therapeutic groin dissection for melanoma: risk factors for short term morbidity. Eur J Surg Oncol 2009; 35(8):877–83.

44. Tonouchi H, Ohmori Y, Kobayashi M, et al. Operative morbidity associated with groin dissections. Surg Today 2004;34:413–8.

45. Beitsch P, Balch C. Operative morbidity and risk factor assessment in melanoma patients undergoing inguinal lymph node dissection. Am J Surg 1992; 164(5):462–5 [discussion: 465–6].

46. Karakousis CP, Driscoll DL. Groin dissection in malignant melanoma. Br J Surg 1994;81(12):1771–4.

47. deVries M, Vonkeman WG, van Ginkel RJ, et al. Morbidity after inguinal sentinel lymph node biopsy and completion lymph node dissection in patients with cutaneous melanoma. Eur J Surg Oncol 2006; 32:785–9.

48. Spillane AJ, Saw RP, Tucker M, et al. Defining lower limb lymphedema after inguinal or ilio-inguinal dissection in patients with melanoma using classification and regression tree analysis. Ann Surg 2008;248(2):286–93.

49. Starritt EC, Joseph D, McKinnon JG, et al. Lymphedema after complete axillary node dissection for melanoma: assessment using a new, objective definition. Ann Surg 2004;240(5):866–74.

50. Erba P, Wettstein R, Rieger UM, et al. A study of the effect of sartorius transposition on lymph node flow after ilioinguinal node dissection. Ann Plast Surg 2008;61(3):310–3.

51. Calabro A, Singletary SE, Balch CM, et al. Patterns of relapse of 1001 consecutive patients with melanoma nodal metastases. Arch Surg 1989;124(9):1051–5.

52. Karakousis CP, Hena MA, Emrich LJ, et al. Axillary node dissection in malignant melanoma: results and complications. Surgery 1990;108(1):10–7.

53. Gadd MA, Coit DG. Recurrence patterns and outcome in 1019 patients undergoing axillary or inguinal lymphadenectomy for melanoma. Arch Surg 1992;127:1412–6.

54. Kretschmer L, Preuer K-PB, Neumann C, et al. Locoregional cutaneous metastasis in patients with therapeutic lymph node dissection for malignant melanoma: risk factors and prognostic impact. Melanoma Res 2002;12(5):499–504.

55. Lawton G, Rasque H, Arivan S, et al. Preservation of muscle fascia to decrease lymphedema after complete axillary and ilioinguinofemoral lymphadenectomy for melanoma. J Am Coll Surg 2002; 195(3):339–51.

56. Nathansohn N, Schachter J, Gutman H, et al. Patterns of recurrence in patients with melanoma after radical lymph node dissection. Arch Surg 2005;140:1172–7.

57. Singletary SE, Shallenberger R, Guinee VF, et al. Surgical management of groin nodal metastases from primary melanoma of the lower extremity. Surg Gynecol Obstet 1992;174(3):195–200.

58. Karakousis CP, Driscoll DL. Prognostic parameters in localized melanoma: gender versus anatomical location. Eur J Cancer 1995;31(3):320–4.

59. Hughes TM, A'Hern RP, Thomas JM, et al. Prognosis and surgical management of patients with palpable inguinal lymph node metastases from melanoma. Br J Surg 2000;87(7):892–901.

60. Ranieri JM, Wagner JE, Azuaje R, et al. Prognostic importance of lymph node tumor burden in melanoma patients staged by sentinel node biopsy. Ann Surg Oncol 2002;9(10):975–81.

61. Meyer T, Merkel S, Gohl J, et al. Lymph node dissection for clinically evident lymph node metastases of malignant melanoma. Eur J Surg Oncol 2002;28:424–30.

Systemic Therapy for Cutaneous Melanoma

Jonathan Treisman, MD[a,b,*], Nina Garlie, PhD[a]

KEYWORDS

- Melanoma • Chemotherapy • Biochemotherapy
- Interferon • Interleukin-2

Cutaneous melanoma is a malignancy of the skin with a propensity for early invasion and widespread metastasis. More than 90% of melanoma is cutaneous, and the principles of treatment of cutaneous melanoma are sometimes applied to other melanomas, (ocular melanoma and so forth). However, the biologic differences between them can significantly alter their outcome and response to treatment. Melanoma is one of the few common cancers with rising incidence in the United States: a steady increase of approximately 3% per year.[1] In 2009, an estimated 68,720 people will be diagnosed with cutaneous melanoma, with 8650 dying from the disease. In the United States, cutaneous melanoma currently ranks sixth in incidence,[1] and 20% of patients will present with regional involvement or distant spread at the time of diagnosis. Melanoma also seems to occur in a younger age group, with most patients presenting between 25 and 65 years old.

Despite the overall advances in the fields of tumor biology and oncology therapeutics, the treatment of metastatic melanoma has remained a challenge, and the prognosis for patients with widely metastatic disease remains poor. The task of treating this malignancy has inspired studies that have dramatically expanded the knowledge of cancer biology. The early suggestion of an immune response, as demonstrated by the regression of lesions injected with Bacillus Calmette Guérin (BCG), has led to numerous studies that have advanced tumor immunology. The study of the immune response to melanoma has led to an understanding of the recognition by the immune system of tumors, and the mechanisms by which the tumor and host interplay. Melanoma has been a model for the study of tumor immunology, and a basis for studies on the recognition of tumor antigens and their presentation by the immune system. Because of the resistance of melanoma to standard treatments, it has been a platform for the study of new agents and has led to the use of cytokine therapies, cellular therapeutics, and gene therapies. In this article, the current systemic therapy for high-risk melanoma and metastatic, cutaneous melanoma is discussed.

ADJUVANT THERAPY FOR MELANOMA

The majority of patients who present with melanoma have early stage disease, with 62.6% presenting with stage 0 or I disease, and an additional 23.1% with stage II disease.[2] The standard therapy for localized melanoma is surgical resection. However, the relatively high rate of recurrence in subgroups of patients with melanoma suggests the need for adjuvant approaches for this disease. Decisions regarding adjuvant therapy for neoplastic diseases represent a balancing of risk of disease recurrence against the relative value of the agent used including its activity, toxicity, and cost. There are several risk

[a] Immunotherapy Program, Aurora St Luke's Medical Center, 2900 West Oklahoma Avenue, Milwaukee, WI 53215, USA
[b] Medical Consultants, Inc, Aurora St Luke's Medical Center, 2901 W Kinnickinnic River Parkway, # 415, Milwaukee, WI 53215-3660, USA
* Corresponding author. Medical Consultants, Inc, Aurora St Luke's Medical Center, 2901 W Kinnickinnic River Parkway, # 415, Milwaukee, WI 53215-3660.
E-mail address: jtreisman@gmail.com (J. Treisman).

Clin Plastic Surg 37 (2010) 127–146
doi:10.1016/j.cps.2009.07.008
0094-1298/09/$ – see front matter © 2010 Elsevier Inc. All rights reserved.

factors that have been associated with melanoma, including primarily the involvement of lymph nodes (LN), the presence of ulceration of the lesion, and the level of invasion, which is best defined by the Breslow depth of invasion but also by the extent of invasion as defined by the Clark level. The staging system for melanoma was revised in 2003[3] to take into account the important risk factors for melanoma, with the goal of increased consistency and identification of various risk groups in patients with resected disease. The up-staging of ulcerated lesions, and the more routine determination of pathologic lymphatic involvement through the use of sentinel node evaluation, has led to better identification of risk in patients. Patients can be stratified into various risk groups: those with stage IA disease who have a very low risk of recurrence, those with stage Ib and IIa disease, who carry an intermediate risk, patients with IIb, IIc, and IIIa disease who have a higher risk, and those with stage IIIb and IIIc disease, who carry a very high risk of recurrence. These groups have a 5-year survival of approximately 95%, 65% to 90%, 45% to 70%, and 25% to 50%, respectively.[3,4] The poor prognosis associated with the recurrent melanoma has led to numerous clinical trials attempting to decrease this risk. These studies have included the use of chemotherapy, immunotherapy including cytokines, vaccines, and cells, and biochemotherapy.

Adjuvant Chemotherapy

Oncologists traditionally have developed adjuvant treatments of malignant disease based on their activity in the metastatic disease.[5] There are several cytotoxic agents that have demonstrated activity in the treatment of melanoma. Despite this, there are limited numbers of phase 3 studies evaluating the effectiveness of these agents in the treatment of high-risk melanoma. Dacarbazine (DTIC) is one of the only Food and Drug Administration (FDA)-approved cytotoxic agents for the treatment of metastatic melanoma, but it has limited benefit in the adjuvant treatment of melanoma. One of a few studies with DTIC given after surgical resection alone showed improvement in relapse-free survival (42% vs 30%), but this was not significant.[6] A small randomized study evaluating the combination of carmustine, actinomycin-D, and vincristine[7] showed an improvement in relapse-free survival at 5 years (29% vs 9%) but not in overall survival, and this regimen has not been pursued. Because of the promising results initially observed with nonspecific immunotherapy using BCG,[8] a subsequent study (E1673) evaluated the activity of this agent

alone or in combination with DTIC. This study, which was one of the largest trials (734 patients) of adjuvant therapy to date, included patients with resected stage I to III disease treated with BCG and DTIC, or BCG alone. There was no benefit seen with adjuvant BCG compared with observation in disease-free survival ($P = .84$) or 5-year overall survival (67% vs 62%, $P = .40$). Nor was there any benefit with DTIC plus BCG over BCG alone.[9]

A study from the German Dermatologic Cooperative Group[7] treated a group of 444 patients with stage III disease with of low-dose subcutaneous interferon-α2B (IFN), the combination of IFN and DTIC 850 mg/m[2], or observation alone. The study found a significant improvement in overall survival in patients treated with IFN alone compared with observation (59% vs 42%, $P = .0045$), yet no benefit was seen in the group of patients treated with the combination of IFN and DTIC (overall survival 45%), suggesting the DTIC actually interfered with the effect of IFN. This study is one of a few studies to indicate a significant benefit of low-dose IFN in the adjuvant setting, and this was seen in overall survival and not just recurrence-free survival. Data from this study and the others discussed here suggest that there is no benefit of chemotherapy in the adjuvant treatment of melanoma.

Adjuvant Immune-based Therapy

Cytokines

The suggestion that there was an immunologic response by the host to tumor led to interest in ways to enhance that response. The recognition of cytokines as mediators of immune signaling led to therapeutic trials in patients with metastatic melanoma. Intriguing cytokine responses observed in the metastatic setting triggered studies to determine their role in adjuvant treatment.

Interferon Interferons are a complex family of proteins with immunomodulatory and antiangiogenic properties that are produced in response to viral infection or after T-cell activation. Their effects include upregulation of the histocompatibility antigen expression on tumor cells, and activation of various effector cells including natural killer (NK) cells, T cells, monocytes, and dendritic cells. IFN is the most extensively studied agent for the adjuvant treatment of melanoma, with several large trials suggesting a benefit for its use.[10] Although there are numerous studies of IFN in the adjuvant setting, it was the pioneering work by Kirkwood using high doses that dramatically advanced the use of this agent.

Three large United States cooperative group trials have shown improvement in disease-free survival, and 2 of these trials showed overall survival benefit with the use of IFN. The cooperative group trial E1684[11] showed a 5-year relapse-free survival improvement (37% vs 26%, P = .002) and suggested an overall survival benefit (40% vs 37%, P = .024). This result corresponded to an increase in disease-free survival from 1 to 1.7 years and an overall survival from 2.8 to 3.8 years. The treatment had the greatest benefit in patients in the patients with node-positive disease. This regimen, which used 20 MIU/m^2, 5 days per week for 4 weeks, followed by 10 $MIU/m^2/d$ 3 days per week for 11 months, is associated with significant toxicities, including flulike symptoms, chronic fatigue, nausea, weight loss, myelosuppression, hepatotoxicity, and depression, requiring dose modification in most patients.[11,12] Despite this, a quality of life analysis suggested that this toxicity was compensated for by the prevention of disease relapse.[13] The data from E1684 led to FDA approval of IFN for the treatment of patients with resected stage IIB and stage III melanoma.

The intriguing results of the E1684 study led to 2 additional studies. The E1690 trial[14] compared high-dose IFN to low-dose IFN and a control. This study also showed an improvement in 5-year relapse-free survival benefit (44% vs 35%, P = .05); however, it failed to show an overall survival benefit. The trial again suggested the importance of dose of the agent, as the low-dose IFN arm had an intermediate relapse-free survival rate, which was not statistically significant. A follow-up analysis of pooled data from the E1684 and E1690 trials[15] showed that patients treated with IFN had continued improvement in relapse-free survival, with a reduction of risk of relapse of 23% (P = .006), but no improvement in overall survival. Qtwist Analysis has shown an improvement in the quality of life associated survival. Finally, the E1694 trial[16] compared high-dose IFN to a ganglioside vaccine, GM2-KLH/QS21, and again showed an improvement in 5-year relapse-free survival (62% vs 49%, P = .0007) and also showed an overall survival benefit (78% vs 73%, P = .015). This result again supported the benefit of IFN, although critics have pointed out that this may have been a negative effect of the vaccine rather than a positive effect of the IFN. However, a small study, E2696,[17] showed that relapse-free survival was better with the combination of IFN plus GM2-KLH vaccine compared with vaccine alone, lending support to the value of IFN. Questions surrounding the use of IFN include the importance of dosing and schedule of administration.

The *European Organization for Research and Treatment of Cancer* (EORTC) 18,952 study[18] evaluated higher dose IFN, using 10 MIU subcutaneous daily 5 days per week for 4 weeks followed by 11 months at 10 MIU 3 days per week for 11 months. Relapse-free survival was improved, but not overall survival. Another trial (E1697)[19] is an ongoing randomized trial that uses only the first 4 weeks of treatment for patients with intermediate and higher-risk disease.

Another question surrounding the use of IFN is the level of benefit related to nodal involvement. In the Sunbelt melanoma trial,[20] 3619 patients underwent sentinel LN staging based on histology or molecular analysis using reverse transcriptase-polymerase chain reaction (RT-PCR). Patients with single LN involvement were randomized to high-dose IFN or observation, and patients with more than one LN or extranodal extension were treated. There was no statistical benefit for patients with a single positive LN who were treated with IFN versus observation in 5-year disease-free survival (70.2% vs 73.2%) or overall survival (75.4% vs 72.9%). As expected, the patients with single LN involvement had significantly better survival than patients with more advanced nodal involvement (44.5% disease-free survival, 52.9% overall survival). No benefit was observed with IFN for patients with LN involvement as detected by RT-PCR.[21]

Potential ways to improve on the results IFN-based therapy include adjustment of the schedule, to improve efficacy as well as to decrease toxicity, and its combination with other agents including other biologic agents, chemotherapy, and vaccines. One of the observations of the data from the E1684[11] was the early separation of the curves between the IFN and observation arms, suggesting the importance of the priming phase of IFN. The E1697 study[19] is a randomized study that compares high-dose IFN for 4 weeks versus observation, that continues to accrue patients with high-risk stage II or early stage III disease. A study from Greece of 364 evaluable patients[22] showed no difference in the disease-free or overall survival in patients treated with induction therapy alone or induction plus 1 year of IFN treatment. The E1697 study randomized patients to 4 weeks of IFN to observation and continues to accrue patients. The Italian melanoma trial[23] is evaluating sequential induction phase versus the standard E1684 regimen, and to date has demonstrated a higher dose achieved, but evaluation is ongoing.

The pegylation of IFN alters its pharmacokinetics, allowing for decreased frequency of administration with the potential for improved toxicity-benefit profile. The EORTC conducted a trial of 1256 patients with resected stage III disease[24] in which patients were randomly assigned to observation or pegylated interferon-α2b (PEG-IFN) 6 μg/kg per week for 8 weeks induction then 3 μg/kg per week. Despite the intended duration of 5 years of treatment, the median length of treatment was only 12 months, with discontinuation in 31% of patients related to toxicity. There was an improvement in 4-year recurrence-free survival in the IFN-treated patients compared with the observation group (45.6% vs 38.9%, hazard ratio 0.82, $P = .01$). The activity of IFN as a monotherapy led to its evaluation in combination therapy. The addition of interleukin-2 to IFN has been studied but did not show a benefit.[25] Although the E2696 trial[17] was not designed to compare the combination of vaccine with IFN to IFN alone, the data were similar to those seen with IFN alone in the previous E1684 and E1690 trials. The combination of IFN with the allogeneic melanoma cell lysate vaccine, Melacine, also failed to show improvement over IFN alone.[26]

Granulocyte-macrophage colony-stimulating factor
Another agent with potential adjuvant activity is granulocyte-macrophage colony-stimulating factor (GM-CSF). In vitro, GM-CSF can activate macrophages to become cytotoxic for melanoma cells and may mediate proliferation, maturation, and migration of dendritic cells (DC). In an early single-arm study,[27] 48 patients with stage III disease received adjuvant GM-CSF, 125 μg subcutaneously for 14 days every 28 days. The data showed an improved survival compared with matched historical controls (37.5 vs 12.2 months, $P<.001$). Overall the drug was well tolerated, with some myalgias, weakness, and fatigue. In a follow-up study presented in abstract form,[28] of 98 patients treated with GM-CSF for 3 years, a melanoma-specific survival rate of 60% was observed, and this was significantly prolonged compared with a group of 142 patients treated for 1 year with GM-CSF (hazard ratio 0.61, $P = .047$). It is noteworthy that 2 patients treated for 3 years with GM-CSF developed acute myeloid leukemia. In a small study[29] of 42 patients with high-risk (stage III B/C, IV), resected melanoma, GM-CSF (125 μg) was administered subcutaneously for 14 days every 28 days. Median overall survival was 65 months. GM-CSF treatment resulted in an increase in mature DC, and was associated with remission or delayed recurrence. Despite the encouraging results in this very high-risk population, randomized phase 3 data are still required to clearly demonstrate the activity of this agent. Data from the E4697 study[30] that has completed accrual should

provide a clearer answer to the value of GM-CSF as a single agent in the adjuvant setting for high-risk melanoma. Studies are already looking at the combination of this agent to try to improve its efficacy.

Adjuvant Vaccines

Although vaccines have been used for the treatment of patients with metastatic disease, they lend themselves to adjuvant therapy in which there is minimal residual disease, there is less tumor heterogeneity, there is more time for the therapy to have its effect, and effects of the tumor on host immune function are minimized. The historic understanding of nonspecific immunotherapies and the viral vaccine production, as well as the brilliant work done to identify the specific antigen recognized by the immune system, has led to an array of vaccine strategies.[31] Vaccines tested in the adjuvant setting include tumor cells, gangliosides, and tumor-associated antigen peptides.

Tumor cell vaccines
Probably the best known and widely studied of the melanoma vaccines is the tumor cell lysate vaccine called Melacine, which is an allogeneic melanoma cell lysate combined with a "detoxified" Freund adjuvant.[32] In the original study by Mitchell and colleagues[33] in stage IV patients, signs of clinical regression were observed in 5 of the 17 patients with measurable disease. Patients with resected stage II melanoma treated with Melacine showed a prolongation of relapse-free survival and overall survival.[34] However, this result occurred only in patients with certain human leukocyte antigen (HLA) types. A phase 3 study compared Melacine to the "Dartmouth" chemotherapy regimen consisting of DTIC, cisplatin, lomustine, and tamoxifen,[35] and showed no significant difference in response rate (7.1% vs 10%). The SWOG-9035 trial[36] was a phase 3 study of patients with T3N0 intermediate risk melanoma. The 600 eligible patients were randomized to receive Melacine or observation. There was a similar relapse-free survival between patients receiving vaccine (65%) and those on the observation arm (63%). On further evaluation, the patients who had matching HLA type to the allogeneic lines were more likely to derive clinical benefit.[34] In a study comparing Melacine and low-dose versus high-dose IFN, there were no differences in clinical outcome, but toxicity was lower in the low-dose IFN arm.[26]

In a recent study testing a modified tumor cell vaccine strategy, patients with early stage melanoma were treated with a mixture of apoptotic/necrotic allogeneic melanoma cell lines loaded onto DC.[37] One patient with stage IIC disease and 7 of 8 patients with stage III disease had disease-free survival at 49.5 months Very few other vaccine strategies using the adjuvant activity of DC have been tested in high-risk patients.[38]

Tumor-antigen peptide vaccines

Several small studies have explored the efficacy of tumor-associated antigenic peptides (gp100 only or gp100 plus tyrosinase) with or without inter-leukin (IL)-2, GM-CSF, Montanide, DC, and incom-plete Freund adjuvant.[39–41] Peptide-specific T cells were induced in most patients. However, the lack of clinical efficacy in these studies promp-ted a recent vaccine study that incorporates a larger number of antigenic epitopes to broaden the antitumor immune response. This prospective, randomized clinical trial (3318)[42] tested the ability of a vaccine with 12 defined, shared melanoma peptides from melanocytic differentiation proteins and cancer testis antigens to induce antitumor immune responses. This vaccine was compared with a 4-peptide vaccine with only melanocytic differentiation peptides. The analysis indicates that patients who developed a T-cell response have a higher probability of longer disease-free survival ($P = .041$), and that the clinical outcome correlates significantly with the T-cell response to certain peptides. Cumulative responses to the 12-peptide vaccine were greater compared with the 4-peptide vaccine ($P = .12$). Preliminary data suggest that median survival for the entire patient population on this trial approaches 3 years, which is a favorable finding compared with published data for this patient population.

Ganglioside vaccines

Gangliosides are immunogenic glycolipids, and the GM2 ganglioside is overexpressed on the surface of the most melanomas. Vaccines were developed in the 1980s, and one of the early studies compared vaccination with a GM2/BCG vaccine compared with BCG alone.[43] The study showed that GM2 antibody was associated with a prolonged disease-free interval and survival. Although the trial failed to show a statistically significant improvement in disease-free or overall survival, it was underpowered, with only 58 patients enrolled to the GM2/BCG arm. More recent studies have used a vaccine with GM2 conjugated to the keyhole limpet hemocyanin protein and QS21 as an adjuvant. The EORTC18961 was the largest adjuvant trial to date, with 1314 patients with stage II disease. Patients were randomized to treatment with

GM2-KLH21 (n = 657) or observation (n = 657), and had no difference in relapse-free survival (75.1% vs 77.8%) or overall survival (89.2% v 92.4%), with a hazard ratio of 1.00.[44] In an Eastern Cooperative Oncology Group (ECOG) study of 880 melanoma patients, there was no difference in outcome between patients treated with GM2-KLH plus BCG versus IFN alone.[16]

Adoptive Immunotherapy

Adoptive immunotherapy for melanoma is based on the transfer of effector cells such as tumor infil-trating lymphocytes (TIL) to mediate cancer regression.[45,46] Most of these studies have evalu-ated their efficacy in patients with large tumor burdens. A recent study evaluated infusions of TIL in combination with IL-2 versus IL-2 alone in patients with regional LN recurrence but no visceral metastasis.[47] Eighty-eight patients were randomized to receive 2 doses of autologous TIL plus IL-2 (n = 44) or IL-2 alone (n = 44). There was no difference in relapse-free survival for the patients who received TIL/IL-2 versus IL-2 alone. However, in patients with 1 tumor-invaded LN (n = 34), the relapse rate was lower in patients who received TIL/IL-2 (30%) versus IL-2 alone (68%) ($P = .0219$). There was no difference in relapse rate in patients with more than 1 tumor-invaded LN. Overall survival was higher in patients who received TIL/IL-2 (73%) versus IL-2 alone (32%) with 1 tumor-invaded LN. Survival was not different in patients with more than one tumor-invaded LN. A current phase 3 study is evaluating the effects of adjuvant TIL in patients with 1 tumor-invaded LN.

Adjuvant Biochemotherapy

Although a benefit for the combination of chemo-therapy and nonspecific immunotherapy had not been observed in previous trials, the high response rates associated with treatment with bi-ochemotherapy (DTIC, cisplatin, velban, IFN, and IL-2) in the metastatic setting[48] led to a comparison of its benefit compared with high-dose IFN in the adjuvant setting.[49] The study enrolled 138 of the intended 200 patients randomized to receive stan-dard high-dose IFN as described in the E1684 study, IFN 10 million units/m^2 subcutaneously for 52 weeks, or biochemotherapy.[50] This study was ended early due to slow accrual. At the time of closure, a futility analysis was performed that showed no difference in 2-year (66% vs 68%) or 5-year (58% vs 59%) disease-free survival or in overall survival. Another study, Intergroup S0008, is similarly studying biochemotherapy versus stan-dard IFN in a randomized phase 3 study.[51]

SUMMARY OF ADJUVANT THERAPY

There remain many unanswered questions regarding the optimal treatment of patients with resected melanoma and the optimal use of these adjuvant therapies available. However, the data with IFN have led to FDA approval of the agent for the adjuvant therapy for patients with intermediate- or high-risk melanoma, and it has now gained acceptance as a standard agent for patients with melanoma larger than 4 mm or with LN involvement. The 2009 National Comprehensive Cancer Network (NCCN) guidelines suggest IFN as a category 2B option for patients with stage IIb or greater disease. Despite this, the recommendation is not universal,[52] and other investigators have concluded that there is currently no standard adjuvant therapy following resection of melanoma.[53,54] Innovation of newer modalities and patient participation in clinical studies will ultimately lead to improvements in the care of patients with increased risk of recurrent disease.

THERAPY FOR METASTATIC MELANOMA

The treatment of metastatic melanoma remains a challenge for the clinician. Although the goal of early systemic adjuvant therapy for melanoma has been a central focus in the systemic management of the disease, there remains a high rate of recurrence. The poor outcomes associated with standard cytotoxic chemotherapeutic agents have led to development of numerous alternative therapies for melanoma treatment, particularly the use of immunotherapeutic treatments. An understanding of tumor biology piloted the development of agents with a more specific target of action on the tumor. The tremendous success of targeted agents in other diseases, such as imatinib (Gleevac) in chronic myelogenous leukemia, and the relative success of other targeted agents in renal cell carcinoma (sorafanib, sutinib, temsirolimus) has prompted trials of such targeted agents in melanoma as well.

In discussing the treatment of metastatic melanoma, it is important to consider outcome measurement. Treatment benefit is usually measured in terms of response rate, and disease-free or overall survival rates. Response rate may overestimate the benefit because these responses may be of only short duration. Overall and disease-free survival may serve to underrepresent the benefit to the individual patient. Measurements of disease stabilization are often used to try to reflect the benefit of some of the newer agents that have antiangiogenic or antiproliferative effects, but do not necessarily induce dramatic tumor shrinkage. In addition, the response rates with immunotherapeutic regimens are often low but may result in prolonged disease-free survival, and thus may actually be very important to the outcome for the individual patient.

Recurrent melanoma is associated with dismal clinical outcomes. Much effort has been extended to improve response rates by evaluating the efficacy of chemotherapy, combination chemotherapy, apoptosis-inducing agents, targeted agents, immune-based therapy, and biochemotherapy.

Chemotherapy

Melanoma is considered a chemotherapy-resistant disease, and systemic chemotherapy has failed to significantly improve the survival of patients with nonresectable metastatic melanoma.[55] The disease frequently becomes refractory to the agents even after initial responses are observed. Despite the lack of curative effect for the patient with advanced metastatic disease, chemotherapy continues to play a role in palliation of the disease. Although many agents have been tested and used for melanoma treatment, single-agent chemotherapy has generally been considered ineffective.[56] One of the challenges in decision-making for the medical oncologist has been the often encouraging results of single-institution trials that are not confirmed by subsequent phase 2 trials,[57] or the conflicting data between studies and their interpretation. Despite the poor overall outcome with these agents, they are still in common use in the clinic.

Alkylating agents

Dacarbazine (DTIC) is the most active single agent, and is the only cytotoxic agent that has been approved for the treatment of advanced melanoma. DTIC is therefore the standard against which other treatments are tested. DTIC is a prodrug of the alkylating agent 5-(3-methyltriazen-1-yl)imidazole-4-carboximide (MTIC). The drug is generally well tolerated, with nausea as its major side effect, which can be controlled with current antiemetic therapy. The response rate for single-agent DTIC in melanoma ranges from 15% to 25%, but these are generally of short duration (3–6 months),[58] and the complete response rate is only 5%. Because of its activity, DTIC has been tested alone or in combination therapy.

Temozolomide (TMZ) is a relatively new alkylating agent. TMZ is similar to DTIC in that it is a prodrug that is converted to MTIC. In contrast to DTIC, TMZ spontaneously converts to MTIC under physiologic conditions.[59] TMZ has the advantage of being 100% bioavailable, and can therefore be administered orally, which significantly improves the ease of use of the agent. In addition, TMZ has extensive tissue penetration including penetration of the blood-brain barrier and the cerebral spinal fluid.[59,60] TMZ was shown to have an objective response rate of 21% (12 of 56 patients) in a phase 2 study, with a median survival time of 5.5 months.[61] In a randomized phase 3 study, TMZ had a slightly higher response rate (13.5% vs 12.1%) and median survival (7.7 vs 6.4 months) than DTIC, neither of which was statistically significant.[62]

Attempts have been made to improve the results with TMZ, primarily through changes in schedule or by the addition of additional agents. A phase 2 study was done to further assess the impact of the extended schedule used in the 2 previous studies (75 mg/m^2/d for 6 weeks every 8 weeks).[63] TMZ cytotoxicity is mediated through methylation of DNA, and a prolonged schedule has the potential to deplete methyl guanine methyltransferase (MGMT) levels, an enzyme that is involved in DNA repair, with improved cell killing. However, the response rate was 12.5% with no complete responses and an estimated 18-month survival of 27%, which was similar to trials with the standard 5-day regimen, and there was no correlation between MGMT and response. A trial with the MGMT inhibitor lomeguatrib similarly did not suggest an improved therapeutic ratio that would warrant its use in melanoma. A study combining TMZ with thalidomide demonstrated a 32% response rate in 38 patients treated.[64] However, a follow up study could not demonstrate an improvement with this regimen.[65] IFN has similarly been administered in combination with TMZ, and a phase 2 study that used a combination of PEG-IFN with TMZ resulted in a 31% response rate in 35 patients with metastatic melanoma, including 3 complete responses.[66] A study by the Dermatologic Oncology Group using TMZ and PEG-IFN showed an 18% response rate and a survival of 9.4 months.[67] The large randomized study by the Dermatologic Cooperative Oncology Group comparing TMZ using the 5-day regimen with or without standard IFN given 3 days per week again showed an improvement in response rate (24% vs 13%) but failed to show a statistical improvement in survival (9.7 vs 8.4 months).[68] Although TMZ has not been approved by the FDA for the treatment of metastatic melanoma, it has become a standard agent for the treatment of patients who are not candidates for cytokine or experimental studies.

The nitrosoureas are a group of alkylating agents that act by cross-linking DNA. Carmustine (BCNU) and lomustine have similar response rates to that of DTIC (10%–20%) but are generally associated with more toxicity, including myelosuppression and alopecia.[69] In clinical practice, these agents have a limited role as single agents, but have been used in combination chemotherapy. Fotemustine is a chloroethyl nitrosourea that more rapidly crosses the blood-brain barrier, which has been more extensively studied in Europe. In a phase 3 trial,[70] fotemustine showed improved response rates over DTIC (15% vs 7%), but this did not translate into a survival advantage (7.3 vs 5.6 months) and although the drug is currently available as first-line therapy in some European countries, it is currently not available in the United States.

The platinum compounds, cisplatin and carboplatin, have a modest activity in patients with melanoma, with a response rate of approximately 15% to 20%.[69] Attempts made to improve the results with cisplatin have resulted in increased toxicity. Cisplatin and carboplatin have found more use in combination with other agents.

Microtubule inhibitors
Microtubular toxins and microtubular disassembly inhibitors have both been used in patients with metastatic melanoma, and have some activity.[69] The vinca alkaloid vinblastine, based on its modest activity and limited toxicity, has primarily been used in combination therapy. In a small study, vinorelbine (Navelbine) was used in combination with tamoxifen, with a 20% response rate, 3 of the 30 patients having a response of longer than 12 months.[71] Other studies with vinorelbine have not demonstrated activity either as first-line[72] or second-line[73] therapy.

Paclitaxel and docetaxel are microtubule disassembly inhibitors with antitumor activity in a variety of neoplastic diseases. Paclitaxel has been evaluated in several phase 1 and 2 studies, and has demonstrated an approximately 12% to 16% response rate in previously untreated patients.[74] Paclitaxel is commonly used in combination with carboplatin in other malignancies, and was similarly tested in melanoma. Rao and colleagues reported a 26% response rate in second-line therapy for patients with melanoma,[75] and this regimen is now being used as a "backbone" for the addition of other agents, despite the limited activity of paclitaxel alone or in combination with carboplatin observed in other studies.[76,77] Docetaxel is another microtubule disassembly inhibitor. A phase 2 docetaxel study showed a 12.5% response rate in melanoma with one of the patients having a durable complete response,[78] and it still being actively studied in other combinations, with some benefit.[79]

The NCCN guidelines for treatment of melanoma in 2009 list several therapies for the treatment of metastatic disease. The recommended agents include the alkylating agents DTIC and TMZ, either as single agents or as combinations, the microtubule inhibitor paclitaxel alone or with a platinum agent, and IL-2. However, all of these recommendations are level 2B, indicating the lack of a regularly effective agent for this disease.

Combination Chemotherapy

A common method to try to improve responses is to combine agents with additive or synergistic activity with nonoverlapping toxicity. There are a numerous combinations of chemotherapy for melanoma that have been and are being developed and studied. These regimens have generally employed DTIC or, more recently, TMZ. The most notable of these regimens is the CVD regimen, which combines cisplatin, velban, and DTIC,[80] and the Dartmouth regimen, which combines cisplatin, carmustine, DTIC, and tamoxifen.[81] In a large phase 3 study comparing the CVD regimen to DTIC alone,[82] there was a trend toward improved response and survival. The Dartmouth regimen originally resulted in a 55% response rate in the initial series of 20 patients with metastatic melanoma. Despite initial promising results, subsequent phase 3 studies have not confirmed an advantage for combination chemotherapy. Although the response rate with combination was improved with the Dartmouth regimen over DTIC alone (18.5% vs 10.2%), this did not translate into an overall improvement in median survival (7.7 vs 6.3 months).[57] Despite these data, the use of combination chemotherapy is still commonly used in the care of patients.

Apoptosis-inducing Agents

Oblimersen is a cytotoxic agent shown to downregulate Bcl-2 and increase apoptosis in human cancer xenografts.[83] In a large clinical study of 771 patients,[84] the combination of oblimersen sodium plus DTIC was shown to increase progression-free survival over DTIC alone (2.6 vs 1.6 months, $P<.001$). Although an improvement in overall survival could not be clearly shown (9.0 vs 7.8 months, $P = .077$), oblimersen did increase survival compared with DTIC alone in patients who had a normal lactate dehydrogenase (LDH) at baseline (11.4 vs 9.7 months, $P = .02$). Oblimersen was well tolerated, with some increase in myelosuppression. In addition to showing a clinical improvement, the study further indicates the heterogeneity of the patients with melanoma and the need to clearly identify patient populations when studying treatments for this disease. The FDA has not approved oblimersen for the treatment of melanoma. One aspect that led to the lack of FDA approval was the delay in follow-up scans in the oblimersen group compared with the group treated with DTIC, which created a time-lag bias, indicating the importance of care in study design and conduction. An additional phase 3 trial is ongoing to further evaluate this agent.

Elesclomol (STA-4783, Synta) is an inducer of reactive oxygen species (ROS), or heat shock proteins, which leads to apoptosis in melanoma. In a double-blind randomized multicenter study,[85] paclitaxel 80 mg/m² weekly was given alone or in combination with elesclomol (213 mg/m²). The combination showed an improvement in objective response rate (15% vs 3.6%), with one complete response in the 53 patients in the combination treatment. This result was also associated with an improvement in progression-free survival (3.7 vs 1.8 months, hazard ratio 0.53, $P = .035$) with a 1-year overall survival rate of 49%. This agent is now undergoing phase 3 testing in the SYMMETRY trial.

Targeted Agents in Melanoma

New cellular and molecular techniques are changing the practice of oncology. These molecular techniques are providing a means for sorting out the heterogeneity inherent in such a complex process as cancer and its interactions with the host.[86] These techniques have provided prognostic information in breast cancer patients using gene array analysis of tumors, as is currently done with the OncoTypeDX analysis[87]; they have also started to allow predictions of tumor response to chemotherapeutic agents. The recent finding that colonic tumors that have a kras mutation are resistant to the EGF-receptor antagonist allows sparing of the patient from the expense and toxicity of the agents. These molecular techniques have allowed for a much more detailed understanding of the cell signaling pathways present in melanoma, which can then be used as targets for therapy.[88] These targeted agents are designed to block cell signaling, to disrupt the pathways involved in angiogenesis, growth, and proliferation, and to enhance tumor apoptosis. These techniques are likely to lead to the individualization of treatment based on assessments of the genetic and epigenetic aspects of the tumor as well as the host.

Tamoxifen

The identification of estrogen receptors in melanoma led to initial trials of hormonal therapy for the disease,[89] and tamoxifen, an estrogen receptor antagonist, might be considered one of the first targeted agents used for the therapy for melanoma. Tamoxifen was initially used as a single agent and then in combination with various chemotherapeutic regimens. Although initial studies suggested a benefit for tamoxifen as a single agent in the treatment of metastatic melanoma, subsequent studies showed a response rate of only 5%.[90–92] In addition, evaluation of melanoma samples using immunostaining failed to demonstrate estrogen receptors. Tamoxifen could have several other effects including effects on angiogenesis, synergic effects with chemotherapy, and reversal of multidrug resistance. A phase 3 study[93] demonstrated an improvement in response (28% vs 12%, $P = .03$) and survival (48 weeks vs 29 weeks, $P = .02$) after DTIC with tamoxifen compared with DTIC alone. In a phase 2 trial of the Dartmouth regimen, the omission of tamoxifen similarly was shown to reduce response rates.[94] A phase 3 study of dacarbazine and carboplatin with or without tamoxifen showed no difference in response or survival.[95] A multi-arm study showed no benefit from the addition of tamoxifen to DTIC or DTIC and IFN.[96] A subsequent study showed no loss of activity to the Dartmouth regimen when tamoxifen was removed.[97] A meta-analysis of the studies with tamoxifen further indicated that, when added to chemotherapy, it did not improve the response rate or survival.[98] Mori and colleagues[99] demonstrated that patients with estrogen receptor α (ER-α) methylation correlated with survival in patients treated with a biochemotherapy regimen containing tamoxifen, suggesting that the variability in the trials may be related to the ER-α methylation status of the patients in the study.

Vascular inhibitors

The production of vascular endothelial growth factor (VEGF) has been implicated in tumor-induced angiogenesis, and inhibition of VEGF-induced angiogenesis can suppress the growth of tumors in murine models. Bevacizumab (Avastin) is a humanized murine monoclonal antibody that binds to VEGF with high affinity, and has been shown in clinical studies to have activity in colon, lung, and breast cancer. In studies in patients with melanoma, some disease stabilization has been observed. In a study by Varker, 25% of treated patients had disease stabilization of 24 to 146 weeks with bevacizumab alone or bevacizumab plus IFN.[100] Bevacizumab has been used in combination with several agents. A study using the combination of paclitaxel and bevacizumab showed an overall survival at 12 months of 43.3%, suggesting some benefit to the regimen.[101]

In a phase 2 study, 53 patients were treated with bevacizumab (given as 10 mg/kg every other week) combined with carboplatin, and weekly paclitaxel (Taxol). This regimen was associated with a 17% response rate (partial remission), and another 30 (57%) achieved stable disease for at least 8 weeks. Median progression-free survival and median overall survival were 6 months and 12 months, respectively.[102] Although a promising agent for control of disease, further randomized studies will be needed to further assess the impact of bevacizumab on the treatment of melanoma.

Axitinib is another antiangiogenic agent that acts by selective inhibitor of the VEGF receptor (VEGFR), which inhibits VEGR-1, -2, and -3. In a single-agent study in 32 patients,[103] Axitinib had an overall response rate of 19% with 1 complete response. An additional 9 patients had stable disease of at least 16 weeks.

Sorafanib

The relative resistance of melanoma to chemotherapy is partly explained by its constitutive activation of cell survival pathways such as the mitogen-activated protein kinase pathway and phosphoinositol-3 kinase, which interfere with the apoptotic pathway. Sorafanib (BAY43-9006, Nexevar) is a tyrosine kinase inhibitor with activity against the RAF serine/threonine kinases, although it is also a multikinase inhibitor with activity against VEGFR-2 and -3. Sorafanib is FDA-approved for the treatment of renal cell carcinoma and hepatocellular carcinoma. In a phase 2 study of 37 patients with metastatic melanoma, no tumor responses were seen although 19% experienced stable disease.[104] Sorafenib was evaluated in combination with paclitaxel and carboplatin in a phase 1 study of 39 patients with advanced cancer (24 with melanoma).[105] Sorafenib-related adverse events were observed in 69% of patients. In patients with melanoma, there was 1 complete response and 9 partial responses. The E2603 study is a phase 3 study randomizing 800 patients to carboplatin and paclitaxel plus sorafanib or a placebo. The results of this study are pending.

Immune-based Therapy

Several observations suggested that the host generates an immunologic response to melanoma, which has inspired the search for an understanding of the biology of the process as well as research aimed at harnessing the response to treatment. This search was originally suggested by the spontaneous regression of melanoma.

Nonspecific immunotherapy studies using intratumoral injections of BCG generated further interest in the concept of immunotherapy for this tumor. The identification of TIL and the characterization of these cells has documented that this immune response can be very specific, and has led to studies of the specific antigens recognized by T lymphocytes in the context of the major histocompatibility complex (MHC). Research has also focused on the escape mechanisms, including ongoing studies of the tolerance to tumor that takes place in the host and methods to overcome this resistance.

Cytokines

The most important therapeutic agent for melanoma treatment has been the T-cell growth factor IL-2. IL-2 has an overall response rate of 16%, with a 6% complete response rate.[106] More importantly, these responses have been durable, with prolonged disease response. Patients with a partial response have a median response duration of 5.9 months, and the median duration of response for patients with a complete response has not been reached. Observations that suggested a role of host immunologic responses has led to the development of cytokine therapy for melanoma, with a focus on IL-2 and IFN.

Interleukin-2 In contrast to IFN, which has both immunologic and antiproliferative properties, IL-2 has no direct antitumor effects, and exerts its function purely through its ability to stimulate an immunologic response by lymphocytes. In early studies with the agent, Grimm and colleagues[107] described the lysis of tumor cells by lymphocytes cultured in T-cell growth factor (IL-2). In addition to its ability to enhance the cytotoxic activity of HLA-specific T cells, IL-2 also induced HLA-unrestricted killing of tumor cells by lymphocytes exposed to the agent in vitro. This lymphokine-activated killer (LAK) activity could be induced in both NK and CD3/CD8+ T cells. In mouse models, IL-2 was able to reduce or eliminate pulmonary metastases in an experimental tumor model using methylcholanthrene-induced sarcomas, and this effect was dose dependent.[108]

The preclinical studies led to the National Cancer Institute Surgery Branch clinical treatment regimen using high-dose IL-2. Patients with metastatic melanoma or renal cell carcinoma were treated with 600,000 to 720,000 units/kg of IL-2 every 8 hours on days 1 to 5 and 15 to 19, and the course was repeated depending on the response. Some patients received concurrent administration of LAK cells. This treatment resulted in a 15% to 20% response rate.[109] Further

studies showed similar responses, and a follow-up report of the 270 patients treated on 8 trials with high-dose IL-2 showed a 16% objective response rate with 10% partial and 6% complete responses, which were durable.[110] Based on these data, IL-2 has been approved by the FDA as a treatment for patients with metastatic melanoma. The median duration of response for complete responders exceeded 59 months, and patients with responses greater than 30 months remained progression-free.[5] A study of 374 patients given high-dose intravenous bolus IL-2 (720,000 IU/kg) from July 1988 to December 1999 in the Surgery Branch of the National Cancer Institute (NCI) reported an overall objective response rate of 15.5%.[111] Some patients received IL-2 with a vaccine. Clinical responses were higher (54%) in patients with only subcutaneous or cutaneous metastases compared with patients with disease at other sites (12.4%) ($P = .000001$).

The toxicities associated with high-dose IL-2 have been the main obstacle to its widespread use in the treatment of patients. Toxicities generally include a capillary leak syndrome manifested by fluid retention, oliguria, and hypoxemia. This syndrome is often associated with cardiac side effects, including arrhythmias. Other common toxicities include gastrointestinal symptoms including diarrhea and nausea, skin irritation and desquamation, confusion, and hematologic toxicities with thrombocytopenia.[112] The availability of guidelines for the use and administration of high dose IL-2 has made consistent delivery of the drug much easier.[113]

Interferon IFN was initially studied in the 1980s for the treatment of metastatic melanoma. Initial phase 1 and 2 studies were associated with an overall response rate of approximately 16%.[114] Up to a third of the responses observed with IFN were complete, with some durable responses. Responses have generally been in patients with small-volume cutaneous or soft tissue disease. IFN has primarily been used in combination with other agents, and a meta-analysis of multiple trials reported a higher overall response in the IFN-containing regimens (24% vs 17%).[69,115] The availability PEG-IFN has allowed better convenience of dosing. Although IFN has a place in the treatment of metastatic disease, it has found much more use as an adjuvant treatment.

Immunomodulatory agents

Studies have slowly elucidated the complex process of immune regulation and have allowed for these pathways to alter the response of the host to tumors. T-cell activation requires the interaction of the costimulatory molecules B7.1 (CD80) and B7.2 (CD86) with the CD28 antigen on the T cells. The interaction of these same costimulatory molecules with cytotoxic T-lymphocyte antigen-4 (CTLA-4) causes inhibition of the lymphocytes, leading to impaired cellular immune functions. These T-cell activation and inhibitory signaling molecules represent potential targets to manipulate the natural immune response to tumors. Antibodies to CTLA-4 may act to enhance the immune response to weak antigens, as seems to be the case with immunogenic tumors. In a murine model, the use of these antibodies in conjunction with a GM-CSF vaccine was able to induce complete regression of B16 tumors in mice.[116] Human anti-CTLA4 antibodies that have been in human clinical testing include ticilimumab (tremelimumab, CP-675,206, Pfizer) and ipilimumab (MDX-020, Bristol-Myers Squibb, Medarex Inc). In the initial phase 1 study of tremelimumab in patients with melanoma,[117] 2 of 29 patients achieved a complete response and 2 experienced partial responses. In addition, 5 others had stabilization of their disease. Patients experienced dose-limiting toxicities, and autoimmune phenomena included diarrhea, dermatitis, vitiligo, panhypopituitarism related to hypophysis, and hyperthyroidism. A subsequent phase 1/2 study showed responses in 8 of 84 patients.[118] The A3671009 phase 3 trial evaluated 630 patients with advanced melanoma, and randomized patients to standard chemotherapy, consisting of DTIC or TMZ. However, the trial was discontinued when interim data found that tremelimumab did not demonstrate superiority over standard chemotherapy. Pfizer has already stated its intention to determine whether tremelimumab showed benefit in any of the advanced melanoma patients who took part in the trial. Analysis of the current phase 3 trial may help identify certain patients who show a better response to tremelimumab, and guide future development. There was no difference in response rate for patients treated with tremelimumab compared with chemotherapy (9.1% vs 10.1%) or progression-free survival (18.6% vs 14.1%). Further study outcomes are expected.[119]

In an early study of the other CTLA4 antibody, ipilimumab was given to 14 patients in conjunction with gp100 210M melanoma peptide vaccine.[120] Responses were seen in 3 patients (2 complete and 1 partial). Treatment was associated with significant immune-related adverse events. In a follow-up study, 139 patients were treated with ipilimumab either alone (85 patients) or in conjunction with a peptide vaccine. A response was observed in 23 patients (17%), with 3 complete responses that were durable (29+, 52+, and 53+ months).[121] In this study and another,[122] 20% to 48% of patients given ipilimumab developed autoimmune toxicity. A meta-analysis of 42 phase 2 studies including 2100 patients reported a 1-year survival rate of approximately 25% for patients with stage III/IV melanoma.[123]

Phase 2 and 3 clinical trials with anti-CTLA-4 antibodies have resulted in 7% to 15% objective response rates in patients with metastatic melanoma. The activity of anti-CDLA-4 antibodies has been explored as monotherapy, and in combination with vaccines, other immunotherapies such as IL-2 and chemotherapy such as DTIC. The response rate in patients who experience grade 3 or 4 autoimmune toxicities is higher (36%) compared with the response rate in patients who do not experience autoimmune toxicity (5%–11%).[124] Current studies with ipilimumab to provide data on efficacy and survival with an active control group include a phase 3 randomized, double-blind study to assess ipilimumab in combination with DTIC versus DTIC alone in patients with stage III/IV melanoma, and a phase 3 study of ipilimumab given as adjuvant therapy in patients with high-risk stage III melanoma. These larger studies will help to demonstrate the utility of anti-CTLA-4 therapy in prolonging clinical responses in patients with melanoma.

New, innovative immune-based treatment strategies for melanoma include those that antagonize receptors that suppress the immune response (CTLA-4, PD-1) and those that activate receptors that amplify the immune response (CD40 on antigen-presenting cells, 4-1BB [CD137] and OX40 on T cells). Development of these new strategies may prove beneficial, especially in increasing the efficacy of standard treatments for melanoma.

Vaccines

Vaccines for melanoma are designed to boost immune reactions against a malignancy that is already established. The review by Rosenberg and colleagues of vaccine therapy in 323 patients with melanoma at the NCI[125] stated an overall objective response rate of 2.6%. When the review was extended beyond the NCI vaccine studies in patients with melanoma to 35 reports of 765 patients with common cancers, the objective response rate was 3.3%. The vaccine with the highest response rate included DC (7.1% objective response rate). In NCI studies combining melanoma vaccines, the overall objective response rate was 13% for patients receiving IL-2 alone (n = 379) and 16% for patients receiving IL-2 and vaccine (n = 305).[126] Higher response rates occurred in vaccinated patients with subcutaneous or cutaneous disease only versus those with visceral disease. Despite low response rates, most vaccines were successful in generating easily detectable, vaccine-specific immune responses. Many groups currently seek to discover the factors that turn a detectable antitumor immune response into an effective antitumor immune response.

DC have been used in vaccination strategies to take advantage of their ability to stimulate T-cell responses and then regulate the response. Generation of DC is technically feasible for most laboratories. However, the most effective method to display the tumor antigen on the DC surface in the appropriate context to induce effective antitumor response remains under investigation. A recent review of 38 DC vaccination studies including 626 patients with metastatic melanoma reported a clinical response rate of 30%, with 3% complete and 6% partial responses, and 21% stable disease.[38] Clinical response correlated with the use of peptide antigens ($P = .03$), the use of any helper antigen/adjuvant ($P = .002$), and induction of antigen-specific T cells ($P = .0004$). Alternative approaches to peptide loading of DC in recent studies include adenoviral transduction, RNA transfection, tumor lysate loading, and tumor cell:DC fusions. Immunizing tumor antigens include melanocyte lineage antigens (Melan-A/MART-1, gp100, tyrosinase), cancer testis antigen (MAGE-A3, NY-ESO-1) and antigens that are overexpressed (p53, survivin). Butterfield and colleagues[127] transduced DC with an adenoviral vector encoding full-length MART-1. Results from this study and 2 others[128,129] support a correlation between clinical benefit and determinant spreading (immune responses to nonvaccine antigens). Two recent studies tested the ability of autologous[130] or allogeneic[131] tumor lysate-loaded DC to induce clinical responses in patients with metastatic melanoma. Responses to the immunizing antigens were observed, but no patients achieved an objective clinical response even with the addition of low-dose or high-dose IL-2.[130]

A potential obstacle to induce effective antitumor immunity in vivo arises from the host immune environment. Most studies immunize with DC in an immunocompetent host, where host immune tolerance can impede antitumor reactivity and negate clinical benefit in patients with advanced disease. Current studies take advantage of homeostatic mechanisms to boost tumor reactivity by lymphodepletion before DC immunization. In a pilot study,[132] 16 patients were treated with a recombinant IL-2/diphtheria toxin conjugate (ONTAK, Denileukin Diftitox). Transient depletion of T cells with subsequent repopulation coincided with de novo appearance of melanoma-specific CD8+ T cells. Objective responses were observed in 4 of 16 patients. A current clinical trial is testing the efficacy of a combination of ONTAK before DC immunization (NCT00056134). Other studies have used lymphodepletion followed by infusion of tumor-reactive T cells with vaccine administration[133] or after a vaccine-priming regimen,[134] with limited clinical benefit.

Adoptive T-cell therapy

The identification in animal tumor models of immunologic control of tumors and. more significantly. the development of tumor immunity led to the search for immune effector cells that are active during cytokine therapy, and those that result in long-term immunity. One of the first cellular therapies was based on finding that lymphocytes develop the capacity to kill tumors in an HLA-independent fashion after exposure to IL-2. These LAK cells were found to kill NK-resistant cell lines, and represented both stimulated NK cells and CD3/CD8 cells. Despite strong preclinical data and preliminary results reported by Rosenberg and colleagues,[109] a prospective randomized trial comparing high-dose IL-2 given with and without LAK showed no significant difference in response or survival.

The observation that immune cells that infiltrate a tumor have reactivity against the tumor and can be expanded has led to a series of clinical trials using TIL for the treatment of melanoma. Clinical responses were observed in these studies, but responses were transient and difficult to contribute to TIL because of concurrent IL-2 administration. The most effective cellular therapy for patients with melanoma has been infusion of TIL after a lymphodepleting chemotherapy preparative regimen.[135] In 3 clinical trials with increasing intensity of lymphodepletion, objective clinical responses were observed in 52 of 93 patients (56%).[136] The ability of the TIL to respond to HLA-matched or autologous melanoma cells has been prerequisite for their clinical use. The long culture time to generate and expand TIL, and to develop antitumor reactivity in TIL is not optimal, because the life expectancy of a patient with advanced melanoma is short. Murine studies have shown that a long culture time and multiple restimulations are inversely correlated with therapeutic efficacy.[137,138] Cells that are cultured longer (older cells) have longer telomeres, and are associated with reduced clinical responses and shorter persistence in vivo.[139,140] A new study by Rosenberg's group[141] demonstrated a similar frequency of tumor-reactive cells in TIL generated via a shorter culture (41%) compared with standard TIL (38%).

The "young" TIL contained a higher frequency of CD4+ cells than standard TIL. Other phenotypic markers expressed on the "young" TIL (CD27, CD28) and longer length of their telomeres were linked in previous studies with T-cell persistence and survival. Rosenberg and colleagues have initiated a clinical trial to test the efficacy of "young" TIL and high-dose IL-2 after nonmyeloablative lymphodepletion in patients with metastatic melanoma. The authors' group and a site in Israel have a similar clinical trial in progress.

It is not always possible to obtain tumor from which to generate TIL for a patient with melanoma, and less likely that melanoma-reactive TIL will be generated. Several techniques have evolved to provide alternatives to the requirement to establish TIL cultures. The discovery and cloning of melanoma-associated antigens has provided a tool with which to generate melanoma-specific T cells from peripheral blood. Dudley and colleagues[142] and Yee and colleagues[143] infused cloned T cells targeting gp100 or MART-1 with and without IL-2 into patients with advanced melanoma. These studies and others involving the transfer of T-cell clones[144,145] and CD8+ T-cell lines[146,147] demonstrated the safety and feasibility of this approach but also a lack of clinical efficacy. In 2008, Hunder and colleagues[148] reported a complete response in a patient with metastatic melanoma infused with cloned CD4+ NY-ESO-1-reactive T cells. The cells persisted for at least 3 months and the response was durable after 22 months. Dudley and colleagues[149] lymphodepleted the patients before T-cell infusion to prolong persistence of the T cells by eliminating the competition for homeostatic cytokines. Patients were treated with an escalating dose of lymphodepleting chemotherapy before adoptive transfer of CD8+ melanoma-reactive T-cell clones and IL-2. No objective responses or persistence of cloned T cells were observed.

The T-cell receptors (TCRs) of highly reactive cells have been cloned and transferred into peripheral blood lymphocytes (PBL), creating a new population of polyclonal T cells with antitumor reactivity. In the first adoptive cell transfer study using genetically engineered autologous T cells, T cells expressing a TCR reactive with MART-1 were shown to persist and express the transgene long-term in vivo.[150] Two of 16 patients underwent regression of metastatic disease. In a follow-up study, 2 of 14 patients underwent regression of disease after being treated with MART-1 TCR-transduced PBL following lymphodepleting chemotherapy.[151] Newer studies will test the efficacy of higher affinity TCRs, and TCRs against cancer antigens present on common epithelial cancers.

Biochemotherapy

The lack of improved survival with combination chemotherapy despite an improved response rate indicates the need to improve the durability of the responses seen. Biochemotherapy regimens combine the chemotherapy agents with immune-based therapy in an effort to improve the responses and durability of the remissions. The initial biochemotherapy studies combined chemotherapy with IFN. A study by Falkson and colleagues reported an improvement in response and response duration when IFN was added to DTIC.[152] However, a follow up study comparing DTIC, DTIC with tamoxifen, DTIC with IFN, or the combination of all 3 drugs showed no significant difference in response or survival.[96]

Because of the durable responses seen with IL-2, biochemotherapy regimens were designed to combine chemotherapy, IL-2, and IFN. In the initial studies a sequential approach was used, and initial studies by Legha and colleagues[48] used an alternating and a sequential approach. The sequential regimen produced an overall response rate of 64% with 21% complete responses. More significant was the duration of response of more than 3 years in those patients who achieved a complete response. Multiple phase 2 studies also observed a high response rate, and suggested survival improvement over CVD alone.[90]

Other studies have not been able to show the benefits of biochemotherapy.[90] In a study of cisplatin, DTIC, and tamoxifen alone or in combination with IL-2 and IFN, there was a similar response with the combination (27% vs 44% $P = .071$), but no improvement in survival (15.8 vs 10.7 months, $P = .052$).[153]

A large phase 3 study, E3695, evaluated 395 patients randomized to CVD or biochemotherapy (BCT) with CVD, IL-2, and IFN. This study showed a modest increase in response rate for BCT over CVD (19.5% vs 13.8%, $P = .140$) and an improved progression-free survival (4.8 vs 2.9 months; $P = .015$), but this did not translate into an overall survival advantage (9.0 vs 8.7 months).[154] A meta-analysis of 18 trials similarly showed that biochemotherapy was associated with an improvement in response rate, but not an improvement in survival.[155] A large review of the M.D. Anderson data, however, comparing patients treated with biochemotherapy versus chemotherapy with or without IFN, showed that biochemotherapy was associated with an improved overall response rate 52% versus 35% as well as improved 5-year survival (17% vs 7%, $P = .0004$) and 10-year survival (15% vs 5%, $P = .0001$), suggesting a benefit for biochemotherapy over chemotherapy.[156] Although the phase 3 data would suggest against an improved survival with biochemotherapy, these regimens are still being developed and studied, and the data suggest some patients will benefit from these aggressive regimens.

SUMMARY OF THERAPY FOR METASTATIC MELANOMA

The optimal management of patients with metastatic melanoma is still being defined. Treatments to date have been unsatisfactory, with median survival in most studies ranging from 6 to 9 months and 5-year survival rates of 1% to 2%.[69] In formulating a treatment plan, patients must be assessed for the relative volume and pace of disease, the presence of brain metastases, and the performance status, as each of these may impact decisions on care. Predictors of poor prognosis include decreased performance status (elevated ECOG score), presence of visceral metastases, increased number of metastatic sites, and elevated serum LDH level.[157] There is no standard management for the disease at this time. The 2009 NCCN guidelines include several agents, but all of these are category 2B recommendations, indicating the lack of activity and documentation of effectiveness. Innovation and clinical trials are probably the optimal management strategies for patients with metastatic melanoma. Despite the drawbacks, each of the agents has its role in current treatment of patients, even with the goal of palliation.

SUMMARY

The medical therapy for melanoma is evolving. The vast knowledge base that is being developed regarding the biology of melanoma is leading to the development of multiple new agents, as well as new strategies for use of existing agents for treatment. The understanding of immune function is providing ways to manipulate and modulate the host response to the tumor either through immunomodulatory agents or cellular therapy. Vaccination strategies to treat or even prevent the disease are still an area of active investigation. Despite these exciting research areas, the current treatment of patients often reverts to therapy with standard chemotherapeutic agents. Although these agents have disappointing overall results, a small group of patients will have significant and sometimes durable responses, providing for their continued use and providing hope to the patient with this severe disease.

ACKNOWLEDGMENTS

The authors thank Ellie Lehmann for reference management.

REFERENCES

1. Jemal A, Siegel R, Ward E, et al. Cancer statistics. CA Cancer J Clin 2008;58:71–96.
2. Chang AE, Karnell LH, Menck HR. The National Cancer Data Base report on cutaneous and noncutaneous melanoma. Cancer 2000;83:1664–78.
3. Balch CM, Buzaid AC, Soong SJ, et al. New TNM melanoma staging system: linking biology and natural history to clinical outcomes. Semin Surg Oncol 2003;21:43–52.
4. Balch CM, Buzaid AC, Atkins MB, et al. Transient T cell depletion causes regression of melanoma metastasis. Cancer 2000;88:1484–91.
5. Slingluff CL, Flaherty K, Rosenberg SA, et al. Cutaneous melanoma. In Cancer. In: DeVita VT, Hellman S, Rosenberg SA, editors. Principles & Practice of oncology. 7th edition. Philadelphia; Lippincott, Williams & Wilkins (LWW) 2005. p. 1897–921.
6. Veronesi U, Adamus J, Aubert C. A randomized trial of adjuvant chemotherapy and immunotherapy in cutaneous melanoma. N Engl J Med 1982;307:913–6.
7. Garbe C, Radny P, Linse R, et al. Adjuvant low-dose interferon 2a with or without dacarbazine compared with surgery alone: a prospective-randomized phase III DeCOG trial in melanoma patients with regional lymph node metastasis. Ann Oncol 2008;19:1195–201.
8. Morton DL, Eilber FR, Holmes EC, et al. BCG immunotherapy as a systemic adjunct to surgery in malignant melanoma. Med Clin North Am 1976;60:431–9.
9. Agarwala SS, Neuberg D, Park Y, et al. Mature results of a phase III randomized trial of bacillus Calmette-Guerin (BCG) versus observation and BCG plus dacarbazine versus BCG in the adjuvant therapy of American Joint Committee on Cancer Stage I-III melanoma (E1673); a trial of the Eastern Oncology Group. Cancer 2004;100:1692–8.
10. Ascierto PA, Kirkwood JM. Adjuvant therapy of melanoma with interferon: lessons of the past decade. J Transl Med 2008;6:62.
11. Kirkwood JM, Strawderman MH, Ernstoff MS, et al. Interferon alfa-2b adjuvant therapy of high-risk resected cutaneous melanoma: the Eastern Cooperative Oncology Group Trial EST 1684. J Clin Oncol 1996;14:7–17.
12. Kirkwood JM, Bender C, Agarwala S, et al. Mechanisms and management of toxicities associated with high-dose interferon alfa-2b therapy. J Clin Oncol 2002;20:3703–18.

13. Cole BF, Gelber RD, Kirkwood JM, et al. Quality-of-life-adjusted survival analysis of interferon alfa-2b adjuvant treatment of high-risk resected cutaneous melanoma: an Eastern Cooperative Oncology Group study. J Clin Oncol 1996;14:2666–73.

14. Kirkwood JM, Ibrahim JG, Sondak VK, et al. High-and low-dose interferon alfa-2b in high-risk melanoma: first analysis of intergroup trial E1690/S9111/C9190. J Clin Oncol 2000;18:2444–58.

15. Kirkwood JM, Manola J, Ibrahim J, et al. Eastern Cooperative Oncology Group. A pooled analysis of eastern cooperative oncology group and intergroup trials of adjuvant high-dose interferon for melanoma. Clin Cancer Res 2004;10:1670–7.

16. Kirkwood JM, Ibrahim JG, Sosman JA, et al. High-dose interferon alfa-2b significantly prolongs relapse-free and overall survival compared with the FM2-KLH/QS-21 vaccine in patients with resected stage IIb-III melanoma: results of intergroup trial 1694/S9512/C509801. J Clin Oncol 2001;19:2370–80.

17. Kirkwood JM, Ibrahim J, Lawson DH, et al. High-dose interferon alfa-2b does not diminish antibody response to GM2 vaccination in patients with resected melanoma: results of the Multicenter Eastern Cooperative Oncology Group Phase II Trial E2696. J Clin Oncol 2001;19:1430–6.

18. Alexander M, Eggermont S, Suciu S, et al. Adjuvant therapy with pegylated interferon alfa-2B versus observation alone in resected stage III melanoma: final results of EORTC 18991, a randomised phase III trial. Lancet 2008;372:117–26.

19. Lawson DH. Choices in adjuvant therapy of melanoma. Cancer Control 2005;12:236–41.

20. McMasters KM. The Sunbelt melanoma trial. Ann Surg Oncol 2001;8:41S–3S.

21. McMasters KM, Ross MI, Reintgen DS, et al. Finals results of the Sunbelt melanoma trial [abstract: 9003]. J Clin Oncol 2008;26.

22. Pectasides D, Dafni U, Bafaloukos D, et al. Randomized phase III study of 1 Mondth versus 1 year of adjuvant high-dose inerferon alfa-2b in patients with resected high-risk melanoma. J Clin Oncol 2009;27:939–44.

23. Chiarion-Sileni V, Del Bianco P, Romanini A, et al. Tolerability of intensified intravenous interferon alfa-2b versus the ECOG 1684 schedule as adjuvant therapy for stage III melanoma: a randomized phase III Italian Melanoma Inter-group trial (IMI-Mel.A. BMC Cancer 2006;6:44.

24. Eggermont AM, Suciu S, Santinami M, et al. Adjuvant therapy with pegylated interferon alfa-2b versus observation alone in resected stage III melanoma: final results of EORTC 18991, a randomized phase III trial. Lancet 2008;372:117–26.

25. Hauschild A, Weichenthal M, Balda BR, et al. Prospective randomized trial of interferon alfa-2b and interleukin-2 as adjuvant treatment for resected intermediate-and high-risk primary melanoma without clinically detectable node metastasis. J Clin Oncol 2003;21:2883–8.

26. Mitchell MS, Abrams J, Thompson JA, et al. Randomized trial of an allogeneic melanoma lysate vaccine with low-dose interferon alfa-2b compared with high-dose interferon alfa-2b for resected stage III cutaneous melanoma. J Clin Oncol 2007;25:2078–85.

27. Spitler LE, Grossbard ML, Ernstoff MS, et al. Adjuvant therapy of stage III and IV malignant melanoma using granulocyte-macrophage colony-stimulating factor. J Clin Oncol 2000;18:1614–21.

28. Spitler LE, Weber RW, Cruickshank S, et al. Granulocyte-macrophage colony stimulating factor (GM-CSF, sargramostim) as adjuvant therapy of melanoma. [Abstract: 20006] In: ASCO Annual Meeting Proceedings. J Clin Oncol 2008;26.

29. Daud AI, Mirza N, Lenox B, et al. Phenotypic and functional analysis of dendritic cells and clinical outcome in patients with high-risk melanoma treated with adjuvant granulocyte macrophage colony-stimulating factor. J Clin Oncol 2008;26:3235–41.

30. Kirkwood JM, Moschos S, Wang W. Strategies for the development of more effective adjuvant therapy of melanoma: current and future explorations of antibodies, cytokines, vaccines, and combinations. Clin Cancer Res 2006;12:2331S–6S.

31. Restifo NP, Lewis JJ. Therapeutic vaccines in cancer. In: DeVita VT, Hellman S, Rosenberg SA, editors. Cancer. 7th edition. Philadelphia: Lippincott, Williams & Wilkins; 2005. p. 2846–56.

32. Sosman JA, Sondak VK. Melacine: an allogeneic melanoma tumor cell lysate vaccine. Expert Rev Vaccines 2003;2:353–68.

33. Mitchell MS, Kan-Mitchell J, Kempf RA, et al. Active specific immunotherapy for melanoma: phase I trial of allogeneic lysates and a novel adjuvant. Cancer Res 1988;48:5883–93.

34. Sosman JA, Unger JM, Liu PY, et al. Adjuvant immunotherapy of resected, intermediate-thickness, node-negative melanoma with an allogeneic tumor vaccine: impact of HLA class I antigen expression on outcome. J Clin Oncol 2002;20:2067–75.

35. Mitchell MS, von Eschen KB. Phase III trial of Melacine melanoma theraccine versus combination chemotherapy in the treatment of stage IV melanoma. Proc Am Soc Clin Oncol 1997;16 [abstract: 494a].

36. Sondak VK, Liu PY, Tuthill RJ, et al. Adjuvant immunotherapy of resected, intermediate-thickness, node-negative melanoma with an allogeneic tumor vaccine: overall results of a randomized trial of the

Southwest Oncology Group. J Clin Oncol 2002;20: 2058–66.

37. von Euw EM, Barrio MM, Furman D, et al. A phase I clinical study of vaccination of melanoma patients with dendritic cells loaded with alloge-neic apoptotic/necrotic melanoma cells. Analysis of toxicity and immune response to the vaccine and of IL-10-1082 promoter genotype as predictor of disease progression. J Transl Med 2008;6:6.

38. Engell-Noerregaard L, Hansen TH, Andersen MH, et al. Review of clinical studies on dendritic cell-based vaccination of patients with malignant mela-noma: assessment of correlation between clinical response and vaccine parameters. Cancer Immu-nol Immunother 2009;58:1–14.

39. Smith JW II, Walker EB, Fox BA, et al. Adjuvant immunization of HLA-A2-positive melanoma patients with a modified gp100 peptide induces peptide-specific CD8+ T-cell responses. J Clin Oncol 2003;21:1562–73.

40. Slingluff CL Jr, Petroni GR, Yamshchikov GV, et al. Clinical and immunologic results of a randomized phase II trial of vaccination using four melanoma peptides either administered in granulocyte-macrophage colony-stimulating factor in adjuvant or pulsed on dendritic cells. J Clin Oncol 2003; 21:4016–26.

41. Slingluff CL Jr, Petroni GR, Yamshchikov GV, et al. Immunologic and clinical outcomes of vaccination with a multiepitope melanoma peptide vaccine plus low-dose interleukin-2 administered either concurrently or on a delayed schedule. J Clin Oncol 2004;22:4474–85.

42. Slingluff CL Jr, Petroni GR, Chianese-Bullock KA, et al. Immunologic and clinical outcomes of a randomized phase II trial of two multipeptide vaccines for melanoma in the adjuvant setting. Clin Cancer Res 2007;13:6386–95.

43. Livingston PO, Wong GY, Adluri S, et al. Improved survival in stage III melanoma patients with GM2 antibodies: a randomized trial of adjuvant vaccina-tion with GM2 ganglioside. J Clin Oncol 1994;12: 1036–44.

44. Eggermont AM, Eggermont S, Suciu W, et al. EORTC 18961: Post-operative adjuvant ganglio-side GM2-KLH21 vaccination treatment vs obser-vation in stage II (T3-T4N0M0) melanoma: 2nd interim analysis led to an early disclosure of the results. J Clin Oncol 2008;26 [abstract: 9004].

45. Rosenberg SA, Spiess P, Lafreniere R. A new approach to the adoptive immunotherapy of cancer with tumor-infiltrating lymphocytes. Science 1986; 233:1318–21.

46. Kawakami Y, Eliyahu S, Jennings C, et al. Recogni-tion of multiple epitopes in the human melanoma antigen gp100 by tumor-infiltrating T lymphocytes

associated with in vivo tumor regression. J Immunol 1995;154:3961–8.

47. Khammari A, Hguyen JM, Pandolfino MC, et al. Long-term follow-up of patients treated by adoptive transfer of melanoma tumor-infiltrating lymphocytes as adjuvant therapy for stage III melanoma. Cancer Immunol Immunother 2007;56:1853–60.

48. Legha SS, Ring S, Bedikian A, et al. Treatment of metastatic melanoma with combined chemo-therapy containing cisplatin, vinblastine and da-carbazine (CVD) and biotherapy using interleukin-2 and interferon-alpha. Ann Oncol 1996;7:827–35.

49. Kim KB, Legha SS, Gonazlez R, et al. A phase III randomized trial of adjuvant biochemotherapy (BC) versus interfernon-alpha-2b (IFN) in patients (pts) with high risk for melanoma recurrence. J Clin Oncol 2006;24:8003.

50. Kevin B, Kima KB, Sewa S, et al. A randomized phase III trial of biochemotherapy versus inter-feron-a-2b for adjuvant therapy in patients at high risk for melanoma recurrence. Melanoma Res 2009;19:42–9.

51. Kim KB, Legha SS, Gonazlez R, et al. A random-ized phase III trial of biochemotherapy versus inter-feron-[alpha]-2b for adjuvant therapy in patients at high risk for melanoma recurrence. Melanoma Res 2009;19:42–9.

52. Kefford RF. Adjuvant therapy of cutaneous mela-noma: the interferon debate. Ann Oncol 2003;14: 358–65.

53. Lens MB, Dawes M. Interferon alpha therapy for malignant melanoma: a systematic review of randomized controlled trials. J Clin Oncol 2002; 20:1818–25.

54. Essner R, Kaushal, A, Flaherty, K, et al. Melanoma and other skin cancers. In: Pazdur R, Coia LR, Hos-kins WJ, et al, editors. Cancer management: a multidisciplinary approach. 11th edition. London: CMP Medica; 2008.

55. Bajetta E, Del Vecchio D, Bernard-Marty C, et al. Metastatic melanoma: chemotherapy. Semin Oncol 2002;29:427–45.

56. O'Day SJ, Kim CJ, Reintgen DS. Metastatic mela-noma: chemotherapy to biochemotherapy. Cancer Control 2002;9:31–8.

57. Chapman PB, Einhorn LH, Meyers ML, et al. Phase III multicenter randomized trial of the Dart-mouth regimen versus dacarbazine in patients with metastatic melanoma. J Clin Oncol 1999; 17:2745–51.

58. Lee SM, Betticher DC, Thatcher N. Melanoma: chemotherapy. Br Med Bull 1995;51:609–30.

59. Stevens MFG, Hickman JA, Langdon SP, et al. Anti-tumor activity and pharmacokinetics in mice of 8-carbomoyl-3-methyl-imidazo[5,1-d]-1,2,3,5-tetra-zin-4(3H)-one (CCCRG81045; M&B 39831), a novel

drug with potential as an alternative to DTIC. Cancer Res 1987;47:5846–52.

60. Newlands ES, Blackledge GR, Slack JA, et al. Phase I trial of temozolomide (CCRG 81045: M&B 39831: NSC 362856). Br J Cancer 1992; 65:287–91.

61. Bleehen NM, Newlands ES, Lee SM, et al. Cancer research campaign phase II trial of temozolomide in metastatic melanoma. J Clin Oncol 1995;13: 910–3.

62. Middleton MR, Grob JJ, Aaronson N, et al. Randomized phase III study of temozolomide versus dacarbazine in the treatment of patients with advanced metastatic malignant melanoma. J Clin Oncol 2000;18:158–66.

63. Rietschel P, Wolchok JD, Krown S, et al. Phase II study of extended-dose temozolomide in patients with melanoma. J Clin Oncol 2008;26:2299–304.

64. Perussia B, Trinchieri G, Jackson A, et al. The Fc receptor for IgG in human natural killer cells: phenotypic, functional, and comparative studies with monoclonal antibodies. J Immunol 1984;133: 180–9.

65. Clark J, Moon J, Hutchins LF, et al. Phase II trial of combination thalidomide (thal) plus temozolomide (TMZ[TT]), in patients with metastatic malignant melanoma (MMM): Southwest Oncology Group S0508. J Clin Oncol 2008;26 [abstract: 9007].

66. Hwu WJ, Panageas KS, Menell JH, et al. Phase II study of temozolomide plus pegylated interferon-alpha-2b for metastatic melanoma. Cancer 2006; 106:2445–51.

67. Spieth K, Kaufmann R, Dummer R, et al. Temozolomide plus pegylated interferon alfa-2b as first-line treatment for stage IV melanoma: a multicenter phase II trial of the Dermatologic Cooperative Oncology Group (DeCOG). Ann Oncol 2008;19: 801–6.

68. Kaufmann R, Spieth K, Leiter U, et al. Temozolomide in combination with interferon-alfa versus temozolomide alone in patients with advanced metastatic melanoma: a randomized, phase III, multicenter study from the Dermatologic Cooperative Oncology Group. J Clin Oncol 2005;23:9001–7.

69. Balch CM, Atkins MB, Sober, AJ. Cutaneous melanoma. In Cancer. In: DeVita VT, Hellman S, Rosenberg SA, editors. Principles & practice of oncology, 7th edition. Philadelphia: Lippincott. Williams & Wilkins; 2005. p. 1754–808

70. Avril MF, Aamdal S, Grob JJ. Fotemustine compared with dacarbazine in patients with disseminated malignant melanoma: a phase III stud. J Clin Oncol 2004;22:1118.

71. Feun LG, Savaraj N, Hurley J, et al. A clinical trial of intravenous vinorelbine tartrate plus tamoxifen in the treatment of patients with advanced malignant melanoma. Cancer 2000;88:584–8.

72. Jimeno A, Hitt R, Quintela-Fandino M, et al. Phase II trial of vinorelbine tartrate in patients with treatment-naive metastatic melanoma. Anticancer Drugs 2005;16:53–7.

73. Whitehead RP, Moon J, McCachren SS, et al. A phase II trial of vinorelbine tartrate in patients with disseminated malignant melanoma and one prior systemic therapy: a Southwest Oncology Group study. Cancer 2004;100:1699–704.

74. Wiernik PH, Einzig AI. Taxol in malignant melanoma. J Natl Cancer Inst Monogr 1993;15:185–7.

75. Rao RD, Holtan SG, Ingle JN, et al. Combination of paclitaxel and carboplatin as second-line therapy for patients with metastatic melanoma. Cancer 2006;106:375–82.

76. Walker L, Schalch H, King DM, et al. Phase II trial of weekly paclitaxel in patients with advanced melanoma. Melanoma Res 2005;15:453–9.

77. Zimpfer-Rechner C, Hofmann U, Figl R, et al. Randomized phase II study of weekly paclitaxel versus paclitaxel and carboplatin as second-line therapy in disseminated melanoma: a multi-centre trial of the Dermatologic Co-operative Oncology Group (DeCOG). Melanoma Res 2003;13:531–6.

78. Bedikian AY, Weiss GR, Legha SS, et al. Phase II trial of docetaxel in patients with advanced cutaneous malignant melanoma previously untreated with chemotherapy. J Clin Oncol 2003;13:2865–8.

79. Kim KB, Hwu WJ, Papadopoulos NE, et al. Phase I study of the combination of docetaxel, temozolomide and cisplatin in patients with metastatic melanoma. Cancer Chemother Pharmacol 2009;64:161–7.

80. Legha SS, Ring S, Papadopoulos N, et al. A prospective evaluation of a triple-drug regimen containing cisplatin, vinblastine, and dacarbazine (CVD) for metastatic melanoma. Cancer 1989;64: 2024–9.

81. Del Prete SA, Maurer LH, O'Donnell J, et al. Combination chemotherapy with cisplatin, carmustine, dacarbazine, and tamoxifen in metastatic melanoma. Cancer Treat Rep 1984;68:1403–5.

82. Buzaid AC, Legha SS, Winn R. Cisplatin (C), vinblastine (V), dacarbazine (D) (CVD) versus dacarbazine alone in metastatic melanoma: preliminary results phase III cancer community oncology program (CCOP). J Clin Oncol 1993;12:1328.

83. Jansen B, Schlagbauer-Sadl H, Brown BD. Bcl-2 antisense therapy chemosensitizes human melanoma in SCID mice. Nat Med 1998;4:232–4.

84. Bedikian AY, Millward M, Pehamberger H, et al. Bcl-2 antisense (oblimersen sodium) plus dacarbazine in patients with advanced melanoma: the Oblimersen Melanoma Study Group. J Clin Oncol 2006;24:4738–45.

85. O'Day S, Gonzalez R, Weber L, et al. Elesclomol (formerly STA-4783) and paclitaxel in stage IV

metastatic melanoma: 2-year overall survival. 33rd European Society of Medical Oncology Congress [abstract]. Stockholm: September 2008.

86. Williams PD, Lee JK, Theodorescu D. Genomancy: predicting tumor response to cancer therapy based on the oracle of genetics. Curr Oncol 2009;16:56–8.

87. Koscielny S. Critical review of microarray-based prognostic tests and trials in breast cancer. Curr Opin Obstet Gynecol 2008;20:47–50.

88. Gray-Schopfer V, Wellbrock C, Marais R. Melanoma biology and new targeted therapy. Nature 2007;445:851–7.

89. Fisher RI, Neifeld JP, Pippman ME. Estrogen receptors in human malignant melanoma. Lancet 1976;2: 337–8.

90. O'Day SJ, Kim CJ, Reintgen DS. Chemotherapy to biochemotherapy. Cancer Control 2002;9: 31–8.

91. Rumke P, Kleeberg UR, MacKie RM, et al. Tamoxifen as a single agent for advanced melanoma in postmenopausal women; a phase II study of the EORTC Malignant Melanoma Cooperative Group. Melanoma Res 1992;2:153–6.

92. Nesbit RA, Woods RI, Tattersall MH, et al. Tamoxifen in malignant melanoma. N Engl J Med 1979; 301:1241–2.

93. Cocconi G, Bella M, Clabresi F. Treatment of metastatic melanoma with dacarbazine plus tamoxifen. N Engl J Med 1992;52:516–23.

94. McClay EF, Mastrangelo MJ, Berd D. Effective combination chemo/hormonal therapy for malignant melanoma: experience with three consecutive trials. Int J Cancer 1992;50:553–6.

95. Agarwala SS, Ferri W, Gooding W, et al. A phase III randomized trial of dacarbazine and carboplatin with and without tamoxifen in the treatment of patients with metastatic melanoma. Cancer 1984; 85:1979–84.

96. Falkson CI, Ibrahim J, Kirkwood JM. Phase II trial of dacarbazine versus dacarbazine with interferon alpha-2b versus dacarbazine with tamoxifen versus dacarbazine with interferon alpha-2b and tamoxifen in patients with metastatic malignant melanoma: an Eastern Cooperative Oncology Group Study. J Clin Oncol 1998;16: 1743–51.

97. Rusthoven JJ, Quirt IC, Isocoe NA, et al. Randomized double-blind, placebo-controlled trial comparing the response rates of carmustine, dacarbazine, and cisplatin with and without tamoxifen in patients with metastatic melanoma. J Clin Oncol 1996;14:2083–90.

98. Lens MB, Reiman T, Husain AF. Use of tamoxifen in the treatment of malignant melanoma: systematic review and meta-analysis. Cancer 2003;98: 1355–61.

99. Mori T, Martinez SR, O'Day SJ, et al. Estrogen receptor-a methylation predicts melanoma progression. Cancer Res 2006;66(13):6692–8.

100. Varker KA, Biber JE, Kefauver C, et al. A randomized phase 2 trial of bevacizumab with or without daily low-dose interferon alfa-2b in metastatic malignant melanoma. Ann Surg Oncol 2007;14: 2367–76.

101. Viteri S, Diaz-Lagares A, Gonzalez A, et al. VEGF serum levels during bevacizumab plus paclitaxel combination in metastatic melanoma. J Clin Oncol 2007;25:8534.

102. Perez DG, Suman VJ, Fitch TR, et al. Phase 2 trial of carboplatin, weekly paclitaxel, and biweekly bevacizumab in patients with unresectable stage IV. Cancer 2009;115:119–27.

103. Fruehauf JP, Lutzky J, McDermott DF, et al. Axitinib (AG-013736) in patients with metastatic melanoma: a phase II study [abstract: 9006] In: ASCO Annual Meeting Proceedings. J Clin Oncol 2008;15S.

104. Eisen T, Ahmad T, Flaherty KT, et al. Sorafenib in advanced melanoma: a Phase II randomized discontinuation trial analysis. Br J Cancer 2006; 95:581–6.

105. Flaherty KT, Schiller J, Schuchter LM, et al. A phase I trial of the oral, multikinase inhibitor sorafenib in combination with carboplatin and paclitaxel. Clin Cancer Res 2008;14:4836–42.

106. Lotze MT, Chang AE, Seipp CA, et al. High dose recombinant interleukin-2 in the treatment of patients with disseminated cancer: responses, treatment related morbidity and histologic findings. JAMA 1986;256:3117.

107. Grimm EA, Mazumder A, Zhang HZ, et al. Lymphokine-activated killer cell phenomenon. Lysis of natural killer-resistant fresh solid tumor cells by interleukin 2- activated autologous human peripheral blood lymphocytes. J Exp Med 1982;155: 1823–41.

108. Rosenberg SA, Mulé JJ, Spiess PJ, et al. Regression of established pulmonary metastases and subcutaneous tumors mediated by the systemic administration of high-dose recombinant interleukin-2. J Exp Med 1985;161:1169–88.

109. Rosenberg SA, Lotze MT, Yang JC, et al. Prospective randomized trial of high-dose interleukin-2 alone or in conjunction with lymphokine-activated killer cells for the treatment of patients with advanced cancer. J Natl Cancer Inst 1993;85: 622–32.

110. Atkins MB, Lotze MT, Dutcher JP, et al. High-dose recombinant interleukin-2 therapy for patients with metastatic melanoma: analysis of 270 patients treated between 1985 and 1993. J Clin Oncol 1999;17:2105–16.

111. Phan GQ, Attia P, Steinberg SM, et al. Factors associated with response to high-dose

interleukin-2 in patients with metastatic melanoma. J Clin Oncol 2001;19:3477–82.

112. Schwartzentruber DJ. Biological therapy with interleukin-2: clinical applications: principles of administration and management of side effects. In: DeVita VT, Hellman S, Rosenberg SA, editors. Biologic therapy of cancer. Bethesda (MD): Lippincott; 1995. p. 235–50.

113. Schwartzentruber DJ. Guidelines for the safe administration of high-dose interleukin-2. J Immunother 2001;24:287–93.

114. Agarwala SS, Kirkwood JM. Interferon in melanoma. Curr Opin Oncol 1996;8:167.

115. Hernberg M, Ryrhonen S, Muhonene T. Regimens with or without interferon-alpha as treatment for metastatic melanoma and renal cell carcinoma: an overview of randomized trials. J Immunother 1999;22(2):145–54.

116. van Elsas A, Hurwitz AA, Allison JP. Combination immunotherapy of B16 melanoma using anti-cytotoxic T lymphocyte-associated antigen 4 (CTLA04) and granulocyte/macrophage colony-stimulating factor (GM-CSF)-producing vaccines induces rejection of subcutaneous and metastatic tumors accompanied by autoimmune depigmentation. J Exp Med 1999;190:355–66.

117. Ribas A, Camacho LH, Lopez-Berestein G, et al. Antitimor activity in melanoma and anti-self responses in a phase I trial with the anti-cytotoxic T lymphocyte-associated antigen 4 monoclonal antibody CP-675.206. J Clin Oncol 2005;23:8968–77.

118. Camacho LH, Antonia S, Sosman J, et al. Phase I/II trial of tremelimumab in patients with metastatic melanoma. J Clin Oncol 2009;27:1075–81.

119. Ribas A, Hauschild A, Kefford R, et al. Phase III, open-label, randomized, comparative study of tremelimumab (CP-675,206) and chemotherapy temozolomide [TMZ] or dacarbazine[DTIC] in patients with advanced melanoma [abstract]. J Clin Oncol 2008;26:LBA 9011.

120. Phan GQ, Yang JC, Sherry RM, et al. Cancer regression and autoimmunity induced by cytotoxic T lymphocyte-associated antigen 4 blockade in patients with metastatic melanoma. Proc Natl Acad Sci U S A 2003;100:8372–7.

121. Downey SG, Klapper JA, Smith FO, et al. Prognostic factors related to clinical response in patients with metastatic melanoma treated by CTL-associated antigen-4 blockade. Clin Cancer Res 2007;13:6681–8.

122. Weber JS, Targan S, Scotland R, et al. Phase II trial of extended dose anti-CTLA-4 antibody ipilimumab (formerly MDX-010) with a multi-peptide vaccine for resected stages IIIC and IV melanoma. J Clin Oncol 2006;24:2510.

123. Korn E. Meta-analysis of Phase 2 cooperative group trials in metastatic Stage IV melanoma to determine progression-free and overall survival benchmarks for future Phase 2 trials. J Clin Oncol 2008;26:526–34.

124. Weber J. Overcoming immunologic tolerance to melanoma: targeting CTLA-4 with ipilimumab (MDX-010). Oncologist 2008;13:16–25.

125. Rosenberg SA, Yang JC, Restifo NP. Cancer immunotherapy: moving beyond current vaccines. Nat Med 2004;10:909–15.

126. Smith FO, Downey SG, Klapper JA, et al. Treatment of metastatic melanoma using interleukin-2 alone or in conjunction with vaccines. Clin Cancer Res 2008;14:5610–8.

127. Butterfield LH, Comin-Anduix B, Vujanovic L, et al. Adenovirus MART-1-engineered autologous dendritic cell vaccine for metastatic melanoma. J Immunol 2008;31:294–309.

128. Butterfield LH, Ribas A, Dissette VB, et al. Determinant spreading associated with clinical response in dendritic cell-based immunotherapy for malignant melanoma. Clin Cancer Res 2003;9:998–1008.

129. Ribas A, Glaspy JA, Lee Y, et al. Role of dendritic cell phenotype, determinant spreading, and negative costimulatory blockade in dendritic cell-based melanoma immunotherapy. J Immunother 2004;27:354–67.

130. Redman BG, Chang AE, Whitfield J, et al. Phase Ib trial assessing autologous, tumor-pulsed dendritic cells as a vaccine administered with or without IL-2 in patients with metastatic melanoma. J Immunother 2008;31:591–8.

131. Bercovici N, Haicheur N, Massicard S, et al. Analysis and characterization of antitumor T-cell response after administration of dendritic cells loaded with allogeneic tumor lysate to metastatic melanoma patients. J Immunother 2008;31:101–12.

132. Rasku MA, Clem AL, Telang S, et al. Transient T cell depletion causes regression of melanoma metastases. J Transl Med 2008;6:12.

133. Appay V, Voelter V, Rufer N, et al. Combination of transient lymphodepletion with busulfan and fludarabine and peptide vaccination in a phase I clinical trial for patients with advanced melanoma. J Immunother 2007;30:240–50.

134. Powell DJ Jr, Dudley ME, Hogan KA, et al. Adoptive transfer of vaccine-induced peripheral blood mononuclear cells to patients with metastatic melanoma following lymphodepletion. J Immunol 2006;177:6527–39.

135. Dudley ME, Wunderlich JR, Robbins PF, et al. Cancer regression and autoimmunity in patients after clonal repopulation with antitumor lymphocytes. Science 2002;198:850–4.

136. Dudley ME, Yang JC, Sherry R, et al. Adoptive cell therapy for patients with metastatic melanoma: evaluation of intensive myeloablative

chemoradiation preparative regimens. J Clin Oncol 2008;26:5233–9.

137. Gattinoni L, Klebanoff CA, Palmer DC, et al. Acquisition of full effector function in vitro paradoxically impairs the in vivo antitumor efficacy of adoptively transferred CD8+ T cells. J Clin Invest 2005;115:1616–26.

138. Klebanoff CA, Gattinoni L, Torabi-Parizi P, et al. Central memory self/tumor-reactive CD8+ T cells confer superior antitumor immunity compared with effector memory T cells. Proc Natl Acad Sci U S A 2005;102:9571–6.

139. Shen X, Zhou J, Hathcock KS, et al. Persistence of tumor infiltrating lymphocytes in adoptive immunotherapy correlates with telomere length. J Immunother 2007;30:123–9.

140. Zhou J, Shen X, Huang J, et al. Telomere length of transferred lymphocytes correlates with in vivo persistence and tumor regression in melanoma patients receiving cell transfer therapy. J Immunol 2005;175:7046–52.

141. Tran KQ, Zhou J, Durflinger KH, et al. Minimally cultured tumor-infiltrating lymphocytes display optimal characteristics for adoptive cell therapy. J Immunother 2008;31:743–51.

142. Dudley ME, Wunderlich J, Nishimura MI, et al. Adoptive transfer of cloned melanoma-reactive T lymphocytes for the treatment of patients with metastatic melanoma. J Immunother 2001;24:363–73.

143. Yee C, Thompson JA, Byrd D, et al. Adoptive T cell therapy using antigen-specific CD8+ T cell clones for the treatment of patients with metastatic melanoma: in vivo persistence, migration, and antitumor effect of transferred T cells. Proc Natl Acad Sci U S A 2002;99:16168–73.

144. Rosenberg SA, Yannelli JR, Yang JC, et al. Treatment of patients with metastatic melanoma with autologous tumor-infiltrating lymphocytes and interleukin-2. J Natl Cancer Inst 1994;86:1159–66.

145. Yee C, Thompson JA, Roche P, et al. Melanocyte destruction after antigen-specific immunotherapy of melanoma: direct evidence of T cell-mediated vitiligo. J Exp Med 2000;192:1637–44.

146. Mitchell MS, Darrah D, Yeung D, et al. Phase I trial of adoptive immunotherapy with cytolytic T lymphocytes immunized against a tyrosinase epitope. J Clin Oncol 2002;20:1075–86.

147. Mackensen A, Meidenbauer N, Vogl S, et al. Phase I study of adoptive T-cell therapy using antigen-specific CD8+ T cells for the treatment of patients with metastatic melanoma. J Clin Oncol 2006;24:5060–9.

148. Hunder NN, Wallen H, Cao J, et al. Treatment of metastatic melanoma with autologous CD4+ T cells against NY-ESO-1. N Engl J Med 2008;358:2698–703.

149. Dudley ME, Wunderlich JR, Yang JC, et al. A phase I study of nonmyeloablative chemotherapy and adoptive transfer of autologous tumor antigen-specific T lymphocytes in patients with metastatic melanoma. J Immunother 2002;25:243–51.

150. Morgan RA, Dudley ME, Wunderlich JR, et al. Cancer regression in patients after transfer of genetically engineered lymphocytes. Science 2006;314:126–9.

151. Dudley ME, Rosenberg SA. Adoptive cell transfer therapy. Semin Oncol 2007;34:524–31.

152. Falkson CI, Falkson G, Falkson HC. Improved results with the addition of interferon alfa-2b to dacarbazine in the treatment of patients with metastatic melanoma. J Clin Oncol 1991;9:1403–8.

153. Rosenberg SA, Yang JC, Schwartzentruber DJ, et al. Prospective randomized trial of the treatment of patients with metastatic melanoma using chemotherapy with cisplatin, dacarbazine, and tamoxifen alone or in combination with interleukin-2 and interferon alfa-2b. J Clin Oncol 1999;17:968–75.

154. Atkins MB, Hsu J, Lee S, et al. Phase III trial comparing concurrent biochemotherapy with cisplatin, vinblastine, dacarbazine, interleukin-2, and interferon alfa-2b with cisplatin, vinblastine, and dacarbazine alone in patients with metastatic malignant melanoma (E3695): a trial coordinated by the Eastern Cooperative Oncology Group. J Clin Oncol 2008;26:5748–54.

155. Ives NJ, Stowe RL, Lorigan P, et al. Chemotherapy compared with biochemotherapy for the treatment of metastatic melanoma: a meta-analysis of 18 trials involving 2,621 patients. J Clin Oncol 2007;25:5426–34.

156. Bedikian AY, Johnson MM, Warneke CL, et al. Systemic therapy for unresectable metastatic melanoma: impact of biochemotherapy on long-term survival. J Immunotoxicol 2008;5:201–7.

157. Manola J, Atkins M, Ibrahim J, et al. Prognosis factors in metastatic melanoma: a pooled analysis of Eastern Cooperative Oncology Group trials. J Clin Oncol 2000;18:3782–93.

Role of Radiation Therapy in Cutaneous Melanoma

Jaime H. Shuff, MD, Malika L. Siker, MD, Mackenzie D. Daly, MD, Christopher J. Schultz, MD*

KEYWORDS

- Radiation therapy • Cutaneous melanoma
- Adjuvant treatment • Postoperative radiation
- Palliative radiation

An estimated 62,480 new cases of cutaneous melanoma were diagnosed in the United States in 2008, approximately 4% of all newly diagnosed cancers.[1] Cutaneous melanoma was also responsible for an estimated 8420 deaths.[1] While incidence is rising, mortality has decreased with a 5-year survival rate of 92% from 1996 to 2003 compared with 82% from 1975 to 1977.[1] This pattern is felt to be due to increased awareness and screening programs leading to earlier detection.[1] Solar ultraviolet (UV) radiation has been linked to the development of cutaneous melanoma, which results from the malignant transformation of epidermal melanocytes.[2,3] A higher incidence of melanoma has been found in areas of the body with high sun exposure, among people with other sun-related skin conditions, within populations dwelling in areas of high ambient sunlight, and among populations with increased sun sensitivity.[4,5] The presence of multiple nevi is also an accepted risk factor.[6,7]

Cutaneous melanoma remains a surgically treated disease for the majority of patients. Most cutaneous melanomas clinically present as visible, pigmented lesions. Approximately 80% of patients present with localized disease, and most are cured by simple excision.[1] However, as lesions grow in size, the risk of locoregional recurrence and distant spread increases dramatically. Lesions may recur at the primary site, as in-transit lesions, or in the neighboring lymphatics. Distant sites such as the lung, liver, brain, and bone are also

at risk. Although surgery retains a role even in patients with advanced disease, adjuvant therapy becomes increasingly important in these patients as well as those at high risk for locoregional or distant spread. Multiple strategies using systemic modalities including cytotoxic agents and immunomodulators have been evaluated, with limited success.[8–13]

Radiotherapy represents an important yet underused modality in the treatment of cutaneous melanoma. The incorporation of radiotherapy into treatment algorithms for patients has been reluctant and controversial. The first use of radiotherapy in the treatment of melanoma may have been by Simpson in 1913, when he successfully treated a large black nevus with radiotherapy. Although there was no histologic confirmation of melanoma, he was able to remove the lesion with radiotherapy without damage to the surrounding normal skin.[14] Throughout the early 1900s, cutaneous melanoma was labeled as a categorically radioresistant tumor despite a paucity of data to support this claim.[15–17] More modern studies have produced evidence to refute this hypothesis, and radiotherapy has gained acceptance in the definitive, adjuvant, and palliative treatment of cutaneous melanoma either alone or combined with other modalities. Treatment planning and techniques must be customized to this unique disease. Acute and late toxicities may manifest with treatment and may be augmented with a multimodality treatment approach. Future

Department of Radiation Oncology, Medical College of Wisconsin, 8701 Watertown Plank Road, Milwaukee, WI 53226, USA

* Corresponding author.

E-mail address: cschultz@mcw.edu (C.J. Schultz).

Clin Plastic Surg 37 (2010) 147–160

doi:10.1016/j.cps.2009.07.007

directions of the use of radiotherapy in cutaneous melanoma include improved treatment conformality resulting from advancements in the technology of treatment delivery and targeting. This review discusses these pertinent issues surrounding the role of radiotherapy in cutaneous melanoma.

MELANOMA AND RADIOBIOLOGIC CONSIDERATIONS
Radioresponse

The putative radioresistance of melanoma was in part based on observations from an early clinical review published in 1936 from Memorial Sloan-Kettering, demonstrating a response rate of 2.5% with radiotherapy in approximately 400 patients with advanced disease.[16] Equipment was poor compared with modern standards, and details describing the type of radiotherapy delivered were not provided. During this era Paterson[17] classified melanoma as a radioresistant disease, with little justification. Despite evidence from clinical reviews demonstrating efficacy and tolerability with treatment with radiotherapy, this misconception was established and propagated in the literature, with data rarely given to support this notion.[18–27]

Renewing interest in this field, in vitro studies in the 1970s using rodent and human melanoma lines suggested that the so-called radioresistance associated with melanoma may instead reflect a broad shoulder in the low-dose portion of the cell survival curve, with enhanced capacity of the melanoma cells for repair of sublethal radiation-induced damage.[28,29] It has been suggested that high radiotherapy doses per fraction may be needed to overcome the cellular repair process. Small clinical trials have provided support for this approach, although results have been mixed.[30–32] This belief has been called into question in view of the improved understanding of the mathematical models to determine radiation response, as well as the need to consider both the tumor and surrounding healthy tissues accounting for the therapeutic ratio.[33] Further confounding this issue is the wide range of radiosensitivities observed with in vitro melanoma cell lines, which remains unexplained.[34,35]

Fraction Size

Overgaard and colleagues[36] have suggested that response rate for melanoma is dependent on fraction size, with complete response rates of 57% with fractions more than 4 Gy compared with 24% with fractions less than 4 Gy (P<.001) from the results of an examination of 204 lesions of melanoma in 114 patients. Bentzen and colleagues[37] found that a fractionation schedule of approximately 6 Gy per fraction was superior for disease control. In this study, tumor size and total dose (after accounting for tumor size) were found to significantly impact tumor control whereas total treatment time was not significant.[37] Patients with multiple lesions had highly correlated response rates as compared with interpatient responses, implying that additional unknown parameters such as patient inherent radiosensitivity or immunologic status may be important.[37]

Clinical response rates with different hypofractionation regimens have been variable. A Danish prospective trial including 35 recurrent or metastatic melanoma lesions in 14 patients randomized treatment to high dose per fraction radiotherapy at either 9 Gy in 3 fractions or 5 Gy in 8 fractions. Complete durable regression was found in 69% of lesions treated in both arms, with an overall response rate of 97%. No difference was found in either arm. The investigators stated that acute and late toxicity in normal tissue was acceptable and similar in both arms.[38] A European multicenter prospective trial showed lower response rates. This trial randomized treatment of 134 metastatic or recurrent lesions of malignant melanoma in 70 patients to radiotherapy (8 or 9 Gy in 3 fractions in 8 days) alone or followed by hyperthermia. Two-year actuarial local control rate was 28% for radiotherapy alone versus 46% with the addition of hyperthermia (P = .008). The higher dose and dose per fraction regimen also resulted in superior local control, with 25% for the 24 Gy patients compared with 56% for the 27 Gy patients on univariate analysis (P = .02). Tumor size was not found to significantly influence outcome.[39]

At the M.D. Anderson Cancer Center (MDACC), Ang and colleagues performed a phase 2 study to assess the efficacy and toxicity of elective adjuvant radiation given in 5 fractions of 6 Gy to patients with cutaneous melanoma of the head at neck who were considered to have high-risk features for locoregional relapse. There were 174 patients enrolled, and 79 of these patients received elective irradiation after wide local excision of lesions 1.5 mm or more thick, or Clark's level IV to V. Thirty-two patients received adjuvant radiation after excision of primary lesion plus a limited neck dissection, and 63 patients received adjuvant radiation after neck dissection for nodal relapse. With a median follow-up of 35 months, the actuarial 5-year locoregional control rate was 88% and the 5-year survival rate was 47% for the entire group. The acute tolerance to the adjuvant hypofractionated regimen was considered to be excellent, with the most frequently observed acute reaction being transient parotid swelling. Moist skin desquamation and confluent mucositis of short duration was noted in less than 5% of patients. Three patients had late radiation complications including moderate neck fibrosis, mild ipsilateral hearing impairment, and transient exposure of external auditory canal cartilage.[40]

Stevens and colleagues from the Royal Prince Alfred Hospital in Sydney, Australia published a retrospective review of 174 patients with local or locoregional melanoma. All patients were treated postoperatively to 30 to 36 Gy in 5 to 7 fractions over 2.5 weeks. Indications for radiation in those with disease limited to the primary site included positive margins, neurotropic desmoplastic histopathology, close margins, tumor satellites, and multiple recurrences. Patients with regional nodal metastases were irradiated for positive surgical margins, extracapsular spread, multiple involved lymph nodes, large lymph nodes, perineural or vascular involvement, and parotid lymph node involvement. The median time to recurrence was 6 months, with recurrence in the radiation field developing in 11% of patients. Median disease-specific survival was 25 months for the entire cohort, 54 months for those with disease limited to primary site, and 23 months in those with locoregional nodal involvement. Few patients developed severe acute side effects. In terms of late complications, arm lymphedema was reported in 58% of patients treated postoperatively to the axilla.[41]

Investigators at the University of Florida published a retrospective review of 56 patients with a median follow-up of 1.7 years who were treated with wide local excision and sentinel node biopsy, or with dissection of regional lymph nodes in those with high-risk features. Patients with residual gross disease, close or positive margins, disease recurrence, satellitosis, and regional node metastases were treated with postoperative radiation. Seventy-three percent of patients were treated with 5 fractions of 6 Gy for a total dose of 30 Gy. Fractions were delivered twice a week over 2.5 weeks. Twenty-five percent of patients were treated to 60 Gy at a median of 2 Gy per fraction. Twelve percent of patients had in-field recurrences and 43% distant relapses. The 5-year in-field locoregional control rate was 87%. There was no difference noted in in-field locoregional control between the hypofractionated and conventional fractionation treatments. Two patients that received hypofractionated treatment had severe late complication of osteoradionecrosis of temporal bone and radiation plexopathy.[42]

When compared with conventional radiotherapy regimens, hypofractionation was not found to improve outcome in the only prospective randomized trial designed to address this question, Radiation Therapy Oncology Group (RTOG) 83-05. In this trial, 137 patients were randomized to treatment with 4 fractions of 8 Gy given in 21 days weekly, and 20 fractions of 2.5 Gy given over 26 to 28 days, 5 days per week. The complete response rate was similar for both arms, 24.2% in the hypofractionated arm and 23.4% in the conventional arm. Partial response rates were also equivalent, with 35.5% in the hypofractionated arm and 34.4% in the conventional arm. There were no reported differences in normal tissue complications.[43] Nevertheless, hypofractionated regimens for cutaneous melanoma remain under investigation.[40,41] Dose fractionation for the treatment of cutaneous melanoma is further discussed later in this article.

In conclusion, enough evidence has emerged to define melanoma as a more radioresponsive tumor than historically indicated. This disease displays a wide range of radiosensitivities and may have an enhanced capacity for repair of radiation-induced damage, as shown in preclinical studies. Hypofractionated delivery of radiotherapy may help to overcome this finding and these regimens have been found to be feasible, with variable response rates. However, hypofractionation has not been shown to result in significantly improved outcomes compared with conventional radiotherapy in a single, prospective randomized trial. The ideal schedule for radiotherapy in cutaneous melanoma is still unknown. The understanding of the radiobiology has improved greatly since the early reports of the 1930s, but further studies are needed to better understand this disease and to define the ideal treatment schedule for radiotherapy in these patients.

ADJUVANT RADIATION THERAPY TO PRIMARY SITE

Surgery has remained the cornerstone of management in most patients with cutaneous melanoma. Primary tumors measuring less than 1 mm in thickness have 5-year survival rates that exceed 90% with surgical resection alone.[44] However, retrospective reviews have revealed prognostic indicators for the likelihood of locoregional recurrence, indicating a role for adjuvant radiation to the primary lesion. High-risk clinicopathologic features include increasing tumor thickness, desmoplastic subtype, ulceration, tumor resection margin, location, and recurrence.

Urist and colleagues reported a review of 3445 patients with stage I cutaneous melanoma. In a single-factor analysis, tumor thickness, tumor ulceration, and increasing patient age were associated with an increased rate of local recurrence. Local recurrence rates at 5 years were 13.2% for patients with lesions of greater than 4 mm in size compared with 0.2% for lesions 0.76 mm. Tumors with ulceration had a local recurrence rate of 11.5% versus 1.9% without the presence of ulceration at 5 years.[45]

Balch and colleagues performed a prospective study evaluating the optimal surgical margin with resection of primary cutaneous melanoma. Four hundred and sixty-eight patients with melanomas of the trunk or proximal extremity were randomized to a 2-cm or 4-cm radial excisional margin. A second group comprised 278 patients with melanoma of the head, neck, or distal extremities who received a 2-cm radial margin. Local recurrence rates were same whether there was a 2-cm or 4-cm margin. Multivariate analysis showed that ulceration and head or neck location were associated with increased local recurrence. Local recurrences were associated with poor survival, with a 5-year survival rate of 9% to 11% compared with 86% for those without a local recurrence.[46]

Ulceration of cutaneous melanoma determined by microscopic evaluation represents a high-risk feature for metastases.[47,48] Survival rates of those with tumors with ulcerated melanoma are significantly lower than those with nonulcerated melanomas of the same thickness.[46] Ulceration is the only prognostic feature of primary melanoma that independently predicts outcomes for melanoma of stages I to III.[44,46,49,50] In the American Joint Committee on Cancer (AJCC) staging system for cutaneous melanoma published by Balch and colleagues[46] in 2001, the 5-year survival rate of patients with T2 nonulcerated melanoma was similar to those with a T1 ulcerated lesion (89% vs 91%), illustrating that an ulcerated lesion has the same survival rate as that of a nonulcerated lesion with a higher T stage.

Surgical resection remains the primary treatment for cutaneous melanoma. After surgical excision, recurrence rates vary between 15% and 24% for lesions 4 mm or larger, and up to 50% in those with head or neck desmoplastic melanoma subtype.[44,45,51] In the setting of high-risk features, adjuvant radiation treatment should be considered for the primary site as well as the regional lymph nodes (**Table 1**).

ADJUVANT RADIATION THERAPY TO REGIONAL LYMPHATICS

Regional lymph nodes are the most common site of metastatic disease for melanoma.[50] For those who present with clinical regional nodal involvement, a lymph node dissection is typically performed. Those without clinical nodal involvement may undergo sentinel lymph node biopsy or elective lymph node dissection. Although the overall survival benefit for sentinel lymph node biopsy is yet unproven, sentinel lymph node biopsy with selective dissection has become the standard of care for melanoma. Many high-risk nodal features have been reported in the surgical literature, including nodal extracapsular extension, 4 or more lymph nodes involved, lymph nodes greater than 3 cm in diameter, positive lymph nodes in the cervical basin, and lymph nodes detected at the time of therapeutic dissection.[52–56] Patients who have any of these high-risk features have a regional recurrence rate of 20% to 80% after nodal dissection.[52–56] Given these high recurrence rates, one must then consider the use of

Table 1	
Indications for adjuvant radiation therapy	
High-risk features	Series
Tumor size >4 mm, ulceration	Urist et al, 1985,[45] Univ. of Alabama at Birmingham
Microscopically positive surgical margins, close excision margins, neurotropic desmoplastic histopathology, multiple involved lymph nodes, large involved lymph nodes with extracapsular spread	Stevens et al, 2000,[41] Royal Prince Alfred Hospital
Cervical lymph node involvement, extracapsular extension, >3 positive lymph nodes, clinically involved lymph nodes, involved lymph node >3 cm	Lee et al, 2000,[53] Roswell Park Cancer Institute
Lymph node extracapsular extension, lymph node ≥3 cm, ≥4 involved lymph nodes, nodal recurrence after previous dissection	Ballo et al, 2003,[80] M.D. Anderson Cancer Center

adjuvant radiation therapy to regional nodes when such high-risk nodal features are present.

In a retrospective review, Creagen and colleagues reviewed 82 patients who had biopsy-proven regional nodal metastases between 1972 and 1977. They compared a control group treated with lymphadenectomy with a group of patients who received adjuvant radiation 4 weeks after lymphadenectomy. No statistically significant difference was seen in disease-free interval or survival for patients with only 1 positive node or those with more than 2 positive nodes. However, there was a significant difference in the time to recurrence, with a median time of 9 months in the control group compared with 20 months in the irradiated group.[57]

Lee and colleagues performed a retrospective analysis of 338 patients with melanoma who had undergone lymph node dissection for pathologically involved lymph nodes at Roswell Park Cancer Institute. Seventy-five percent of patients underwent therapeutic lymph node dissection, whereas the remainder had elective node dissection. No patients were treated with adjuvant radiation to the nodal basin. Overall, nodal basin recurrence was 30% at 10 years. Patients with extracapsular extension had a 10-year nodal recurrence much higher than those without (63% vs 23%, respectively). Nodal basin failure rate was 80% for lymph nodes measuring greater than 6 cm compared with 42% for those 3 to 6 cm in size. Failure rate was 24% in the nodal basin for nodes smaller than 3 cm. They also found that the number of nodes involved predicted for nodal basin failure, with a failure rate of 63% for those with more than 10 nodes involved. Eighty-seven percent of patients with nodal basin failure developed distant metastases compared with 54% of those without nodal failure. The recommendation of these investigators was the consideration of adjuvant radiation if there was cervical lymph node involvement, extracapsular extension, more than 3 positive lymph nodes, clinically involved nodes, or nodal involvement size greater than 3 cm in diameter.[53]

Investigators at the MDACC retrospectively reviewed patients with axillary metastases treated with axillary dissection followed by adjuvant hypofractionated radiation (30 Gy at 6 Gy per fraction over 2.5 weeks). Patients treated with adjuvant radiation had high-risk features including lymph node size 3 cm or larger, 4 or more positive lymph nodes, extracapsular extension, or recurrent disease after initial surgical resection alone. A total of 89 patients were reviewed, with a median follow-up of 63 months. Sixty-six patients were treated for their first axillary disease and 22 patients for recurrent axillary disease after prior surgery. At 5 years, they found an actuarial overall survival of 50%, disease-free survival of 46%, distant metastasis-free survival of 49%, and axillary control rate of 87%. Univariate analysis showed that axillary control was inferior if axillary disease was greater than 6 cm in size (72% vs 93%). It was also found that the distant metastasis-free and disease-free survivals were less if there were more than 2 nodes positive for metastatic disease or if the primary tumor had a Breslow thickness greater than 4 mm.[58]

At MDACC, elective irradiation to regional lymphatics after local excision of primary cutaneous head and neck melanomas that are 1.5 mm or more thick or Clark level IV or higher has been used as an alternative to prophylactic neck dissection. In 2004, Bonnen and colleagues reported a retrospective review of 157 patients with stage I or II cutaneous melanoma of the head and neck who received elective regional radiotherapy after wide local excision of the primary lesion. The elective radiation therapy was delivered to the primary tumor site and the ipsilateral draining lymph nodes, including the supraclavicular fossa. The median prescribed dose was 30 Gy at 6 Gy per fraction delivered twice weekly to the primary site and draining lymphatics. Actuarial 5-year local control and overall survival were 94% and 58%, respectively. Actuarial 5-year regional control was 89% and distant metastasis-free survival was 63%. All local disease recurrences occurred within the radiation field, and 11 of the 15 regional recurrences also occurred within the radiation field.[59]

In conclusion, the standard of care for patients with lymph node metastases is therapeutic lymph node dissection. Patients who have high-risk primary tumors without clinical lymph node metastases should be considered for sentinel lymph node biopsy. Such patients may also be considered as candidates for elective nodal irradiation. Postoperative nodal irradiation is indicated in those patients with high-risk clinicopathologic features including lymph node size, number of involved lymph nodes, and the presence of extracapsular extension. Unfortunately, patients with cutaneous melanoma with high-risk features have a high risk of distant metastases and overall poor prognosis. Therefore, it is appropriate to weigh potential benefits of radiation therapy in the context of the entire burden of treatment, which often also includes the possibility of systemic adjuvant therapy for patients at high risk of local and distant recurrent disease (see **Table 1**).

SYSTEMIC THERAPY COMBINED WITH RADIATION THERAPY

Retrospective studies have identified an apparent improvement in locoregional control with the addition of adjuvant radiation therapy in patients with high-risk clinicopathologic features. However, despite improved locoregional control, many patients develop distant metastases that ultimately lead to their demise. A systematic review of systemic adjuvant therapy for patients at high risk for recurrent melanoma was reported by Verma and colleagues.[60] This review concluded that none of the systemic therapies evaluated has improved overall survival; however, high-dose interferon led to improvement in disease-free survival and reduction in 2-year mortality.[60]

Overall, results with the use of high-dose interferon have been mixed. A North Central Cancer Treatment Group study compared high-dose interferon-α2a to observation, and found no significant difference noted in survival.[61] In Eastern Cooperative Oncology Group (ECOG) 1684, investigators compared high-dose interferon-α2b to observation in patients with lesions 4 mm or larger, with 61% of patients with recurrent disease having lymph node involvement. There was a significant improvement in survival in the high-dose interferon group, with a reduction in mortality at 5 years compared with the nontreated patients (63% vs 54%). However, this difference was no longer statistically significant at 12.6 years. The recurrence-free survival benefit was significant at both 5 and 12.6 years, favoring the high-dose interferon arm.[8]

ECOG 1690 was designed to confirm the results of ECOG 1684 and assess the toxicity of low-dose interferon. Patients were randomized to high-dose interferon-α, low-dose interferon, or observation. There was no survival difference between the 3 arms at a median follow-up of 4.3 years, but patients treated with high-dose interferon had improved disease-free survival.[9] ECOG 1694 randomized patients to GM ganglioside-keyhole limpet hemocyanin vaccine or high-dose interferon. At 16 months, an interim analysis was performed showing a statistically significant overall and disease-free survival benefit for high-dose interferon, with this improvement persisting at a median follow-up of 2.1 years.[10]

Conill and colleagues performed a retrospective review to assess the efficacy and toxicity of the combination of interferon-α2b and adjuvant radiation. A total of 18 patents with high-risk features (extracapsular spread, 3 lymph nodes or more involved, nodal size 3 cm or greater, or nodal recurrence) were treated with therapeutic lymph node dissection for clinically positive lymph nodes followed by adjuvant radiation therapy. Sixteen of 18 patients received adjuvant radiation at 6 Gy per fraction, twice weekly, to a total of 30 Gy in 5 fractions (n = 8) or 36 Gy in 6 fractions (n = 8). Two patients were treated with fractions of 2 Gy 5 times a week to total dose of 50 Gy in 25 fractions. All patients received adjuvant interferon-α2b, mostly at high dose (n = 15). Ten patients received interferon-α2b concurrent with radiation, 5 patients more than 30 days after completing radiation, and 3 patients less than 30 days after completing radiation. Disease-free survival at 3 years was 88%. Radiation therapy was well tolerated, with all patients experiencing only grade 1 acute skin reaction. Late radiation toxicity was seen in only 3 patients, including a single patient with grade 3 telangiectasia and 2 patients with grade 4 myelopathy.[62]

Hazard and colleagues reviewed the results of 10 patients with cutaneous melanoma who received interferon-α2b therapy given concomitantly (n = 6) or within 1 month of completion of radiation therapy (n = 4). Five of the 10 patients (3 patients treated concurrently and 2 patients treated adjuvantly) experienced severe subacute/late complications. Three patients received 2 Gy per fraction to 50 Gy, and developed complications including peripheral neuropathy at 4 and 8 months, lymphedema at 8 months, and radiation necrosis of subcutaneous tissue at 7 months. One patient received 2.5 Gy per fraction to 52.5 Gy, and developed radiation necrosis of the brain 15 months after treatment for a scalp melanoma. One patient received 4 Gy per fraction 3 times a week for 2 weeks and then 6 Gy per fraction 2 times a week for 2 weeks, for a total dose 36 Gy, and developed radiation necrosis of the subcutaneous tissue and severe lymph edema at 8 months.[63]

Gyorki and colleagues performed a retrospective review of 18 patients treated with interferon-α2b based on the protocol published by Kirkwood and colleagues[8,9] whereby patients received adjuvant radiotherapy during the maintenance phase of their treatment. Radiation therapy consisted of 40 to 50 Gy in 15 to 25 fractions to nodal basins. Seven patients started radiation therapy later than 1 month after completion of induction phase, and 11 patients started within 1 month. Seven patients developed grade 3 skin reactions. Severe radiation-induced toxicity was seen in 3 patients in the form of severe oral mucositis, radiation pneumonitis, and wound dehiscence that took 10 months to heal.[64]

In summary, the retrospective reviews described here demonstrate increased acute and late toxicity when patients are treated with radiation therapy and interferon, given either concomitantly or sequentially. However, no prospective studies have been performed to better evaluate the toxicity and efficacy of this combination of treatment modalities. Patients treated with this approach should be closely monitored for potential toxicities.

PALLIATIVE RADIATION THERAPY: NON–CENTRAL NERVOUS SYSTEM SYSTEMIC METASTASIS

The aggressive nature of melanoma and its unpredictable behavior often results in both locoregional and systemic recurrence. Systemic therapy remains the mainstay of treatment for systemic disease. However, due to the location of metastatic disease (ie, brain metastasis) or further disease progression in the face of systemic therapy, many patients will benefit from palliative radiation therapy. Patients are frequently not referred for palliative radiation therapy because of the false belief that melanoma is relatively radioresistant and therefore radiation therapy is likely to be ineffective. Whereas there are no prospective studies examining the role of radiation therapy in the palliative setting for non–central nervous system (CNS) metastasis, retrospective reviews have been reported investigating the potential benefits of palliative radiation.

Olivier and colleagues performed a retrospective review of 84 patients with 114 metastatic lesions that were treated with palliative radiation for metastatic disease in the bone, subcutaneous tissue, and viscera. The median total dose was 30 Gy, with a median dose per fraction of 3 Gy. Nine percent of patients had a complete response in their presenting symptoms, 75% with a partial response, 11% with stable disease, and 5% with no improvement in symptoms. The median freedom from progression was 6 months after radiation therapy. Patients who were treated with more than 30 Gy were noted to have a significantly longer freedom from progression. Patients with a biologic effective dose (BED) greater than 39 Gy_{10} had a longer freedom from progression compared with those with a lower BED (7 vs 4 months). Survival also appeared to be significantly associated with total dose of radiation, BED, and site of metastatic disease. The median survival was 8 months in those treated to more than 30 Gy or more than 39 Gy_{10}.[65]

Seegenschmiedt and colleagues reviewed the results of 121 patients treated with radiation therapy for advanced melanoma (International Union Against Cancer [UICC] stages IIB/III/IV). Most patients were treated with 2 to 6 Gy daily fractions to median total radiation dose of 48 Gy. Median survival was 15.3 months with a 5-year cumulative survival of 21%±8%. Seven patients had a complete response to radiation, whereas tumor progression was noted in 25 (21%) patients. Those who had a complete response to radiation survived longer, with a median survival of 40 months compared with a median of 10 months in those without complete response. Prognostic factors for complete response and long-term survival by univariate analysis included UICC stage and primary location in head and neck. On multivariate analysis, radiation dose of greater than 40 Gy was also prognostic.[66]

Retrospective reviews show the potential benefit of palliative radiation therapy in patients with metastatic melanoma. Despite the historical belief that melanoma is a radioresistant tumor, data have shown that both in the adjuvant and palliative setting, partial and even complete response to the irradiated disease may occur. At their institution the authors have elected to treat at a standard dose per fraction. **Fig. 1** illustrates objective radioresponse of in-transit metastases treated at 2 Gy per fraction to 50 Gy, delivered with concurrent temozolomide.

CENTRAL NERVOUS SYSTEM METASTASES

Nearly half of patients with advanced melanoma develop CNS metastases.[67] After lung and breast malignancies, melanoma represents the third most common cause of brain metastases.[68] brain metastases typically occur late in the course of disease, with widespread extracranial metastases. While systemic therapy is the mainstay of treatment for metastatic disease, it produces an objective response in 10% to 25% of patients.[69] The brain represents a sanctuary site as systemic agents may have difficulty crossing the blood-brain barrier. Because melanoma typically leads to the development of multiple brain metastases with a propensity for hemorrhage, whole brain radiation therapy is typically employed because the majority of patients are unresectable.[70] With palliative whole brain radiation therapy, median survival is 3 to 5 months.[71–73] For those with a solitary brain metastasis, resection may be done first, followed by radiation therapy.[74] Stereotactic radiosurgery is a technique that delivers a focused high dose of radiation therapy to a small volume of disease. This approach has been evaluated in patients with melanoma, and may be radiobiologically superior.[28,29,75,76]

Samlowski and colleagues performed a retrospective review of 44 patients with melanoma, including 156 intracranial metastases treated

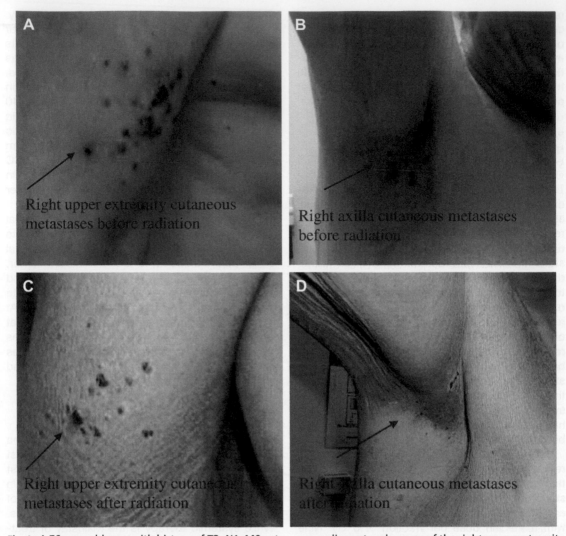

Fig. 1. A 76-year-old man with history of T3aN1aM0 cutaneous malignant melanoma of the right upper extremity, treated with wide local excision and axillary lymph node dissection with 1/56 LN positive for microscopic meta-static. Nine months later he developed in-transit metastases involving the lateral right upper extremity (*A*) and right axilla (*B*). He was treated with radiation therapy to 50 Gy delivered in 25 fractions of 2 Gy each with concurrent Temodar. Tumor regression is noted at 6 months after completion of radiation therapy (*C* and *D*). (*Courtesy of J. Frank Wilson, MD, Medical College of Wisconsin.*)

with stereotactic radiosurgery. Primary treatment was stereotactic radiosurgery for those with 5 brain metastases or less, and whole brain radiation for those with more than 5 metastases followed by stereotactic boost to large lesions. Dose with stereotactic radiosurgery was based on maximal diameter of the metastasis, with 22 Gy for lesions less than 2 cm, 18 Gy for lesions 2 to 3 cm, and 15 Gy for lesions 3 cm or grater. Lesions larger than 4 cm were generally not considered for stereotactic radiosurgery. Local control was 65.6%, and stereotactic radiosurgery failed to control 45 lesions. Median survival time was 11.1 months, and the 2-year survival was 17.7%.

Patients who had resection before radiation had improved survival compared with those who did not have resection (14.4 vs 6.5 months).[75]

A retrospective study was performed by Mathieu and colleagues of 244 patients with melanoma treated with gamma-knife radiosurgery for brain metastases. Ninety-eight patients had a single metastasis, whereas multiple metastases were present in 146 patients. The mean time to develop brain metastases was 49.4 months. Intracranial metastases were asymptomatic in 48.8% of patients. Radiosurgery alone was the treatment for brain metastases in 45.1% of patients, whereas radiosurgery was used as a boost in combination with whole brain radiation in 37.7% of patients. The isodose line used to deliver gamma-knife radiosurgery varied between 30% and 90%. The median margin dose delivered was 18 Gy, and the median maximum dose was 32 Gy. The median survival time after radiosurgery was found to be 5.3 months, with a median survival from diagnosis of brain metastases of 7.8 months. The 6-month actuarial survival was 42.8%. Progression of at least one metastasis after radiosurgery was noted in 30.9% of patients. Progression of CNS disease was the cause of death in 40.5% of patients compared with 50.9% of patients who succumbed to progression of systemic disease. There was no difference in survival for patients treated with radiosurgery alone or those who had radiosurgery as salvage to other failed therapy. Median survival was 4.5 months for those with 2 to 3 metastases, 3.2 months for those with 4 to 6 metastases, and 2.4 months for those with more than 6 metastases.[76]

Boogerd and colleagues evaluated the efficacy of temozolomide in the treatment of brain metastases from melanoma, and whether whole brain radiotherapy could be deferred. They evaluated 52 patients from 3 prospective studies of temozolomide. Patients with brain metastases 2 cm or larger, extensive edema, tumor localized in brain stem, or previous stereotactic radiosurgery were excluded. Systemic metastases were stabilized in 7 patients (13%), in addition to 5 partial responses and 1 complete response. Six patients had stabilization of brain metastases, whereas 2 had partial responses and 3 had complete responses. Radiation for cerebral recurrence was required in 2 patients. The median time to neurologic progression was 7 months, and the median survival was 5.6 months.[77]

The Cytokine Working Group recently published a phase 2 study evaluating temozolomide, thalidomide, and whole brain radiation therapy for patients with brain metastases from metastatic melanoma. Thirty-nine patients with melanoma who had magnetic resonance imaging-proven CNS metastases and no previous systemic therapy were treated with whole brain radiation to 30 Gy in 10 fractions on days 1 to 5 and days 8 to 12, temozolomide (75 mg/m^2/d) during weeks 1 to 6, and thalidomide (100 mg/d) during weeks 1 to 4, then increased by 100 mg/d during weeks 5, 7, and 9 to a maximum of 400 mg/d. Those patients without CNS or extracranial disease progression received additional temozolomide at 10-week intervals. The response rate was 7.6%, with 1 complete response and 2 partial responses. At 10-weeks, 7 patients had stable CNS disease. The median time to progression

was 7 weeks, and the median overall survival was 4 months. Forty-five percent of patients required admission for side effects or symptomatic disease progression.[78]

Although whole brain radiotherapy has been the standard of care for palliation of brain metastases in patients with melanoma, retrospective studies have suggested that these patients can be safely and effectively treated with stereotactic radiosurgery, either up front or as salvage, reserving whole brain radiation, resection, or further stereotactic radiosurgery for recurrent brain metastases. Systemic treatments, used alone or in combination with radiation therapy, represent another potential approach that is still under investigation. However, there are no randomized data to define treatment guidelines for patient selection and sequencing of these modalities.

TOXICITY

In general, radiation treatment side effects are broadly divided into acute and long-term toxicity. Acute toxicity is defined as toxicity that occurs during or within 90 days of the completion of treatment. Anticipated acute reactions when treating cutaneous melanoma with radiation therapy typically include erythema of the skin corresponding to the treatment field, dry or moist desquamation of the skin, and potential discomfort. In head and neck locations, mucositis and transient parotiditis often develop.[79] Long-term or "late" toxicity is toxicity that develops later than 90 days following completion of radiation therapy. Treatment toxicity varies with the intent of irradiation, definitive versus adjuvant versus palliative. The location of the radiation treatment field and the adjacent normal tissues largely determine the toxicity profile. Taking these factors into consideration, the following discussion of radiation toxicity for the treatment of cutaneous melanoma is organized anatomically and focuses on cervical, axillary, and inguinal nodal regions.

When evaluating complications secondary to adjuvant irradiation for cervical nodal metastases from melanoma, investigators at the MDACC published one of the largest retrospective series. Of the 160 patients in their study, treatment complications were reported in 27 patients. Eighteen patients (12%) were found to have grade 1 late complications, including slight induration, due to the loss of subcutaneous fat or slight atrophy of the irradiated skin or mucous membranes. Nine patients (10%) experienced grade 2 toxicity: 3 required treatment for hearing impairment, 2 were diagnosed with thyroid dysfunction, 2 had wound breakdown, 1 developed bone exposure, and 1 experienced ear pain. In this series, a hypofractionated radiation scheme, median total dose of 30 Gy in fractions of 6 Gy, was employed.[80]

The Trans Tasman Radiation Oncology Group (TROG) performed a phase 2 prospective trial to evaluate late toxicity following standard fractionation adjuvant radiation therapy. Of a total of 130 patients, 41 had disease in the head and neck region. Most patients experienced no long-term toxicity from their radiation. A modest amount of grade 1 toxicity was reported. Twenty-two percent of the head and neck patients reported grade 2 toxicity of the skin. Grade 2 mucositis, subcutaneous changes, and joint changes were reported in 5%, 10%, and 2% of patients, respectively. Two percent of the head and neck patients were found to have grade 3 neurologic changes, including neuralgia, paresis, or objective neurologic findings at or below the treated cord level. Another 2% of patients treated to the head and neck experienced severe induration and loss of subcutaneous tissue, or neck fibrosis.[81] However, surgery alone may cause long-term deficits. In one study of melanoma patients treated with cervical lymphadenectomy, 7% were found to have functional deficits and 6% of patients had long-term pain.[44]

Considering axillary nodal regions, the risk of arm edema with axillary dissection alone has been reported to be 1% to 3%.[44,55] With the addition of external beam radiation therapy, the risk of developing lymphedema has been reported as high as 58%.[41] In an MDACC series, the 5-year actuarial rates of developing grade 1, grade 2, or grade 3 arm edema following hypofractionated adjuvant radiation therapy were 21%, 19%, and 1%, respectively. No significant joint, soft tissue, or neurologic complications were seen.[56] Using a fractionation scheme of 48 Gy in 20 fractions over 4 weeks, the prospective TROG trial reported upper extremity lymphedema in 39% of treated patients. Seven percent of patients were documented to have grade 3 arm lymphedema. In addition, this series reported grade 3 bone and joint complications in 2% of treated patients.[81] A recently published retrospective review evaluating field extent, axilla only versus axilla and supraclavicular fossa, indicated that equivalent axillary control of disease may be obtained, with decreased treatment complications. Although arm edema remained the most common treatment toxicity, there were no grade 3 complications seen in this series. Upper extremity lymphedema was reported to be 21%.[82]

Regarding inguinal and pelvic nodal regions, a surgical review of regional nodal dissection in the treatment of metastatic melanoma, published in the *Journal of Surgical Oncology*, nicely delineated how surgical technique impacted long-term complications. The investigators concluded that the most commonly used surgical techniques for inguinal and pelvic nodal dissections resulted in 5% to 15% wound infection rates, 2% to 8% skin edge necrosis, and 21% to 40% risk of lymphedema.[83] With the addition of adjuvant radiation therapy, the prospective TROG study described earlier also indicated that the incidence of significant lymphedema at 4 years rose to 48%, with grade 3 leg edema occurring in 18% of patients. Grade 4 toxicity resulting in complications such as skin ulceration, mucous membrane ulceration, and subcutaneous tissue necrosis was seen in 3% of patients treated to the groin.[81] In contrast, retrospective data from an MDACC series indicated that the 3-year actuarial rate of any grade 2 or 3 lymphedema following adjuvant irradiation of the inguinal nodes is 40% (27% for grade 2 alone).[84] The investigators also found that one-half of the patients who were scored as grade 2 lymphedema had evidence of lymphedema before radiation therapy. In addition, an association between long-term complications (wound healing and lymphedema) and patient body mass index (BMI; calculated as the weight in kilograms divided by height in meters squared) was identified. A BMI equal to or exceeding 30 kg/m^2 correlated with an 83% risk of clinically significant long-term complication.[84]

With sparse prospective data and known limitations of retrospective reviews, it is difficult to draw definitive conclusions about long-term toxicity. Current series suggest that when treating patients to the cervical and axillary nodal regions, the long-term complications are mild to moderate but overall are acceptable in the setting of adverse disease characteristics.[80,82] When treating the inguinal nodes in the postoperative setting, careful consideration of adverse pathologic factors, risk of systemic involvement, and individual patient characteristics is important. Nevertheless, the risk of severe long-term toxicity is minimal. Despite the anticipated acute and potential long-term complications associated with adjuvant radiation therapy following lymph node dissection for melanoma, the benefits most often outweigh the morbidity of a regional recurrence with appropriate patient selection.

FUTURE DIRECTIONS

Significant and appropriate emphasis has been placed on advanced surgical techniques and new systemic therapies in the treatment of metastatic melanoma. However, in recent years there have also been tremendous technological advances in radiation oncology. Highly conformal techniques such as intensity-modulated radiation therapy (IMRT) enable conformal avoidance of normal tissues while delivering the desired radiation dose to the tumor. Increased normal tissue sparing ultimately translates to a wider therapeutic index and may allow for radiation dose escalation, which in turn may increase the odds of achieving long-term tumor control. Image-guided radiation therapy (IGRT) has enhanced the ability to confirm the position of the patient and the treatment target before each fraction. It is anticipated that IGRT will allow adaptive therapy by which treatment delivery can be modified during the course of treatment to account for changes in tumor size or physiology. At their institution, in selected melanoma cases the authors are using tomotherapy-based IMRT with daily image guidance. With the avoidance of larger volumes of normal tissues and adjacent organs, dose escalation to the tumor has become feasible, as has the safe delivery of more aggressive combined modality treatments.

SUMMARY

Cutaneous melanoma has long been thought to be radioresistant; however, it is now believed that melanoma can demonstrate a broad range of radiosensitivity. Given this radiobiologic characteristic, many fractionation schemes have been used to treat cutaneous melanoma, including standard fractionation and hypofractionation. No randomized, prospective studies have shown one method to be superior to the other. What is known is that those individuals with high-risk features benefit from adjuvant treatment, but continue to be at high risk of distant failure, and thus often have a poor prognosis. The tolerance of radiation therapy varies with treatment site, and can be influenced by prior, concurrent, and future treatments. Thus, multiple factors must be taken into consideration in the delivery of radiation therapy to primary lesions, sites of occult nodal disease, or distant metastasis sites. When delivered appropriately, radiation therapy can enhance local and regional control of gross or occult metastatic disease and can be a useful therapy to palliate sites of metastatic disease.

REFERENCES

1. Jemal A, Siegal R, Ward E, et al. Cancer statistics, 2008. CA Cancer J Clin 2008;58:71–96.
2. Beral V, Evans S, Shaw H, et al. Cutaneous factors related to the risk of malignant melanoma. Br J Dermatol 1983;109:165–72.
3. Gellin GA, Kopf AW, Garfinkel L. Malignant melanoma. A controlled-study of possibly associated factors. Arch Dermatol 1969;99:43–8.
4. English DR, Armstrong BK, Kricker A, et al. Sunlight and cancer. Cancer Causes Control 1997;8:271–83.
5. Tucker MA, Goldstein AM. Melanoma etiology: where are we? Oncogene 2003;22:3042–52.
6. Cho E, Rosner BA, Feskanich D, et al. Risk factors and individual probabilities of melanoma for whites. J Clin Oncol 2005;23:2669–75.
7. Bliss JM, Ford D, Swerdlow AJ, et al. Risk of cutaneous melanoma associated with pigmentation characteristics and freckling: systematic overview of 10 case controlled studies. The International Melanoma Analysis Group (IMAGE). Int J Cancer 1995;62:367–76.
8. Kirkwood JM, Strawderman MH, Ernstoff MS, et al. Interferon-alfa-2b adjuvant therapy of high-risk resected cutaneous melanoma: the Eastern Cooperative Oncology Group Trial EST 1684. J Clin Oncol 1996;14:7–17.
9. Kirkwood JM, Ibrahim JG, Sondak VK, et al. High- and low-dose interferon alpha-2b in high-risk melanoma: first analysis of intergroup trial E1690/s9111/c9190. J Clin Oncol 2000;18:2444–58.
10. Kirkwood JM, Ibrahim JG, Sosman JA, et al. High-dose interferon alpha-2b significantly prolongs relapse-free and overall survival compared with the GM2-KLH/QS-21 vaccine in patients with resected stage IIB-III melanoma: results of intergroup trial E1694/S9512/C509801. J Clin Oncol 2001;19:2370–80.
11. Perales M, Wolchok JD. Melanoma vaccines. Cancer Invest 2002;20:1012–26.
12. Morton DL, Hsueh EC, Essner R, et al. Prolonged survival of patients receiving active immunotherapy with canvaxin therapeutic polyvalent vaccine after complete resection of melanoma metastatic to regional lymph nodes. Ann Surg 2002;236:438–49.
13. Tsao H, Atkins MB, Sober AJ. Management of cutaneous melanoma. N Engl J Med 2004;351:998–1012.
14. Simpson FE. Radium in skin diseases. JAMA 1913;61:80–3.
15. Coley WB, Hoquet JP. Metastatic cancer, with a report of 91 patients. Ann Surg 1916;64:206–41.
16. Adair FE. Treatment of melanoma. Surg Gynecol Obstet 1936;62:406–9.
17. Paterson R. Classification of tumours in relation to radiosensitivity. Br J Radiol 1933;6:218–33.
18. Ellis F. The radiosensitivity of malignant melanoma. Br J Radiol 1939;12:327–52.
19. Nitter L. The treatment of malignant melanoma with special reference to the possible effect of radiotherapy. Acta Radiol 1956;46:547–62.
20. Tod MC. Radiological treatment of malignant melanoma. Br J Radiol 1946;19:223–9.

21. Dickson RJ. Malignant melanoma. A combined surgical and radiotherapeutic approach. Am J Roentgenol 1958;79:1063–70.

22. Hellriegel W. Radiation therapy of primary and metastatic melanoma. Ann N Y Acad Sci 1963;100:132–41.

23. Owen AK. A case of melanosarcoma treated with roentgen rays. Am J Roentgenol 1924;11:335–6.

24. Evans WA, Leucutia T. The treatment of metastatic tumors of skin: pigmented moles and melanomas. Am J Roentgenol 1931;26:236–59.

25. Anderson HF, Simpson CA. Pigmented moles and their treatment. Am J Roentgenol 1935;33:54–8.

26. Harwood AR, Cummings BJ. Radiotherapy for malignant melanoma: a re-appraisal. Cancer Treat Rev 1981;8:271–82.

27. Jenrette JM. Malignant melanoma: the role of radiation therapy revisited. Semin Oncol 1996;23:759–62.

28. Dewey DL. The radiosensitivity of melanoma cells in culture. Br J Radiol 1971;44:816–7.

29. Barranco SC, Romsdahl MM, Humphrey RM. The radiation response of human malignant melanoma cells grown in vitro. Cancer Res 1971;31:830–3.

30. Hornsey S. The relationship between total dose, number of fractions and fraction size in the response of malignant melanoma in patients. Br J Radiol 1978;51:905–9.

31. Habermalz HJ, Fischer JJ. Radiation therapy of malignant melanoma: experience with high individual treatment doses. Cancer 1976;38:2258–62.

32. Adams JS, Habeshw T, Kirk J. Response rate of malignant melanoma to large fraction irradiation. Br J Radiol 1982;55:605–7.

33. Stevens G, McKay MJ. Dispelling the myths surrounding radiotherapy for treatment of cutaneous melanoma. Lancet Oncol 2006;7:575–83.

34. McKay MJ, Kefford RF. The spectrum of in vitro radiosensitivity in four human melanoma cell lines is not accounted for by the differential induction or rejoining of DNA double strand breaks. Int J Radiat Oncol Biol Phys 1995;31:345–52.

35. Rofstad EK. Radiation sensitivity in vitro of primary tumors and metastatic lesions of malignant melanoma. Cancer Res 1992;52:4453–7.

36. Overgaard J, Overgaard M, Hansen PV, et al. Some factors of importance in the radiation treatment of malignant melanoma. Radiother Oncol 1986;5:183–92.

37. Bentzen SM, Overgaard J, Thames HD, et al. Clinical radiobiology of malignant melanoma. Radiother Oncol 1989;16:169–82.

38. Overgaard J, von der Maase H, Overgaard M. A randomized study comparing two high-dose per fraction radiation schedules in recurrent or metastatic malignant melanoma. Int J Radiat Biol Phys 1985;11:1837–9.

39. Overgaard J, Gonzalez Gonzalez D, Hulshof MC, et al. Randomized trial of hyperthermia as adjuvant to radiotherapy for recurrent or metastatic malignant melanoma. Lancet 1995;345:540–3.

40. Ang KK, Peters LJ, Weber RS, et al. Postoperative radiotherapy for cutaneous melanoma of the head and neck region. Int J Radiat Oncol Biol Phys 1994;30:795–8.

41. Stevens G, Thompson JF, Firth I, et al. Locally advanced melanoma: results of postoperative hypofractionated radiation therapy. Cancer 2000;88:88–94.

42. Chang DT, Amdur RJ, Morris CG, et al. Adjuvant radiotherapy for cutaneous melanoma: comparing hypofractionation to conventional fractionation. Int J Radiat Oncol Biol Phys 2006;66(4):1051–5.

43. Sause WT, Cooper JS, Rush S, et al. Fraction size in external beam radiation therapy in the treatment of melanoma. Int J Radiat Oncol Biol Phys 1991;20:429–32.

44. Balch CM, Soong SJ, Smith T, et al. Long term results of a prospective surgical trial comparing 2 cm vs. 4 cm excision margins for 740 patients with 1-4 mm melanomas. Ann Surg Oncol 2001;8(2):101–8.

45. Urist MM, Balch CM, Soong S, et al. The influence of surgical margins and prognostic factors predicting the risk of local recurrence in 3445 patients with primary cutaneous melanoma. Cancer 1985;55(6):1398–402.

46. Balch CM, Soong SJ, Gershenwald JE, et al. Prognostic factors analysis of 17,600 melanoma patients: validation of the American Joint Committee on Cancer melanoma staging system. J Clin Oncol 2001;19:3622–34.

47. Balch CM, Wilkerson JA, Murad TM, et al. The prognostic significance of ulceration of cutaneous melanoma. Cancer 1980;45:3012–7.

48. McGovern VJ, Shaw HM, Milton GW, et al. Ulceration and prognosis in cutaneous malignant melanoma. Histopathology 1982;6:399–407.

49. Buzaid AC, Ross MI, Balch CM, et al. Critical analysis of the current American Joint Committee on Cancer staging system for cutaneous melanoma and proposal of a new staging system. J Clin Oncol 1997;15:1039–51.

50. Balch CM, Soong SJ, Murad TM, et al. A multifactorial analysis of melanoma: prognostic factors in melanoma patients with lymph node metastases (stage II). Ann Surg 1981;193:377–88.

51. O'Brien CJ, Coates AS, Peterson-Schaefer K, et al. Experience with 998 cutaneous melanomas of the head and neck over 30 years. Am J Surg 1991;162:310–4.

52. Calabro A, Singletary SE, Balch CM. Patterns of relapse in 1001 consecutive patients with melanoma nodal metastases. Arch Surg 1989;124:1051–5.

53. Lee RJ, Gibbs JF, Proulx GM, et al. Nodal basin recurrence following lymph node dissection for

melanoma: implications for adjuvant radiotherapy. Int J Radiat Oncol Biol Phys 2000;46(2):467–74.

54. Monsour PD, Sause WT, Avent JM, et al. Local control following therapeutic nodal dissection for melanoma. J Surg Oncol 1993;54:18–22.

55. Shen P, Wanek LA, Morton DL. Is adjuvant radiotherapy necessary after positive lymph node dissection in head and neck melanoma? Ann Surg Oncol 2000;7:554–9.

56. Bowsher WG, Taylor BA, Hughes LE. Morbidity, mortality, and local recurrence following regional node dissection for melanoma. Br J Surg 1986;73: 906–8.

57. Creagan ET, Cupps RE, Ivins JC, et al. Adjuvant radiation therapy for regional nodal metastases from malignant melanoma. Cancer 1978;42:2206–10.

58. Ballo MT, Strom EA, Zagars GK, et al. Adjuvant irradiation for axillary metastases from malignant melanoma. Int J Radiat Oncol Biol Phys 2002;52(4): 964–72.

59. Bonnen MD, Ballo MT, Garden AS, et al. Elective radiotherapy provides regional control for patients with cutaneous melanoma of the head and neck. Cancer 2004;100(2):383–9.

60. Verma S, Quirt I, McCready D, et al. Systematic review of systemic adjuvant therapy for patients at high risk for recurrent melanoma. Cancer 2006; 106(7):1431–42.

61. Creagan ET, Dalton RJ, Ahmann DL, et al. Randomized, surgical adjuvant clinical trial of recombinant interferon alfa 2a in selected patients with malignant melanoma. J Clin Oncol 1995;13:2776–83.

62. Conill C, Jorcano S, Domingo-Domenech J, et al. Toxicity of combined treatment of adjuvant irradiation and interferon alpha2b in high-risk melanoma patients. Melanoma Res 2007;17(5):304–9.

63. Hazard LJ, Sause WT, Noyes RD. Combined adjuvant radiation and interferon-alpha 2B therapy in high- risk melanoma patients: the potential for increased radiation toxicity. Int J Radiat Oncol Biol Phys 2002;52(3):796–800.

64. Gyorki DE, Ainslie J, Joon ML, et al. Concurrent adjuvant radiotherapy and interferon-alpha 2b for resected high risk stage III melanoma—a retrospective single centre study. Melanoma Res 2004;14:223–30.

65. Olivier KR, Schild SE, Morris CG, et al. A higher radiotherapy dose is associated with more durable palliation and longer survival in patients with metastatic melanoma. Cancer 2007;110(8):1791–5.

66. Seegenschmiedt MH, Ludwig K, Altendorf-Hofmann A, et al. Palliative radiotherapy for recurrent and metastatic malignant melanoma: prognostic factors for tumor response and long-term outcome: a 20-year experience. Int J Radiat Oncol Biol Phys 1999;44(3):607–18.

67. Douglas JG, Margolin K. The treatment of brain metastases from malignant melanoma. Semin Oncol 2002;29(5):518–24.

68. Schouten LJ, Rutten J, Huveneers HA, et al. Incidence of brain metastases in a cohort of patients with carcinoma of the breast, colon, kidney, and lung and melanoma. Cancer 2002;94:2698–705.

69. Atkins MB. Cytokine-based therapy and biochemotherapy for advanced melanoma. Clin Cancer Res 2006;12(7):2353s–8s.

70. Wen PY, Black PM, Loeffler JS. Metastatic brain cancer. In: Devita VT, Hellman S, Rosenberg SA, editors. Cancer: principles and practice of oncology. 6th edition. Philadelphia: Lippincott, Williams & Wilkins; 2001. p. 2655–70.

71. Broadbent AM, Hruby G, Tin MM, et al. Survival following whole brain radiation treatment for cerebral metastases: an audit of 474 patients. Radiother Oncol 2004;71:259–65.

72. Lagerwaard FJ, Levendag PC, Nowak PJ, et al. Identification of prognostic factors in patients with brain metastases: a review of 1292 patients. Int J Radiat Oncol Biol Phys 1999;43:795–803.

73. Meier S, Baumert BG, Maier T, et al. Survival and prognostic factors in patients with brain metastases from malignant melanoma. Onkologie 2004;27: 145–9.

74. Brega K, Robinson WA, Winston K, et al. Surgical treatment of brain metastases in malignant melanoma. Cancer 1990;66:2105–10.

75. Samlowski WE, Watson GA, Wang M, et al. Multimodality treatment of melanoma brain metastases incorporating stereotactic radiosurgery (SRS). Cancer 2007;109(9):1855–62.

76. Mathieu D, Kondziolka D, Cooper PB, et al. Gamma knife radiosurgery in the management of malignant melanoma brain metastases. Neurosurgery 2007; 60:471–82.

77. Boogerd W, de Gast GC, Otilia D. Temozolomide in advanced malignant melanoma with small brain metastases. Cancer 2007;109(2):3106–212.

78. Atkins MB, Sosman JA, Agarwala SA, et al. Temozolomide, thalidomide and whole brain radiation therapy for patients with brain metastasis from metastatic melanoma. Cancer 2008;113(8):2139–45.

79. Bastiaannet E, Beukema JC, Hoekstra HJ. Radiation therapy following lymph node dissection in melanoma patients: treatment, outcome and complications. Cancer Treat Rev 2005;31:18–26.

80. Ballo MT, Bonnen MD, Garden AS, et al. Adjuvant irradiation for cervical lymph node metastases from melanoma. Cancer 2003;97:1789–96.

81. Burmeister BH, Smithers BM, Spry N, et al. Radiation therapy following nodal surgery for melanoma: an analysis of late toxicity. ANZ J Surg 2002;72: 344–8.

82. Beadle BM, Guadagnolo BA, Ballo MT, et al. Radiation therapy field extent for adjuvant treatment of axillary metastases from malignant melanoma. Int J Radiat Oncol Biol Phys 2009;73(5):1376–82.

83. Mack LA, McKinnon JG. Controversies in the management of metastatic melanoma to

regional lymphatic basins. J Surg Oncol 2004;86: 189–99.

84. Ballo MT, Gunar KZ, Jeffery EG, et al. A critical assessment of adjuvant radiotherapy for inguinal lymph node metastases form melanoma. Ann Surg Oncol 2004;11:1079–84.

Surgical Treatment of Advanced Melanoma

Christopher J. Hussussian, MD

KEYWORDS

- Metastatic melanoma • Metastectomy
- Surgery • Resection • Outcomes

Indications for surgical treatment of metastatic melanoma include palliation and prolongation of life. Palliative surgery is considered for patients who have surgically resectable metastases that are either symptomatic or anticipated to cause significant symptoms before the patient dies of the disease. Surgical resection of metastases can also significantly prolong survival from stage IV melanoma, and has been documented in some cases to provide long-term disease-free survival. Considerable clinical judgment, combined with an understanding of the natural history of metastatic melanoma and knowledge of treatment alternatives, is required to determine whether the potential benefits of surgery outweigh the risks in any individual patient.

The prognosis for American Joint Committee on Cancer (AJCC) stage IV melanoma is less than 10%[1] and systemic chemotherapy, immunotherapy, biochemotherapy, or local radiation therapy is usually offered as treatment. Cures are uncommon and these modalities have, almost without exception, been unable to significantly prolong survival. Surgery, however, has the potential to render a patient clinically disease-free in a minimally morbid, cost-effective manner. In selected patients significant improvement in quality of life as well as prolonged survival can be expected.

Morton and colleagues[2] recently reported the results of a randomized prospective trial of Canvaxin (CancerVax Corp, Carlsbad, CA), a whole cell melanoma vaccine. This study (Malignant Melanoma Active Immunotherapy Trial, Stage IV) compared Canvaxin plus bacillus Calmette-Guérin (BCG) versus BCG alone as adjuvant therapy for patients with stage IV melanoma. Of note, all patients underwent complete surgical excision of their metastatic disease as a condition for inclusion in the study. The study was terminated early by the data safety monitoring committee for lack of beneficial effect of the Canvaxin. However, an important outcome was the relatively high 5-year survival rates of both study groups. The combined overall 5-year survival rate in the 496 patients examined was more than 40% despite the inclusion of patients with brain metastases. A similar result occurred in a published trial that studied 41 patients who received a melanoma vaccine after undergoing resection of melanoma metastases.[3] This strategy resulted in a 5-year survival of 46%. In comparison, a recent review of studies including 50 or more patients[4] indicates that overall survival for stage IV melanoma that is not surgically resected clusters around 21% at 5 years. These data seem to support an aggressive surgical approach to localized stage IV melanoma.

PATIENT SELECTION

The clinical course of systemic melanoma can vary widely among patients.[5] Decisions regarding surgical resection of metastatic melanoma depends on several factors including the sites and numbers of metastases, their rate of growth, types and responses to previous treatment, and the age, overall condition, and desires of the patient. The number of different organs or tissues containing metastases is the most significant factor predicting survival. The median survival for a patient with melanoma metastases in one site is 7 months, for a patient with disease at 2 sites it is 4 months, and when 3 sites are involved median survival is 2 months. The location of the

Department of Plastic and Reconstructive Surgery, Medical College of Wisconsin, Milwaukee, Plastic Surgery Associates, 22370 Bluemound Road, Waukesha, WI 53005, USA
E-mail address: cjhussussian@mac.com

Clin Plastic Surg 37 (2010) 161–168
doi:10.1016/j.cps.2009.07.004
0094-1298/09/$ – see front matter © 2010 Published by Elsevier Inc.

metastasis is also important, with short survival times associated with liver and brain metastases compared with skin, subcutaneous tissue, distant lymph nodes, lung, and bone. The rate of growth of metastatic melanoma is difficult to know, although the time to recurrence can be measured and has a significant impact on survival. Median survival for patients who progress from regional to distant metastasis is 5.6 months if the disease-free interval is less than 18 months, and 8 months if the interval is greater than 18 months.[6] Martinez and Young have recommended criteria for melanoma metastectomy including 1 or 2 visceral sites, 8 or fewer lesions, good functional status, and life expectancy of 3 months or greater.[7] If complete resection cannot be expected, then surgical intervention should be limited to palliation only (ie, relief of gastrointestinal obstruction or management of bleeding). Patients with metastatic melanoma typically initially present with disease at a single site,[6,8] and this disease is usually amenable to surgical resection. In this case, surgery should be considered the treatment of choice.

Complete staging is important in determining a patient's eligibility for surgical resection of metastatic melanoma. Whereas routine use of advanced imaging in following patients with early-stage melanoma is generally not advocated,[9,10] ultrasonography, computed tomography (CT), magnetic resonance imaging (MRI), and ^{18}F-fluorodeoxyglucose positron emission tomography (FDG-PET) help to accurately stage the patient with advanced disease.[11–17] Ultrasonography has a high sensitivity and specificity for melanoma metastatic to the lymph nodes.[12] A recent comparison of FDG-PET and whole body MRI demonstrated an 86.7% accuracy rate for FDG-PET versus 78.8% for MRI.[17] MRI, however, was more accurate in specific organ sites including the brain and liver, and high-quality spiral

CT scans may be better in the detection of small pulmonary metastases.

Although some centers routinely use ultrasound for follow-up surveillance of nodal basins, most practitioners use it to examine a lesion for resectability or to confirm a diagnosis of suspected metastatic disease. There are ultrasonographic findings specific for lymph nodes involved with melanoma, and ultrasonography can help guide fine-needle aspiration for histologic confirmation. When distant metastases have been confirmed and definitive surgery is being considered, patients should be staged with MRI of the brain, CT scan of the thorax abdomen, and pelvis with oral and intravenous contrast, and whole body PET/CT scan. This combination of studies should detect 80% to 90% of early metastatic deposits, and enable clinicians to determine resectability and plan an appropriate surgical procedure that completely removes all detectable disease.

MANAGEMENT OF SPECIFIC METASTATIC SITES
Skin, Lymph Nodes, Subcutaneous Tissues

Skin, soft tissue, and distant lymph node metastases represent the most common sites of initial distant recurrence, occurring in up to 40% of patients with stage IV disease.[18] Metastases to these sites have better prognoses than those to other tissues, and this is reflected in the revised AJCC staging, which classifies them as M1a disease.[19] Five-year survival rates for resection of melanoma metastases to these tissues ranges from 11% to 49%[6,20–23] (**Table 1**). Favorable prognostic indicators include involvement of skin (versus lymph node), low number of lesions, and long disease-free interval. One particularly favorable group is the small subset of patients (0.61%) who present with solitary cutaneous metastatic melanoma from an unknown primary.

Table 1
Survival after complete resection of skin, soft tissue, and remote lymph node metastases in patients with melanoma

Study	Year	N	Median Survival (Months)	5-Year Survival (%)	Site
Markowitz et al[20]	1991	72	24	38	Lymph nodes
	—	60	50	49	Soft tissue
Gadd and Coit[21]	1992	199	20	11	Lymph nodes
Karakousis et al[22]	1994	23	29	22	Lymph nodes
	—	27	24	33	Subcutis
Barth et al[6]	1995	281	15	14	All sites
Meyer et al[23]	2000	45	18	20	Lymph nodes
	—	30	17	17.8	Skin

One study demonstrated an 8-year survival estimate of 83% following complete resection of their metastatic disease.[24]

Resection margins of 1 cm are generally adequate to ensure compete resection. Multiple resections are possible, and subsequent resections may be done for recurrent disease. For clusters of individual metastases that are resectable, adjuvant radiotherapy should be considered. Clinically evident or biopsy-proven lymph node metastases should be managed by complete dissection of the affected basin. In the axilla this should include level II and in the neck, levels I to V. Disease in the parotid should include parotidectomy and neck dissection.

When soft tissue metastases are localized to the lower extremity and are too locally advanced or too numerous to completely resect without unacceptable morbidity, isolated limb perfusion (ILP) should be considered as an alternative to amputation. ILP is a surgical procedure for regional delivery of chemotherapeutic agents to an extremity. ILP consists of vascular cannulation of an arm or leg and mechanical perfusion with blood containing high doses of various cytotoxic agents. Because the vasculature of the limb is isolated from the rest of the body, the normal toxicity of the agents to visceral organs is minimized, allowing for otherwise lethal doses to be regionally administered. Whereas the use of a variety of agents has been described, the most common regimen used currently consists of melphalan with or without tumor necrosis factor. In addition, hyperthermia may be used to potentiate their effect.[25] Although complete responses can only be expected in about 50% of patients, those with a complete response have a 40% 5-year survival.[26]

ILP is contraindicated in patients with significant peripheral vascular disease, and is limited to treatment of the lower extremity. Alternative treatments for local control of cutaneous metastatic melanoma include carbon dioxide laser as well as direct injection of various immune system modulating agents including BCG, interleukin-2, and interferon-a. Partial responses may allow for conversion of unresectable disease to that which is resectable.

Pulmonary Metastases

The lungs are the most common visceral organ to which melanoma metastasizes, with reports of 15% to 36% prevalence.[5,27,28] Although there is significant variation in reported prevalence, this may be due to variation in subject follow-up. At least one author has reported a 10% annual probability of developing pulmonary metastases at 5 years, increasing to 30% at 20 years.[28] Symptoms of cough, hemoptysis, or chest pain generally correlate with advanced disease, underscoring the importance of screening chest radiographs at routine intervals to detect asymptomatic disease. Any suspicious finding on a radiograph should be further evaluated by CT or biopsy as indicated.

Median survival in patients with melanoma metastatic to the lung is approximately 8 months in patients treated without surgery.[6] Complete surgical resection may extend median survival up to 40 months (**Table 2**).[27–33] Harpole and colleagues[28] found that patients not considered amenable to surgical therapy due to bilateral lesions, and hilar or mediastinal disease had a 5-year survival of 4% versus 20% for those who could be completely resected. Tafra and colleagues[30] similarly reported a 27% 5-year survival for patients with pulmonary disease who underwent surgery versus 3% in those who did not. More recently, Neuman and colleagues[33] reported a median survival of 40 months in patients undergoing metastectomy for pulmonary disease versus 13 months in patients who were not selected for surgery. Whereas patients undergoing surgery tended to have more favorable prognostic

Table 2
Survival after complete resection of pulmonary metastases in patients with melanoma

Study	Year	N	Median Survival (Months)	5-Year Survival (%)
Karp et al[29]	1990	29	10	5
Gorenstein et al[27]	1991	59	18	25
Harpole et al[28]	1992	98	20	20
Karakousis et al[22]	1994	39	14	14
Tafra et al[30]	1995	106	18	27
Leo et al[31]	2000	282	19	22
Andrews et al[32]	2006	86	35	33
Neuman et al[33]	2007	26	40	29

indicators such as a solitary lesion and absence of extrapulmonary metastases, complete surgical resection remained an independent predictor of increased survival.

Patient selection plays a critical role in treatment of melanoma patients with pulmonary disease. Although patients with solitary nodules have the best prognosis, those with multiple lesions that can be completely resected also have a survival advantage.[30,31] Surgeon judgment must include pulmonary reserve and predicted postoperative pulmonary status. In addition, whereas some patients may benefit from palliative resections to alleviate pain or bleeding, only complete resection offers a survival benefit.[29]

Although complete resection is the most important prognostic factor, longer disease-free interval, negative lymph nodes, and presence of a solitary lesion are also noted.[28,31] Long disease-free interval is a correlate to high tumor doubling time (TDT), which has been studied as a prognostic factor in metastatic pulmonary disease.[34] A TDT greater than 60 days (estimated from preoperative chest radiographs) correlated with a median survival improvement from 16 to 29 months. Similar studies may help to define objective criteria to help guide decisions regarding which patients might benefit from pulmonary metastectomy.

Gastrointestinal Metastases

Although almost 50% of patients who die of metastatic melanoma have involvement of their gastrointestinal (GI) tract detected at autopsy,[35] clinical antemortem diagnosis is made in less than 5%.[36] The most common GI tract site of involvement is the small bowel (75%–90%), followed by the colon (20%–25%) and stomach (3%–16%).[37] Symptoms from GI tract involvement include anemia, pain, bleeding, obstruction, palpable mass, and weight loss.

Patients with GI tract metastases generally have a poor prognosis, with a median survival of 5 to 11 months. However, patients who are able to undergo complete metastectomy have an increase in their median survival to 15 to 28 months (**Table 3**).[37–40] In one study, the number of metastatic sites did not matter for prognosis as long as complete resection could be obtained.[41] Because patients with melanoma metastatic to the GI tract are often symptomatic, surgery for palliation is often indicated even if complete resection is not possible. Surgery for symptomatic melanoma metastatic to the GI tract is palliative in more than 90% of cases.[38,39]

Table 3 Survival after complete resection of gastrointestinal metastases in patients with melanoma				
Study	Year	N	Median Survival (Months)	5-Year Survival (%)
Ricaniadis et al[37]	1995	23	28	28
Ollila et al[38]	1996	46	49	41
Agrawal et al[39]	1999	19	15	38
Gutman et al[40]	2001	35	17	—

Adrenal Metastases

There is evidence from multiple studies demonstrating improved survival following complete resection of melanoma metastatic to the adrenal gland.[41–43] The largest study from the John Wayne Cancer Center identified 83 patients with adrenal metastases, of whom 27 underwent surgical treatment with complete resection possible in 18. Those undergoing complete resection had an improved median survival of 28 months versus 12 months for the nonoperative group.[43] In general, resection of adrenal metastases from melanoma compares favorably with resection of metastatic disease from other sites. Careful selection of patients with resectable adrenal disease and limited extra-adrenal involvement may be associated with improved survival.

Hepatic Metastases

Liver metastases from melanoma occur in 10% to 20% of patients with stage IV melanoma. These patients have a median survival of 4 to 9 months, and traditionally they have not been considered for surgical management. A prospective database review of 1750 melanoma patients at the John Wayne Cancer Institute and the Sydney Melanoma Unit identified 34 patients who underwent exploration for hepatic metastases.[44] Of these patients, 24 underwent resection with complete resection possible in 18. Median survival was 28 months for the patients who underwent complete resection versus 4 months for those who underwent exploration only. In a separate report examining the John Wayne Cancer Institute data alone, median survival was 28 months in the 9 out of 654 patients with liver metastases who were able to undergo complete resection of their lesions, compared with 9 months in the nonoperative group and 10 months in the group undergoing exploration alone.[41]

Whereas resection of liver metastases due to melanoma is associated with improved median survival, interpretation of these data is difficult because only 2% of eligible patients in these studies underwent complete resection. This statistic demonstrates the importance of patient selection in obtaining satisfactory patient outcomes. Whereas the occasional patient may benefit from resection of isolated metastatic melanoma, the large majority seem to present with disease that is unresectable.

Intracranial Metastases

Melanoma brain metastases are common, and melanoma represents the third most common type of brain metastases in the United States after lung and breast cancer. In autopsy studies approximately 50% of patients with disseminated melanoma had evidence of brain metastases,[35] whereas rates in clinical studies vary between 9% and 18% of patients with stage IV melanoma.[45,46] Patients present clinically with symptoms of headache, neurologic deficit, or behavioral changes, and workup should consist of MRI. The mainstay of initial treatment is corticosteroids, with dexamethasone being particularly effective in reducing edema and temporarily relieving symptoms.

Surgical excision followed by cranial radiation is the treatment of choice for solitary lesions that can be resected with minimal morbidity. Prospective randomized studies of metastectomy for other tumors have generally demonstrated an advantage in combining surgery with adjuvant whole brain radiation as opposed to surgery alone.[47] Retrospective studies investigating this question specifically for melanoma have also suggested that survival may be improved with additional whole brain radiation,[48–50] and most investigators have advocated this approach. Whereas median survival for melanoma metastatic to the brain varies between 2.75 and 4 months,[49,51] median survival following surgical resection and adjuvant whole brain radiation ranges from 8.9 to 18 months (**Table 4**).[48–50,52]

Optimizing results following metastectomy for melanoma metastatic to the brain requires careful patient selection. Negative prognostic factors include the presence of more than one metastatic brain lesion,[49,50] the need for repeat surgery for recurrence,[50] incomplete resection of tumor,[50,52] and infratentorial lesions.[52] In these reports, surgery was accomplished with minimal morbidity and was effective in relieving neurologic symptoms.

Whereas whole brain radiation therapy alone has been demonstrated to be less effective at achieving local control or significantly prolonging survival for metastatic melanoma patients,[53] stereotactic radiosurgery (SRS) is increasingly being studied as an alternative to craniotomy in patients with small brain metastases.[53–57] Median survival following SRS is roughly equivalent to that following surgical resection, but the local control is worse, with only 65% to 75% of patients achieving resolution of symptoms.[56,57] In addition, approximately 20% of patients develop postradiation intracerebral hemorrhage with significant neurologic deterioration,[55,56] perhaps because brain metastases from melanoma are known to be particularly prone to bleeding. Total intracranial tumor volume and number of intracranial lesions are important predictors of local control and survival.[54] SRS seems to be a viable alternative for patients who are unable or unwilling to undergo surgical resection for melanoma metastatic to the brain, especially when the lesions are small.

Bone Metastases

Patients presenting with bone metastases from melanoma have a median survival of 4 to 6 months.[5] Treatment of bone metastases depends

Table 4
Survival after complete resection of intracranial metastases in patients with melanoma

Study	Year	N	Median Survival (Months)	Comment
Skibber et al[48]	1996	12	6	Surgery only
		22	18	Surgery plus WBRT
Sampson et al[49]	1998	52	6	Surgery only
	—	87	9	Surgery plus WBRT
Wroński et al[52]	2000	91	7	Postoperative WBRT in some patients
Zacest et al[50]	2002	12	1	Surgery only
	—	135	10	Surgery plus WBRT

Abbreviation: WBRT, adjuvant whole brain radiation therapy.

on the degree of symptoms, the location and number of lesions, the overall condition of the patient, and the expected survival. Palliation is usually the goal of treatment, although some investigators advocate resection for cure in selected patients with solitary lesions to the appendicular skeleton.[58]

Palliative goals include relief of pain and maximization of function including ambulation. Symptomatic metastases in weight-bearing bones require special consideration. If the lesion is large, and especially if there is evidence of cortical destruction, prophylactic stabilization or radiation are sometimes used. Pathologic fractures should be stabilized unless the risk of surgery is high or the expected life span short.

SUMMARY

In the absence of effective nonsurgical treatments, surgical resection should be considered for patients with stage IV melanoma. There are no prospective trials to help guide clinical decisions about metastectomy, nor are any likely to be completed soon. Decisions must therefore be made based on a thorough understanding of the variable nature of the disease, the patient's goals and desires, and the potential risks and benefits of intervention. Cure is usually not a realistic aim, and treatment must reflect a carefully considered judgment that attempts to improve or preserve the quality of life while potentially prolonging survival. Satisfactory outcomes are only obtained with careful patient selection. Because patients with limited disease burden do best with surgical treatment, thorough preoperative staging with appropriate imaging is important. Accurate preoperative assessment of resectability is critical because any benefit of surgery in these patients depends on complete resection of the disease. Although patients generally can be expected to eventually succumb to their disease, many reports of long-term survival following resection of metastatic melanoma from a variety of soft tissue sites demonstrate that this approach can be extremely successful. Unlike chemotherapy or radiation therapy, surgical resection of metastatic disease can quickly render a patient free of detectable disease, with a quick return to normal activities. Novel adjuvant therapies to help augment the benefits of surgical treatment of advanced melanoma in the future are under development. This approach emphasizes the continued strong collaboration between surgeon and oncologist, and is the likeliest route to improving treatment options for this difficult disease.

REFERENCES

1. Balch CM, Soong SJ, Gershenwald JE, et al. Prognostic factors analysis of 17,600 melanoma patients: validation of the American Joint Committee on Cancer melanoma staging system. J Clin Oncol 2001;19(16):3622–34.
2. Morton DL, Mozzillo N, Thompson JF, et al. An international, randomized, phase III trial of bacillus Calmette-Guérin (BCG) plus allogeneic melanoma vaccine (MCV) or placebo after complete resection of melanoma metastatic to regional or distant sites [abstract]. J Clin Oncol 2007;25(18S):474s.
3. Tagawa S, Cheung E, Banta W, et al. Survival analysis after resection of metastatic disease followed by peptide vaccines in patients with stage IV melanoma. Cancer 2006;106(6):1353–7.
4. Mosca PJ, Teicher E, Nair S, et al. Can surgeons improve survival in stage IV melanoma? J Surg Oncol 2008;97(5):462–8.
5. Balch CM, Soong SJ, Murad TM, et al. A multifactorial analysis of melanoma. IV. Prognostic factors in 200 melanoma patients with distant metastases (stage III). J Clin Oncol 1983;1(2):126–34.
6. Barth A, Wanek LA, Morton DL. Prognostic factors in 1,521 melanoma patients with distant metastases. J Am Coll Surg 1995;181(3):193–201.
7. Martinez S, Young S. A rational surgical approach to the treatment of distant melanoma metastases. Cancer Treat Rev 2008;34:614–20.
8. Essner R, Lee JH, Wanek LA, et al. Contemporary surgical treatment of advanced-stage melanoma. Arch Surg 2004;139(9):961–6 [discussion: 966–7].
9. Hofmann U, Szedlak M, Rittgen W, et al. Primary staging and follow-up in melanoma patients—monocenter evaluation of methods, costs and patient survival. Br J Cancer 2002;87(2):151–7.
10. Tsao H, Feldman M, Fullerton JE, et al. Early detection of asymptomatic pulmonary melanoma metastases by routine chest radiographs is not associated with improved survival. Arch Dermatol 2004;140(1):67–70.
11. Dalrymple-Hay MJ, Rome PD, Kennedy C, et al. Pulmonary metastatic melanoma—the survival benefit associated with positron emission tomography scanning. Eur J Cardiothorac Surg 2002;21(4):611–4 [discussion: 614–5].
12. Voit C, Schoengen A, Schwürzer-Voit M, et al. The role of ultrasound in detection and management of regional disease in melanoma patients. Semin Oncol 2002;29(4):353–60.
13. Garbe C, Paul A, Kohler-Späth H, et al. Prospective evaluation of a follow-up schedule in cutaneous melanoma patients: recommendations for an effective follow-up strategy. J Clin Oncol 2003;21(3):520–9.
14. Finkelstein S, Carrasquillo J, Hoffman J, et al. A prospective analysis of positron emission

tomography and conventional imaging for detection of stage IV metastatic melanoma in patients undergoing metastasectomy. Ann Surg Oncol 2004; 11(8):731–8.

15. Horn J, Lock-Andersen J, Sjøstrand H, et al. Routine use of FDG-PET scans in melanoma patients with positive sentinel node biopsy. Eur J Nucl Med Mol Imaging 2006;33(8):887–92.

16. Akcali C, Zincirkeser S, Erbagcý Z, et al. Detection of metastases in patients with cutaneous melanoma using FDG-PET/CT. J Int Med Res 2007;35(4):547–53.

17. Pfannenberg C, Aschoff P, Schanz S, et al. Prospective comparison of 18F-fluorodeoxyglucose positron emission tomography/computed tomography and whole-body magnetic resonance imaging in staging of advanced malignant melanoma. Eur J Cancer 2007;43(3):557–64.

18. Balch C, Buzaid A, Soong SJ, et al. New TNM melanoma staging system: linking biology and natural history to clinical outcomes. Semin Surg Oncol 2003;21(1):43–52.

19. Balch CM, Buzaid AC, Soong SJ, et al. Final version of the American Joint Committee on Cancer staging system for cutaneous melanoma. J Clin Oncol 2001; 19(16):3635–48.

20. Markowitz JS, Cosimi LA, Carey RW, et al. Prognosis after initial recurrence of cutaneous melanoma. Arch Surg 1991;126(6):703–7 [discussion: 707–8].

21. Gadd MA, Coit DG. Recurrence patterns and outcome in 1019 patients undergoing axillary or inguinal lymphadenectomy for melanoma. Arch Surg 1992;127(12):1412–6.

22. Karakousis CP, Velez A, Driscoll DL, et al. Metastasectomy in malignant melanoma. Surgery 1994; 115(3):295–302.

23. Meyer T, Merkel S, Goehl J, et al. Surgical therapy for distant metastases of malignant melanoma. Cancer 2000;89(9):1983–91.

24. Bowen GM, Chang AE, Lowe L, et al. Solitary melanoma confined to the dermal and/or subcutaneous tissue: evidence for revisiting the staging classification. Arch Dermatol 2000;136(11):1397–9.

25. Kroon BB, Noorda EM, Vrouenraets BC, et al. Isolated limb perfusion for melanoma. Surg Oncol Clin N Am 2008;17(4):785–94, viii–ix.

26. Sanki A, Kam PC, Thompson J. Long-term results of hyperthermic, isolated limb perfusion for melanoma: a reflection of tumor biology. Ann Surg 2007;245(4): 591–6.

27. Gorenstein LA, Putnam JB, Natarajan G, et al. Improved survival after resection of pulmonary metastases from malignant melanoma. Ann Thorac Surg 1991;52(2):204–10.

28. Harpole DH, Johnson CM, Wolfe WG, et al. Analysis of 945 cases of pulmonary metastatic melanoma. J Thorac Cardiovasc Surg 1992;103(4):743–8 [discussion: 748–50].

29. Karp NS, Boyd A, DePan HJ, et al. Thoracotomy for metastatic malignant melanoma of the lung. Surgery 1990;107(3):256–61.

30. Tafra L, Dale PS, Wanek LA, et al. Resection and adjuvant immunotherapy for melanoma metastatic to the lung and thorax. J Thorac Cardiovasc Surg 1995;110(1):119–28 [discussion: 129].

31. Leo F, Cagini L, Rocmans P, et al. Lung metastases from melanoma: when is surgical treatment warranted? Br J Cancer 2000;83(5):569–72.

32. Andrews S, Robinson L, Cantor A, et al. Survival after surgical resection of isolated pulmonary metastases from malignant melanoma. Cancer Control 2006;13(3):218–23.

33. Neuman H, Patel A, Hanlon C, et al. Stage-IV melanoma and pulmonary metastases: factors predictive of survival. Ann Surg Oncol 2007;14(10):2847–53.

34. Ollila DW, Stern SL, Morton DL. Tumor doubling time: a selection factor for pulmonary resection of metastatic melanoma. J Surg Oncol 1998;69(4):206–11.

35. Patel JK, Didolkar MS, Pickren JW, et al. Metastatic pattern of malignant melanoma. A study of 216 autopsy cases. Am J Surg 1978;135(6):807–10.

36. Reintgen DS, Thompson W, Garbutt J, et al. Radiologic, endoscopic, and surgical considerations of melanoma metastatic to the gastrointestinal tract. Surgery 1984;95(6):635–9.

37. Ricaniadis N, Konstadoulakis MM, Walsh D, et al. Gastrointestinal metastases from malignant melanoma. Surg Oncol 1995;4(2):105–10.

38. Ollila DW, Essner R, Wanek LA, et al. Surgical resection for melanoma metastatic to the gastrointestinal tract. Arch Surg 1996;131(9):975–9, 979–80.

39. Agrawal S, Yao TJ, Coit DG. Surgery for melanoma metastatic to the gastrointestinal tract. Ann Surg Oncol 1999;6(4):336–44.

40. Gutman H, Hess K, Kokotsakis J, et al. Surgery for abdominal metastases of cutaneous melanoma. World J Surg 2001;25(6):750–8.

41. Wood TF, DiFronzo LA, Rose DM, et al. Does complete resection of melanoma metastatic to solid intra-abdominal organs improve survival? Ann Surg Oncol 2001;8(8):658–62.

42. Branum GD, Epstein RE, Leight GS, et al. The role of resection in the management of melanoma metastatic to the adrenal gland. Surgery 1991;109(2):127–31.

43. Haigh PI, Essner R, Wardlaw JC, et al. Long-term survival after complete resection of melanoma metastatic to the adrenal gland. Ann Surg Oncol 1999; 6(7):633–9.

44. Rose DM, Essner R, Hughes TM, et al. Surgical resection for metastatic melanoma to the liver: the John Wayne Cancer Institute and Sydney Melanoma Unit experience. Arch Surg 2001;136(8):950–5.

45. Mendez IM, Del Maestro RF. Cerebral metastases from malignant melanoma. Can J Neurol Sci 1988; 15(2):119–23.

46. Tarhini AA, Agarwala SS. Management of brain metastases in patients with melanoma. Curr Opin Oncol 2004;16(2):161–6.

47. Patchell R. Postoperative radiotherapy in the treatment of single metastases to the brain: a randomized trial. JAMA 1998;280(17):1485–9.

48. Skibber JM, Soong SJ, Austin L, et al. Cranial irradiation after surgical excision of brain metastases in melanoma patients. Ann Surg Oncol 1996;3(2):118–23.

49. Sampson JH, Carter JH, Friedman AH, et al. Demographics, prognosis, and therapy in 702 patients with brain metastases from malignant melanoma. J Neurosurg 1998;88(1):11–20.

50. Zacest AC, Besser M, Stevens G, et al. Surgical management of cerebral metastases from melanoma: outcome in 147 patients treated at a single institution over two decades. J Neurosurg 2002;96(3):552–8.

51. McWilliams RR, Brown PD, Buckner JC, et al. Treatment of brain metastases from melanoma. Mayo Clin Proc 2003;78(12):1529–36.

52. Wroński M, Arbit E. Surgical treatment of brain metastases from melanoma: a retrospective study of 91 patients. J Neurosurg 2000;93(1):9–18.

53. Ballo MT, Ang KK. Radiation therapy for malignant melanoma. Surg Clin North Am 2003;83(2):323–42.

54. Yu C, Chen JC, Apuzzo ML, et al. Metastatic melanoma to the brain: prognostic factors after gamma knife radiosurgery. Int J Radiat Oncol Biol Phys 2002;52(5):1277–87.

55. Radbill AE, Fiveash JF, Falkenberg ET, et al. Initial treatment of melanoma brain metastases using gamma knife radiosurgery: an evaluation of efficacy and toxicity. Cancer 2004;101(4):825–33.

56. Mathieu D, Kondziolka D, Cooper PB, et al. Gamma knife radiosurgery in the management of malignant melanoma brain metastases. Neurosurgery 2007;60(3):471–81 [discussion: 481–2].

57. Samlowski W, Watson G, Wang M, et al. Multimodality treatment of melanoma brain metastases incorporating stereotactic radiosurgery (SRS). Cancer 2007;109(9):1855–62.

58. DeBoer DK, Schwartz HS, Thelman S, et al. Heterogeneous survival rates for isolated skeletal metastases from melanoma. Clin Orthop Relat Res 1996;(323):277–83.

Future Advances in Melanoma Research

Thomas J. Hornyak, MD, PhD

KEYWORDS

- Melanoma • Melanocyte • Nevus • Senescence
- Oncogene • Cancer stem cell

Although there have been no recently developed, widely implemented therapeutic advances in melanoma in increasing the survival of patients with advanced disease, considerable advances have been made within the past decade highlighting the molecular, cellular, and genetic determinants of malignant melanoma,[1] which have promoted a more detailed understanding of melanoma development and behavior to suggest new therapeutic approaches. High-throughput sequencing efforts of targeted regions of the cancer genome have unexpectedly yielded important findings in the somatic genetics of melanoma, leading to the identification of newly recognized molecular targets.[2] Future comprehensive DNA sequencing efforts using melanoma genetic material should reveal additional characteristic genetic lesions associated with precise clinical subtypes of melanoma as well as their frequencies of occurrence. These findings will suggest novel therapeutic targets. Comparative genome hybridization (CGH) has been used to reveal aberrations of the melanoma genome correlating with the activation of specific cell cycle and signaling genes. In addition to providing more insights into therapeutic mechanisms, these findings will enable the diagnosis of indeterminate pigmented lesions to be made with more precision. As a counterpart to future genetic advances, the application of findings about the histone code and DNA methylation to melanoma will reveal which epigenetic modifications occurring in melanoma cells lead to malignant progression and resistance to therapy. Future findings relating epigenetic markers to tumor formation and prognosis may rival the importance of genetic markers in the future.

Oncogene-induced senescence, regarded as a cellular mechanism protecting against malignant progression following genetic alterations predisposing to cancer, seems to account for the growth arrest of melanocytic nevi[3,4] despite the presence of an oncogenic mutation in these lesions.[5,6] Understanding its determinants in melanocytes may be important for devising strategies to revert malignant lesions to a more benign state. Initial findings describing melanoma stem cells,[7,8] examples of cancer stem cells that have been identified previously in hematologic and nonhematologic malignancies, may lead eventually to the identification of a highly specific subpopulation of melanoma tumor cells, responsible for tumor self-renewal during metastasis, which could be targeted with appropriate agents. Systems biology, a merging of computational techniques and dynamic analyses enabling prediction of the complex effects of changes in cellular states, also represents a technique that could be harnessed to increase the understanding of malignant melanoma. Traditional melanoma immunotherapy has recently incorporated creative introduction of conventional chemotherapy with the use of tumor-infiltrating lymphocytes and gene therapy to boost the success rate of this cell-based therapeutic approach.[9,10] The need for access to melanoma tumor tissue, primary and metastatic, has been a roadblock to progress in melanoma

This activity was supported by the Intramural Research Program of the NIH, National Cancer Institute, Center for Cancer Research.
Dermatology Branch, Center for Cancer Research, National Cancer Institute, National Institutes of Health, 10 Center Drive, Building 10/12N242, Bethesda, MD 20892, USA
E-mail address: hornyakt@mail.nih.gov

Clin Plastic Surg 37 (2010) 169–176
doi:10.1016/j.cps.2009.07.005

research, and initiatives undertaken by the National Cancer Institute and other organizations have addressed this in a formal way.

This review concentrates on describing 5 areas in which future advances are likely to impact on the ability to understand, prognosticate, and treat human melanoma: (1) germline mutations, (2) somatic mutations and DNA sequencing, (3) CGH, (4) oncogene-induced senescence, and (5) melanoma stem cells.

INHERITED MUTATIONS AND MELANOMA SUSCEPTIBILITY

The description of hereditary germline mutations accounting for increased melanoma susceptibility not only has had important implications for patient management but also has revealed important determinants, stimulating additional discoveries in melanocyte and melanoma cell biology. The gene CDKN2A at chromosome 9p21, encoding the p16 and p14 tumor suppressor proteins, is the most frequently mutated gene in hereditary melanoma syndrome.[11–13] Identification of CDKN2A as a major melanoma susceptibility gene led to recognition of the importance of p16 loss or inactivation in the development of sporadic melanoma[14] and melanocyte immortalization.[15,16] This identification has also resulted in the successful development of mouse models to study melanoma experimentally.[17,18]

In contrast to the high penetrance of CDKN2A mutations for familial melanoma, another melanoma susceptibility gene that has been identified has low penetrance, and is present widely throughout certain populations of European continental ancestry. This gene is MC1R, encoding a G-protein coupled receptor, the type 1 melanocortin receptor, transducing intracellular signals on binding by its ligand, melanocortin 1 or α-melanocyte stimulating hormone (α-MSH), that facilitates the production of eumelanin (dark or brown-black melanin), inside the melanocyte. The MC1R gene was identified as the "red hair gene," and certain variants of the gene are associated both with a red-haired, freckled phenotype and an increased susceptibility to melanoma (and nonmelanoma skin cancer) development.[19–21]

The International Melanoma Genetics Consortium (GenoMEL; www.genomel.org) was formed to evaluate further the risk of melanoma and other cancers in families with variations in known melanoma susceptibility genes, to identify additional susceptibility genes, and to explore gene-environment interactions in the development of melanoma and other relevant malignancies. A recent report from this initiative[11] confirmed the association of

CDKN2A mutations with pancreatic cancer[22]; it also reported that mutations in the p16 component of CDKN2A accounted for only 38% of the total cases in the study, with mutations in the p14 component of CDKN2A and the CDK4 gene, another rare melanoma susceptibility gene, contributing another 3%. Hence, the majority of variations responsible for familial melanoma in these consortium cases have not yet been identified. Although some of these unaccounted cases may be the result of occult CDKN2A mutations in more distant regulatory regions of the gene, it is likely that mutations in currently unrecognized melanoma susceptibility genes account for many of these cases. Identification of these genes, using consortia of affected families in conjunction with laboratory-based analyses of genetic linkage and additional candidate genes, will identify additional genes that, like CDKN2A and CDK4, yield greater insights into the biology of melanoma development.

SOMATIC MUTATIONS IN MELANOMA AND INTENSIVE SEQUENCING-BASED ANALYSES OF THE MELANOMA GENOME

As described earlier, the discovery of inherited mutations in the germline can reveal important determinants of tumor development in individuals with hereditary tumor predisposition syndromes. However, most melanomas occur sporadically, in individuals without a significant family history of melanoma. To identify important molecular factors contributing to the development of sporadic melanoma, a different approach was necessary, one based on examining the DNA of melanoma tissue to discover genetic alterations that determine malignant transformation and cancer development. For example, members of the RAS family of proto-oncogenes, which transmit intracellular signals following the binding of growth factors to their cellular receptors, are frequently mutated in human cancer. An HRAS mutation in a bladder tumor was the first described somatic mutation in human cancer.[23] Mutations in NRAS were described nearly 2 decades ago in human melanoma,[24] suggesting that activation of RAS-dependent intracellular signaling was also an important characteristic of cutaneous melanoma.

An intensive sequencing-based approach to discover cancer-specific alterations in the RAS-RAF-MEK-ERK signaling pathway (mitogen-activated protein or MAP kinase pathway) led to the discovery that mutations in the BRAF gene, encoding the BRAF serine/threonine kinase, were present in 66% of melanomas analyzed in the study.[2] Eighty percent of BRAF mutations in human cancer occur at a specific site in the

BRAF coding sequence, resulting in the substitution mutation BRAF^{V600E} in the protein. This discovery has generated much excitement in melanoma research because of the possibility that BRAF might represent a viable target for molecular-based therapy. Since the initial report, a variety of additional analyses have elaborated on these findings. In melanomas, activating mutations in BRAF and NRAS are frequent but mutually exclusive.[25] Mutations in BRAF are most closely associated with melanomas that develop on skin not chronically exposed to sunlight, such as the skin of the trunk, which receives intermittent, but high-intensity, sunlight exposure.[26] Melanomas occurring on chronically sun-exposed skin, such as the skin of the face, as well as acral and mucosal melanomas, have infrequent activating mutations in BRAF. In contrast, activating mutations in NRAS, usually at codon 61, are nearly equally distributed between melanomas occurring on chronically sun-exposed, nonchronically sun-exposed, acral, and mucosal surfaces.[27] Site-specific differences in mutational frequencies suggest that the intensity and amount of ultraviolet exposures results in cellular changes, promoting the development of distinct genetic lesions within melanocytes and ultimately leading to malignant progression.

In the future, expansive DNA sequencing analyses of melanoma specimens will reveal additional mutations that contribute to melanoma development and pathogenicity. An instructive example to consider is the set of mutations that have been described from intensive DNA sequencing of colorectal carcinomas. A targeted sequencing effort, focusing on the sequencing of genes encoding kinases in the phosphatidylinositol 3-kinase (PI3K) signaling pathway, revealed multiple mutations in the PIK3CA gene, encoding the p110α subunit of PI3K, in colorectal carcinomas at high frequency (32%).[28] These mutations were found to promote growth and invasiveness of colorectal cancer cells,[29] confirming their pathogenicity. A more extensive analysis, the sequencing of important catalytic domains of 340 genes encoding cellular serine/threonine kinases, revealed mutations in 8 additional genes in colorectal carcinoma cells, including 3 genes that contribute to the PI3K signaling pathway that were also implicated in the previous study.[30] The complete cancer genome of an individual patient with acute myelogenous leukemia has been sequenced, revealing 8 previously undescribed mutations that are likely to contribute to cancer progression.[31] Similar efforts to explore novel mutations in kinases controlling intracellular signaling pathways as well as other critical sets of genes, such as the matrix metalloproteinases,[32] in melanoma tissues will define currently unrecognized genes that could represent viable therapeutic targets. These efforts will be particularly important because strategies to inhibit BRAF, though frequently mutated and important for governing melanoma cell growth and survival in vitro,[33,34] have thus far yielded disappointing results. The use of sorafenib, a multikinase inhibitor that inhibits both BRAF and BRAF^{V600E} activity, in melanoma has not been found to be more effective than current therapies in initial clinical trials.[35] Evaluation of additional molecular targets and signaling pathways identified by DNA sequencing-based approaches is urgently needed.

ONCOGENE-INDUCED SENESCENCE: CONVERTING MELANOMA CELLS INTO A DORMANT STATE

Oncogene-induced senescence is a cellular response, characterized by a cessation of cell division, resistance to death, and other morphologic and gene expression changes, to the expression of an activated oncogene.[36,37] Oncogene-induced senescence was first demonstrated as an in vitro response of fibroblasts to the expression of an activated RAS-family oncogene, and is thought to represent a protective response against the development of actual malignancy. Additional genetic and epigenetic changes in the senescent cell are required for malignant progression, and may convert the activity of the oncogene from mediating cell cycle arrest to fostering malignant progression. Cellular mechanisms enforcing oncogene-induced senescence may thus represent viable targets for therapeutic intervention.

In addition to melanomas, BRAF^{V600E} mutations are found at high frequency in melanocytic nevi.[6] The presence of activating mutations in a RAS signaling pathway member suggested that BRAF activation in melanocytes might induce oncogene-induced senescence. In laboratory-based experiments, introduction of BRAF^{V600E} into cultured human melanocytes was found to result in an arrest of cell division and the induction of characteristic markers of cellular senescence. Some of these same markers are expressed in vivo by melanocytic nevi.[4] All of this evidence suggests that melanocytic nevi result from oncogene-induced senescence in human melanocytes, with an arrest in cell proliferation following an initial stimulus from activation of an oncogene, resulting in the stability of this benign neoplasm. This insight leads to a follow-up question: what are mechanisms that maintain a melanocytic nevus in a senescent state in the presence of an activated oncogene which, in melanoma cells, is capable of driving their tumorigenicity?

A recent set of studies has defined a set of novel determinants of oncogene-induced senescence that may represent opportunities for future intervention against malignant melanoma. Screening of BRAF^{V600E}-expressing melanocytes led to the identification of insulinlike growth factor binding protein 7 (IGFBP7) as a determinant of oncogene-induced senescence in human melanocytes. In this study, administration of IGFBP7 to mice xenografted with BRAF^{V600E} human melanoma cells induced a significant regression of these tumors.[38] In another study, expression of interleukin (IL)-6 along with associated cytokines IL-8 and IL-1α were found to mediate an oncogene-induced senescence response.[39] A third report implicated expression of the chemokine receptor CXCR2, which binds IL-8 along with other cytokines, for reinforcing cellular senescence responses. As summarized in **Fig. 1**, the use of these and other mediators of senescence that have yet to be characterized may be useful in the future for reverting melanoma cells in patients toward a senescentlike state. Although this strategy may not cure melanoma, administration of soluble proteins and cytokines that have the potential for inducing a state of dormancy could be important for achieving long-term control of this malignancy in patients with advanced disease.

LARGE-SCALE MELANOMA GENOME ANALYSIS: THE USE AND FUTURE OF COMPARATIVE GENOMIC HYBRIDIZATION

CGH is a molecular technique that is used to survey an entire genome for changes in copy number, such as amplifications or deletions, of specific regions of the genome.[40] CGH can be used to compare genetic material from tumor cells with that of normal cells by hybridizing tumor cell DNA to either normal metaphase chromosomes or to fragments of DNA arrayed on a microchip. Amplifications or deletions of regions of tumor DNA can be systematically detected. Appraisal of these changes can provide a global picture of the aberrations of a particular cancer genome and reveal genomic regions commonly amplified or deleted in particular cancers, such as melanoma. Identification of these genomic regions can be useful for specifying genes commonly amplified or deleted in melanoma that participate in melanoma progression.

CGH has been used to great benefit in revealing aberrations in genomes of melanomas and other pigmented lesions. CGH has been used recently to reveal significant differences between the degree of DNA copy number changes in melanomas compared with melanocytic nevi, with 96% of melanomas examined exhibiting chromosomal aberrations and only 13% of benign melanocytic nevi exhibiting copy number alterations. All of the nevi with chromosomal aberrations

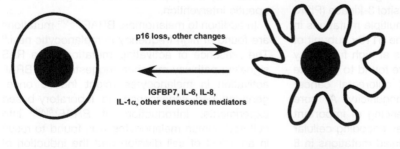

p16 loss, other changes

IGFBP7, IL-6, IL-8, IL-1α, other senescence mediators

senescent melanocytic nevus cell

malignant melanoma cell

Fig. 1. Oncogene-induced senescence and melanocytic nevi. Both nevi and melanoma cells often have mutations in BRAF. Loss of p16 and other factors results in progression of nevus cells to malignant melanoma. Recent studies suggest that factors such as insulinlike growth factor binding protein 7 (IGFBP7), interleukin-6 (IL-6), IL-8, IL-1α, and other secreted factors may be capable of reverting melanoma cells toward a "senescentlike" state.

were Spitz nevi, with an isolated gain of the short arm of chromosome 11 the common finding.[41] This aberration has been associated with HRAS amplifications and mutations in Spitz nevi.[42] In another study, CGH was useful in distinguishing between benign and malignant proliferative nodules in large congenital melanocytic nevi,[43] whose distinctions can be difficult to make on clinical and histopathological grounds alone. A comprehensive study of genomic alterations in different clinical subtypes of melanoma has revealed striking differences in the patterns of chromosomal aberrations. Amplifications are more common in acral and mucosal melanoma than in melanomas occurring on either chronically sun-exposed or nonchronically sun-exposed skin. Acral melanomas commonly have amplifications at chromosomal units 5p, 11q, 12q, and 15, whereas gains at 1q, 6p, and 8q are characteristic of sinonasal mucosal melanomas. Amplifications of the CCND1 and CDK4 genes, encoding the cyclin D1 and cyclin-dependent kinase 4 cell cycle-related proteins, are found more commonly in these types of melanoma, which typically do not contain the BRAF mutation found in melanomas occurring elsewhere.[27]

CGH analysis has detected aberrations in the KIT gene, encoding a receptor tyrosine kinase important for melanocyte function. Careful DNA sequencing of this gene in melanomas has revealed examples of activating mutations in KIT, including mutations known to be sensitive to the kinase inhibitor imatinib.[44] KIT amplifications and mutations have been detected predominantly in mucosal (including anal) and acral melanomas and melanomas arising on chronically sun-damaged skin. Recent examples have described melanoma patients with activating mutations in KIT responding dramatically to imatinib treatment.[45,46]

In the future, CGH may be used routinely for diagnostic evaluation of pigmented lesions, such as the atypical Spitz nevus, recurrent melanocytic nevi, and proliferative nodules in congenital nevi[47] that today are difficult to classify solely on clinical and histopathological grounds. Finer discrimination of amplifications and deletions within genomic regions using dense DNA microarrays will reveal additional melanoma oncogenes, such as MITF,[48] which contribute to tumorigenicity of small subsets of melanomas. Careful clinical correlations will be necessary to take maximum advantage of these discoveries, which will further enhance the understanding of the biology of melanoma development.

MELANOMA STEM CELLS IN TUMOR INITIATION AND PROPAGATION

The concept of cancer stem cells (CSCs) is grounded in an attempt to account for the immense proliferative properties of many tumors with evidence that only certain cells comprising heterogeneous tumors possess the greatest proliferative capacity. According to the CSC hypothesis, tumor initiation and development is driven by a subset of tumor cells, cancer stem cells, with self-renewal and differentiation properties similar to those of normal stem cells that are responsible for renewing tissues such as the skin and the colonic epithelium. These properties may account both for metastatic disease and for tumor heterogeneity, explaining why some, but not all, cells within the tumor are capable of regenerating the tumor at a distant site. CSCs were first demonstrated in a hematopoietic system malignancy, acute myelogenous leukemia.[49] Their existence and properties were subsequently demonstrated in breast adenocarcinoma[50] and other solid malignancies. Although experimental results provide impressive evidence of the ability of CSCs, isolated by their expression of specific cell surface markers using fluorescence-activated cell sorting, to initiate tumors, one important limitation (**Fig. 2**) has been the reliance on interspecies xenograft assays to demonstrate the tumor-initiating properties of CSCs. Hence, it is possible that the growth of CSCs in immunocompromised mice is due in part to favorable interactions between the selected human tumor cells and murine stroma rather than simply the intrinsic tumor initiation properties of CSCs.

Recent studies have pointed to the existence of a subpopulation of cells in melanoma tumors with differentiation, self-renewal, and tumor-initiating properties similar to those of CSCs. In experiments with primary melanoma tumor tissue, melanoma cells that were enriched in expression of the cell surface marker CD20 differentiated into multiple cell lineages under appropriate culture conditions, and exhibited enhanced properties of tumor formation when xenografted into immunocompromised mice.[7] In another study, the expression of the cancer stem cell marker CD133 in melanoma cells correlated with tumor-initiating properties.[51] CD133 was found to be coexpressed with the ATP-binding cassette (ABC) superfamily transporter ABCB5 in human melanoma specimens,[52] and ABCB5 was found to be a cell surface marker of human melanoma cells enriched in tumor-initiating capability that is functionally important for melanoma growth as xenografts.[8]

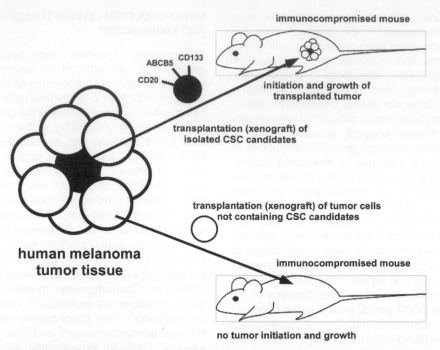

Fig. 2. Experimental system for studying human melanoma stem cells. Human melanoma tumor tissue is obtained and cells are separated, based on their expression of cell surface proteins that are candidates for specific markers of melanoma stem cells (such as CD20, ABCB5, and CD133). Separated tumor cells are implanted into immuno-compromised mice subcutaneously. Tumor cell subsets enriched for melanoma stem cells produce tumors with relatively small numbers of cells, whereas tumor cells depleted of melanoma stem cells do not produce tumors, even with relatively large numbers of cells.

Although melanoma tumor-initiating cells were found to be uncommon in the above studies, a more recent study using mice additionally immunodeficient for the gamma-subunit of the interleukin-2 receptor found that approximately one-quarter of cells from advanced primary and metastatic melanoma specimens possessed tumor-initiating capacity, without any prior selection for cell surface markers.[53] This finding challenges the specificity of melanoma tumor-initiating cells identified in the previous studies, and demonstrates how details of the xenograft system utilized can impact upon experimental results.

The variability of result obtained in an attempt to define a melanoma tumor-initiating cell, or melanoma stem cell, renders it unclear whether these cells will demonstrate characteristics of CSCs in other solid tumors such as breast[50] and colon[54] cancers. In the future, comprehensive efforts using substantial numbers of samples obtained from primary human melanoma tissue are likely to be used, with a variety of immunodeficient and humanized xenograft systems, to analyze melanoma tumor cell heterogeneity. These efforts may lead to the identification of highly specific markers for subsets of cells within certain metastatic melanomas and, especially, early primary

melanomas capable of tumor initiation and propagation. Targeting melanoma stem cells with specific therapeutic agents may be important and, in fact, necessary for eradicating their tumor-initiating potential to achieve durable remission of metastatic melanoma. Different types of melanoma stem cells conceivably will be shown to exist, each requiring a distinctive therapeutic approach based on its active intracellular signaling pathways. Variations between different types of melanoma stem cells may determine their propensity and location of metastasis. Comprehensive research studies on melanoma stem cells and, more generally, melanoma tumor heterogeneity will be important in devising a set of rational, broad strategies to treat this malignancy in the future.

SUMMARY

Important efforts to understand, classify, diagnose, and treat human melanoma better are ongoing. This article tries to provide a picture of how some current research initiatives in melanoma genetics and tumor biology may be applied to this effort to yield specific beneficial future results. Additional approaches that have not been addressed in detail will be just as important. Gene expression profiling is a method that has been used to demonstrate previously unrecognized distinctions between follicular lymphomas that have important prognostic significance.[55] This technique has been applied initially to human melanoma specimens[56,57] with prognostic results comparable with those achieved from Breslow thickness. Future efforts with a greater number and diversity of primary tumor specimens should reveal molecular signatures, facilitating the identification of thin melanomas likely to metastasize and, conversely, thick melanomas unlikely to recur. Advances in immunotherapy will benefit from precise targeting of cellular immunoregulatory molecules capable of enhancing intrinsic antitumor immunity.[58] The role of clinicians as supporters of melanoma research will be essential as scientists seek greater access to primary tumor tissue and clinical insights that can provide a context for the application of laboratory advances.

REFERENCES

1. Chin L, Garraway LA, Fisher DE. Malignant melanoma: genetics and therapeutics in the genomic era. Genes Dev 2006;20:2149–82.
2. Davies H, Bignell GR, Cox C, et al. Mutations of the BRAF gene in human cancer. Nature 2002;417: 949–54.
3. Gray-Schopfer VC, Cheong SC, Chong H, et al. Cellular senescence in naevi and immortalisation in melanoma: a role for p16? Br J Cancer 2006;95: 496–505.
4. Michaloglou C, Vredeveld LC, Soengas MS, et al. BRAFE600-associated senescence-like cell cycle arrest of human naevi. Nature 2005;436:720–4.
5. Papp T, Pemsel H, Zimmermann R, et al. Mutational analysis of the N-ras, p53, p16INK4a, CDK4, and MC1R genes in human congenital melanocytic naevi. J Med Genet 1999;36:610–4.
6. Pollock PM, Harper UL, Hansen KS, et al. High frequency of BRAF mutations in nevi. Nat Genet 2003;33:19–20.
7. Fang D, Nguyen TK, Leishear K, et al. A tumorigenic subpopulation with stem cell properties in melanomas. Cancer Res 2005;65:9328–37.
8. Schatton T, Murphy GF, Frank NY, et al. Identification of cells initiating human melanomas. Nature 2008; 451:345–9.
9. Dudley ME, Wunderlich JR, Robbins PF, et al. Cancer regression and autoimmunity in patients after clonal repopulation with antitumor lymphocytes. Science 2002;298:850–4.
10. Morgan RA, Dudley ME, Wunderlich JR, et al. Cancer regression in patients after transfer of genetically engineered lymphocytes. Science 2006;314:126–9.
11. Goldstein AM, Chan M, Harland M, et al. High-risk melanoma susceptibility genes and pancreatic cancer, neural system tumors, and uveal melanoma across GenoMEL. Cancer Res 2006;66:9818–28.
12. Hussussian CJ, Struewing JP, Goldstein AM, et al. Germline p16 mutations in familial melanoma. Nat Genet 1994;8:15–21.
13. Kamb A, Shattuck-Eidens D, Eeles R, et al. Analysis of the p16 gene (CDKN2) as a candidate for the chromosome 9p melanoma susceptibility locus. Nat Genet 1994;8:23–6.
14. Walker GJ, Flores JF, Glendening JM, et al. Virtually 100% of melanoma cell lines harbor alterations at the DNA level within CDKN2A, CDKN2B, or one of their downstream targets. Genes Chromosomes Cancer 1998;22:157–63.
15. Bennett DC, Cooper PJ, Hart IR. A line of non-tumorigenic mouse melanocytes, syngeneic with the B16 melanoma and requiring a tumour promoter for growth. Int J Cancer 1987;39:414–8.
16. Sviderskaya EV, Hill SP, Evans-Whipp TJ, et al. p16(Ink4a) in melanocyte senescence and differentiation. J Natl Cancer Inst 2002;94:446–54.
17. Chin L, Pomerantz J, Polsky D, et al. Cooperative effects of INK4a and ras in melanoma susceptibility in vivo. Genes Dev 1997;11:2822–34.
18. Noonan FP, Recio JA, Takayama H, et al. Neonatal sunburn and melanoma in mice. Nature 2001;413: 271–2.
19. Box NF, Duffy DL, Chen W, et al. MC1R genotype modifies risk of melanoma in families segregating CDKN2A mutations. Am J Hum Genet 2001;69: 765–73.
20. Rees JL. Genetics of hair and skin color. Annu Rev Genet 2003;37:67–90.
21. Valverde P, Healy E, Sikkink S, et al. The Asp84Glu variant of the melanocortin 1 receptor (MC1R) is associated with melanoma. Hum Mol Genet 1996; 5:1663–6.
22. Goldstein AM, Fraser MC, Struewing JP, et al. Increased risk of pancreatic cancer in melanoma-prone kindreds with p16INK4 mutations. N Engl J Med 1995;333:970–4.
23. Parada LF, Tabin CJ, Shih C, et al. Human EJ bladder carcinoma oncogene is homologue of Harvey sarcoma virus ras gene. Nature 1982;297:474–8.
24. van 't Veer LJ, Burgering BM, Versteeg R, et al. N-ras mutations in human cutaneous melanoma from sun-exposed body sites. Mol Cell Biol 1989;9:3114–6.
25. Tsao H, Goel V, Wu H, et al. Genetic interaction between NRAS and BRAF mutations and PTEN/MMAC1 inactivation in melanoma. J Invest Dermatol 2004;122:337–41.
26. Maldonado JL, Fridlyand J, Patel H, et al. Determinants of BRAF mutations in primary melanomas. J Natl Cancer Inst 2003;95:1878–90.

27. Curtin JA, Fridlyand J, Kageshita T, et al. Distinct sets of genetic alterations in melanoma. N Engl J Med 2005;353:2135–47.

28. Samuels Y, Wang Z, Bardelli A, et al. High frequency of mutations of the PIK3CA gene in human cancers. Science 2004;304:554.

29. Samuels Y, Diaz LA Jr, Schmidt-Kittler O, et al. Mutant PIK3CA promotes cell growth and invasion of human cancer cells. Cancer Cell 2005;7:561–73.

30. Parsons DW, Wang TL, Samuels Y, et al. Colorectal cancer: mutations in a signalling pathway. Nature 2005;436:792.

31. Ley TJ, Mardis ER, Ding L, et al. DNA sequencing of a cytogenetically normal acute myeloid leukaemia genome. Nature 2008;456:66–72.

32. Palavalli LH, Prickett TD, Wunderlich JR, et al. Analysis of the matrix metalloproteinase family reveals that MMP8 is often mutated in melanoma. Nat Genet 2009;41:518–20.

33. Hingorani SR, Jacobetz MA, Robertson GP, et al. Suppression of BRAF (V599E) in human melanoma abrogates transformation. Cancer Res 2003;63: 5198–202.

34. Wellbrock C, Ogilvie L, Hedley D, et al. V599EB-RAF is an oncogene in melanocytes. Cancer Res 2004; 64:2338–42.

35. Eisen T, Ahmad T, Flaherty KT, et al. Sorafenib in advanced melanoma: a Phase II randomised discontinuation trial analysis. Br J Cancer 2006;95:581–6.

36. Campisi J, d'Adda di Fagagna F. Cellular senescence: when bad things happen to good cells. Nat Rev Mol Cell Biol 2007;8:729–40.

37. Serrano M, Lin AW, McCurrach ME, et al. Oncogenic ras provokes premature cell senescence associated with accumulation of p53 and p16INK4a. Cell 1997; 88:593–602.

38. Wajapeyee N, Serra RW, Zhu X, et al. Oncogenic BRAF induces senescence and apoptosis through pathways mediated by the secreted protein IGFBP7. Cell 2008;132:363–74.

39. Kuilman T, Michaloglou C, Vredeveld LC, et al. Oncogene-induced senescence relayed by an interleukin-dependent inflammatory network. Cell 2008; 133:1019–31.

40. Bauer J, Bastian BC. Distinguishing melanocytic nevi from melanoma by DNA copy number changes: comparative genomic hybridization as a research and diagnostic tool. Dermatol Ther 2006;19:40–9.

41. Bastian BC, Olshen AB, LeBoit PE, et al. Classifying melanocytic tumors based on DNA copy number changes. Am J Pathol 2003;163:1765–70.

42. Bastian BC, LeBoit PE, Pinkel D. Mutations and copy number increase of HRAS in Spitz nevi with distinctive histopathological features. Am J Pathol 2000; 157:967–72.

43. Bastian BC, Xiong J, Frieden IJ, et al. Genetic changes in neoplasms arising in congenital melanocytic nevi: differences between nodular proliferations and melanomas. Am J Pathol 2002; 161:1163–9.

44. Curtin JA, Busam K, Pinkel D, et al. Somatic activation of KIT in distinct subtypes of melanoma. J Clin Oncol 2006;24:4340–6.

45. Hodi FS, Friedlander P, Corless CL, et al. Major response to imatinib mesylate in KIT-mutated melanoma. J Clin Oncol 2008;26:2046–51.

46. Lutzky J, Bauer J, Bastian BC. Dose-dependent, complete response to imatinib of a metastatic mucosal melanoma with a K642E KIT mutation. Pigment Cell Melanoma Res 2008;21:492–3.

47. Murphy MJ, Jen M, Chang MW, et al. Molecular diagnosis of a benign proliferative nodule developing in a congenital melanocytic nevus in a 3-month-old infant. J Am Acad Dermatol 2008;59:518–23.

48. Garraway LA, Widlund HR, Rubin MA, et al. Integrative genomic analyses identify MITF as a lineage survival oncogene amplified in malignant melanoma. Nature 2005;436:117–22.

49. Lapidot T, Sirard C, Vormoor J, et al. A cell initiating human acute myeloid leukaemia after transplantation into SCID mice. Nature 1994;367:645–8.

50. Al-Hajj M, Wicha MS, Benito-Hernandez A, et al. Prospective identification of tumorigenic breast cancer cells. Proc Natl Acad Sci U S A 2003;100: 3983–8.

51. Monzani E, Facchetti F, Galmozzi E, et al. Melanoma contains CD133 and ABCG2 positive cells with enhanced tumourigenic potential. Eur J Cancer 2007;43:935–46.

52. Frank NY, Margaryan A, Huang Y, et al. ABCB5-mediated doxorubicin transport and chemoresistance in human malignant melanoma. Cancer Res 2005;65:4320–33.

53. Quintana E, Shackleton M, Sabel MS, et al. Efficient tumour formation by single human melanoma cells. Nature 2008;456:593–8.

54. O'Brien CA, Pollett A, Gallinger S, et al. A human colon cancer cell capable of initiating tumour growth in immunodeficient mice. Nature 2007;445:106–10.

55. Dave SS, Wright G, Tan B, et al. Prediction of survival in follicular lymphoma based on molecular features of tumor-infiltrating immune cells. N Engl J Med 2004;351:2159–69.

56. Winnepenninckx V, Lazar V, Michiels S, et al. Gene expression profiling of primary cutaneous melanoma and clinical outcome. J Natl Cancer Inst 2006;98: 472–82.

57. Winnepenninckx V, van den Oord JJ. Gene expression profiling and clinical outcome in melanoma: in search of novel prognostic factors. Expert Rev Anticancer Ther 2007;7:1611–31.

58. Kirkwood JM, Tarhini AA, Panelli MC, et al. Next generation of immunotherapy for melanoma. J Clin Oncol 2008;26:3445–55.

Index

Note: Page numbers of article titles are in **boldface** type.

A

Abdomen, imaging of, in melanoma, 60

Adrenal glands, metastases of advanced melanoma to, 164

Alkylating agents, in metastatic melanoma, 132–133

American Joint Committee on Cancer (AJCC), staging of melanoma, 55–56, 79, 80

Apoptosis-inducing agents, in metastatic melanoma, 134

Axilla, dissection of, in sentinel lymph nodes, 114–116, 119, 121

B

B-K mole, as problematic diagnosis, 6–8

Biochemotherapy, adjuvant, in melanoma, 131
    in metastatic melanoma, 139–140

Blue nevus(i), cellular, atypical, diagnosis of, 2
        diagnosis of, 11
            malignant, 11–12

Brain, imaging of, in melanoma, 60
    metastases of advanced melanoma to, 165

C

Canvaxin, in advanced melanoma, 161

Central nervous system, metastasis of melanoma to, 153–155

Children, melanoma in, surgical management of, 69
    Spitz nevus in, 69

Completion lymph node dissection, 57

Cryotherapy, in lentigo maligna, 38–39

Cytokines, in melanoma, 128–130
    in metastatic melanoma, 136

D

Dysplastic nevus, as problematic diagnosis, 6–8

E

Ear, melanoma on, surgical management of, 68

Elderly, melanoma in, management of, 69–70

Eyelid, melanoma on, surgical management of, 68

F

Face, melanoma on, surgical management of, 67–68

Fraction size, of radiation therapy, in melanoma, 148–149

G

Gamma probe, for localization of radioactive node, 94, 95

Gangliosides, in melanoma, 131

Gastrointestinal tract, metastases of advanced melanoma to, 163, 164

Genitalia, melanoma on, surgical management of, 68–69

Genomic hybridization, comparative, use and future of, 172–173

Granulocyte-macrophage colony-stimulating factor, in melanoma, 130

Groin, dissection of, in sentinel lymph nodes, 116–117, 120, 121

Grossing, of sentinel lymph nodes, 102, 103, 107, 109

H

Hand, melanoma on, surgical management of, 68

Head and neck, melanoma of, **73–77**
        adjunctive therapy for, 76
        follow-up and surveillance of, 76
        patient workup in, 73
        primary, management of, 74–75
        risk factors for, 74
        types of, 73–74
        suspicious lesion of, biopsy of, principles of, 74

I

Immune-based therapy, in metastatic melanoma, 135–136

Immunomodulation, in lentigo maligna, 39–40

Immunomodulatory agents, in metastatic melanoma, 136–137

Immunotherapy, adoptive, in melanoma, 131

Interferons, in melanoma, 128–130
    in metastatic melanoma, 136

Interleukin-2, metastatic melanoma, 136

L

Laser therapy, in lentigo maligna, 39

Lentigo maligna, and lentigo maligna melanoma, 35
        differential diagnosis of, 36–37
    clinical presentation/diagnosis of, 36–37
    cryotherapy in, 38–39
    diagnosis and treatment of, **35–46**
    epidemiology and patient demographics of, 35–36
    histology of, 37
    immunomodulation in, 39–40
    laser therapy in, 39

Clin Plastic Surg 37 (2010) 177–180
doi:10.1016/S0094-1298(09)00138-2

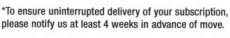

Moving?

Make sure your subscription moves with you!

To notify us of your new address, find your Clinics Account Number (located on your mailing label above your name), and contact customer service at:

Email: journalscustomerservice-usa@elsevier.com

800-654-2452 (subscribers in the U.S. & Canada)
314-447-8871 (subscribers outside of the U.S. & Canada)

Fax number: 314-447-8029

Elsevier Health Sciences Division
Subscription Customer Service
3251 Riverport Lane
Maryland Heights, MO 63043

*To ensure uninterrupted delivery of your subscription,
please notify us at least 4 weeks in advance of move.*

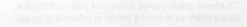

Printed and bound by CPI Group (UK) Ltd, Croydon, CR0 4YY

03/10/2024

01040362-0016